TEACHING ABOUT
SEXUALITY AND HIV

TEACHING ABOUT SEXUALITY AND HIV

PRINCIPLES AND METHODS FOR EFFECTIVE EDUCATION

*Evonne Hedgepeth, Ph.D. and
Joan Helmich, M.A.*

NEW YORK UNIVERSITY PRESS
New York and London

NEW YORK UNIVERSITY PRESS
New York and London

Library of Congress Cataloging-in-Publication Data
Hedgepeth, Evonne.
    Teaching about sexuality and HIV : principles and methods for
effective education / Evonne Hedgepeth and Joan Helmich.
        p.   cm.
    Includes bibliographical references and index.
    ISBN 0-8147-3515-0 (alk. paper).—ISBN 0-8147-3535-5 (pbk. :
alk. paper)
    1. Sex instruction—United States.   2. AIDS (Disease)—Study and
teaching—United States.   3. HIV (Viruses)—Study and teaching—
United States.   I. Helmich, Joan.   II. Title.
HQ57.5.A3H43   1996
613.9'07—dc20   96-13431
                          CIP

New York University Press books are printed on acid-free
paper, and their binding materials are chosen for strength
and durability.

Manufactured in the United States of America

10 9 8 7 6 5

IN LOVING MEMORY OF
Dodie Bielka, Becky Minas, John Parker,
Mary Lee Tatum, and Lester Kirkendall.

CONTENTS

Both of us have been teaching about sexuality and training sexuality educators since the early 1970s—in public schools, community health settings, and colleges. Evonne's academic background is in psychology, history, education, and human sexuality; Joan's is in education, applied behavioral sciences, language arts, and family planning. Evonne currently serves as part-time faculty at The Evergreen State College in Olympia, Washington, in addition to working as a private consultant and trainer in sexuality education and in various topics within human sexuality. Joan is the training director for The Center for Health Training in Seattle and also works independently as a consultant and trainer.

Evonne served as the primary author of Part I; Joan, of Part II. Each contributed significantly to the other section.

ACKNOWLEDGMENTS

We are deeply appreciative of the people who have helped us with this book. Many sexuality education specialists, community health educators, and classroom teachers reviewed part or all of the text in its early stages and made substantive suggestions; we particularly thank Betty Freund, Katie Meyer, and Beth Reis. Many others gave us valuable ideas, input, perspectives, stories, and feedback, including Carol Cassell, Ann Castel Davis of Macmillan Publishing, Maureen Considine, Andy Darring, Teresa Fritz, Caroline Haskell, Doug Kirby, Judith McKoy, Carole Miller, Wayne Pawlowski, Irene Peters, Lisa Schwartz, Anne Terrell, John Thompson, Teri Tomatich, and participants and core staff of the Northwest Institute for Community Health Educators; we are extremely thankful for their continuing efforts and creativity in this field.

We also recognize the assistance and support of Karen McMillan Hicks and Denise DeLisle, who did our graphics; Sophia Verongos, our research assistant; the staff of The Center for Health Training; the staff of The Evergreen State College Library; Niko Pfund, our ever-patient and helpful editor at New York University Press as well as his colleague, Despina Papazoglov Gimbel.

Very special thanks goes to Peggy Brick, who spent many hours reviewing the final draft and made invaluable suggestions.

Finally, our deepest gratitude goes to Andy McMillan and Gail Stringer for their love, support, and patience as they sustained us emotionally and physically through this long project.

INTRODUCTION

Teachers often ask us:

"What can I do about my own discomfort with sexuality?"

"How do I deal with inappropriate student questions?"

"How can we expect students to learn what they need when we have so little time to spend on sexuality/HIV education?"

"How should I respond to concerned parents or organized opposition?"

"Should I be open with students about my own sexual values and experiences?"

"Students hate doing role plays. Why are they so important for sexuality education?"

"Is there a good book I can read to learn more about this stuff?"

When the subject is sexuality, an educator's usual concerns—comfort with the material, selecting effective methods and curricula to engage learners, working with administrators and parents—are magnified. Whether you are an experienced sexuality educator or not, whether you approach teaching about the subject with relish or reluctance, you may share some of these concerns. Even if you have been doing this work for some time, you may wonder if you handle some situations appropriately or if you can be more effective.

We wrote this book on sexuality education principles and methodology with two main audiences in mind: *classroom teachers* who address sexuality topics within their regular teaching, and *community health educators* who specialize in teaching about sexual health, HIV prevention, or family planning. This book also may be useful to those who teach about sexuality or HIV as part of their job responsibilities: school nurses, childbirth and parenting educators, clinicians and counselors, trainers in sexuality topics (e.g., sexual harassment), religious educators, teacher educators, and college professors of human sexuality.

Professionals in this field have learned a lot about what works in sexuality education and how it differs from teaching other subjects. Educators have come a long way from the simple "telling" methods of the 1960s and 1970s, when they covered a few "essential" subjects (e.g., pregnancy prevention and STDs), hoping they would affect student behaviors. Some "sex education" programs (as they were called then) included exploration of values and attitudes, but even this broader approach had little impact on risk-taking behavior. In recent years, research and experience have revealed more about what works in sexuality education, and *why*.

In this book, we focus on the "how" and "why" of effective sexuality and HIV education rather than on the "what." The basic principles of such education have much in common with effective education in general; however, some issues and situations are unique or especially salient to this profession. Knowing how to create productive learning environments and use interactive and practice methods, for example, are useful skills for teaching any subject; they are *absolutely critical* to teaching about sexuality and HIV, as is dealing with student discomfort.

Our purposes are twofold: (1) to review guiding principles and address concerns relevant to effective sexuality and HIV education (Part I); and (2) to review specific teaching methods and their application in sexuality and HIV education (Part II). Throughout the book, we share stories and learning activities to illustrate these principles and methods; we also highlight some of the best curricula currently available.

This book is *not* content based: it does not provide updated information on sexuality topics (such as HIV/AIDS) except incidentally within illustrations of principles and methods. Nor is it a "recipe book" of teaching activities; many such resources are available elsewhere.

ESTABLISHING A COMMON LANGUAGE FOR SEXUALITY EDUCATION

Sexuality educators must be explicit about the meanings they attribute to sexuality and gender terms to avoid confusing learners. The word "sex," for example, can be used to describe heterosexual intercourse, sexual activity of any kind, or the condition of being male or female (one's "sex"). The term "gender" can mean "male" and "female," or socialized roles for men and women ("masculine" and "feminine"). To understand how we use sexuality terminology in this book, please consult our glossary of key vocabulary.

KEY VOCABULARY FOR THIS BOOK

TERMS REFERRING TO FAMILY

Family: Two or more individuals (one of whom must be legally an adult) who live together with a commitment to care for each other. Our diverse culture recognizes many possible family configurations.

Family of origin: The family into which an individual was born or adopted (either legally or informally).

Family of choice: A group of individuals chosen by a person to substitute for or supplement his/her family of origin.

TERMS REFERRING TO GENDER

Gender: Physical characteristics associated with being female, male, or a chromosomal, hormonal, or developmental variation. These characteristics are the result of several factors: chromosomal patterns (XX, XY, or variations, such as XYY, XO); hormonal release patterns (cyclic or continuous); brain organization; response of target tissues to hormones; pubertal development; and influence of maternal disorders or drugs that affected the development of primary characteristics (such as fetal genitalia) or secondary characteristics (such as breast development).

Gender identity: An individual's self-perception of being male or female (i.e., "I am male" or "I am female"). A person's *gender identity* may or may not be congruent with the person's actual *gender* (e.g., the case of a transsexual person, whose gender identity does not match his/her gender at birth).

Gender roles: Cultural values and messages regarding differential expectations for males and females (*if* the culture differentiates between them): for example, the "feminine role" refers to the set of characteristics and behaviors expected of females and the "masculine role" to characteristics and behaviors considered appropriate for males.

Gender role identity: The extent to which a female or male individual accepts or rejects the cultural expectations *(gender role)* for his/her gender. A person's *gender role identity* may or may not be congruent with the *gender role* prescribed for him/her: that is, both males and females may be more or less "masculine," "feminine," or "androgynous" (some combination of both).

TERMS REFERRING TO SEXUAL ORIENTATION

Sexual orientation (also known as *affectional* or *erotic orientation*): An individual's actual feelings of attraction to other individuals in order to fulfill his/her sexual, affectional, social, emotional, and/or spiritual needs. Persons attracted primarily to the other gender are called *heterosexual;* to the same gender, *homosexual* (or *gay* and *lesbian*); and to both genders, *bisexual.*

Sexual orientation identity: An individual's self-perception regarding his/her own sexual orientation, that is, "I am heterosexual," "I am homosexual," or "I am bisexual." A person's actual *sexual orientation* may be incongruent with his/her *sexual orientation identity,* for example, a man who identifies as heterosexual but has sex with other men, or a woman who is sexually attracted to both genders but identifies as "lesbian."

Heterosexism: A belief in the superiority of, and privileges afforded to, heterosexual orientation and relationships.

Homophobia: Stereotyping, prejudice, discrimination, and hatred directed toward gays, lesbians, and bisexual people. Homophobia, much like racism and sexism, is expressed on individual, institutional, and cultural levels.

Biphobia: Stereotyping, prejudice, discrimination, and distrust directed specifically toward bisexual people.

TERMS REFERRING TO SEX AND SEXUALITY

Abstinence: Not engaging in any activity that puts one at risk for sexually transmitted diseases or pregnancy.

Sex or *sexual activity:* Physical acts of genital intimacy between persons of the same (homosexual) or different (heterosexual) genders. (Confusion often arises because many people, including educators and clinicians, use *sexually active* to mean exclusively "having heterosexual intercourse.")

Sexual intercourse or *coitus:* Heterosexual sex. (*Note:* Some people use this term also to mean homosexual sex.)

Safer sex: Sexual behavior that puts one at less risk of unwanted or undesirable consequences of sexual activity.

Prophylactic: Any product or object, such as latex condoms, spermicides, or dental dams, that reduces the likelihood of disease transmission or unwanted pregnancy.

Sexuality: A significant aspect of a person's life consisting of many interrelated factors: sexual anatomy, physiology, growth and development; gender, gender identity, and gender role identity; sexual orientation and sexual orientation identity; sexual behaviors and life-styles; sexual beliefs, attitudes, and values; body image and self-esteem; sexual health; sexual fantasies and dreams; relationship to others; life experiences; and spirituality as it relates to sexuality.

PART ONE

GENERAL PRINCIPLES AND SPECIAL ISSUES FOR TEACHING ABOUT SEXUALITY AND HIV

CHAPTER 1

The Modern Context for Teaching about Sexuality and HIV

"What does your mother do?" asked the older gentleman, making conversation with the seven-year-old occupying the seat next to him on a cross-country flight. The boy had moved to this location behind his mother, who was busy preparing a presentation for the next day.

"Well, she teaches about sexuality."

"Your mom teaches about *sex?*"

"No, not *sex,*" the boy replied, "*sexuality.* There's a difference, you know."

"Oh, really," said the man, perplexed. "Could you tell me what it is?"

"Well . . . sex is about things people can *do.* But sexuality is just part of who you *are.*"

The man thought for a moment, and said, "You know, I'm a lot older than you and until just now I've never known the difference between *sex* and *sexuality.* Thank you very much!"

> (Condensation of a conversation overheard
> by Maureen Considine, sexuality educator)

TEACHING SEXUALITY (NOT "SEX") EDUCATION

"Sex education," to many people, means teaching the basics of sexual "plumbing" and perhaps a few other rudimentary topics such as puberty, HIV, STDs, and pregnancy prevention. Since most adults have never experienced formal education about sexuality, they view the topic with a narrow, often distorted lens. Some fear it means teaching youngsters "how to have sex." But as one adolescent in a television audience observed recently, "We don't need anyone to teach us that—we figure it out all by ourselves!"

Sexuality education, by contrast, describes a much broader approach, addressing *all* aspects of becoming and being a sexual, gendered person including biological, psychological, and social perspectives. The main objectives of such *comprehensive* sexuality education are to help people feel good about themselves and their bodies, remain healthy, and build positive, equitable loving relationships—to be "sexually healthy" (see box). Sexual behavior is only a small part of the total picture.

The Goal of Comprehensive Sexuality Education

Sexually healthy people . . .
- Appreciate their own bodies.
- Interact with both genders in appropriate and respectful ways.
- Express love and intimacy in appropriate ways.
- Avoid exploitative relationships.
- Recognize their own values and show respect for people with different values.
- Recognize what is personally "right" and act on these values.
- Take responsibility for and understand the consequences of their own behavior.
- Enjoy sexual feelings without necessarily acting on them.
- Communicate effectively with family, friends, and partners.
- Talk with a partner about sexual activity before it occurs, including sexual limits (theirs and their partner's), contraceptive and prophylactic use, and meaning in the relationship.
- If sexually active, use contraception and prophylaxis effectively.
- Practice health prevention, such as regular checkups, breast or testicular self-exams.
- Understand the impact of media and peer messages on thoughts, feelings, values, and behaviors related to sexuality.
- Seek further information about sexuality as needed.

(Source: Adapted and revised from "Life Behaviors of a Sexually Healthy Adult," *Guidelines for Comprehensive Sexuality Education: Kindergarten–12th Grade*, National Guidelines Task Force, Sexuality Information and Education Council of the U.S. [SIECUS] [1992]. Author of original adaptation unknown.)

A comprehensive sexuality education program addresses everything from growth and development to self-esteem, to gender roles and stereotypes, to understanding the media, to resisting peer pressure, to being a sexual person throughout life, to prevention and treatment of sexual health problems, to knowing the difference between love and lust, to communication and other relationship skills and parenting.

School-based comprehensive sexuality education ideally begins in preschool or kindergarten, building upon key concepts each year until graduation from high school. It is best offered within the context of a comprehensive health curriculum and most effective when its messages are reinforced by parents and the community.

Sex-positive sexuality education is distinguished from "prophylactic sex education," which concentrates mainly on the prevention of undesirable sexual consequences such as sexually transmitted diseases, sexual abuse, unplanned pregnancy,

HIV, and sexual violence and harassment. While prevention topics are an important component of a comprehensive sexuality education program, discussing only the "dangers of sex" without also addressing the pleasures and joys of sexual relationships promotes a predominantly "sex-negative," fear-based view of human sexuality.

The full potential of comprehensive sexuality education is still unknown. Most sexuality education programs have not been truly comprehensive in either scope or sequence due to many limiting factors, including organized opposition. Researchers estimate that less than 10 percent of students in this country receive comprehensive sexuality education.[1] In its place, schools teach what Debra Haffner of the Sexuality Information and Education Council of the U.S. (SIECUS) calls "organ recitals and disaster prevention."[2]

Nonetheless, research reveals that sexuality education is correlated with the following significant changes in sexual knowledge, attitudes, comfort and behavior:

- Increases in sexual knowledge and personal comfort with sexuality.[3, 4]
- Increased tolerance toward the behaviors and personal values of others.[5]
- Delay in the onset of sexual intercourse and increased likelihood of using contraception when individuals do begin having intercourse.[6, 7]
- Increased communication with parents about sexual matters,[8] which correlates with more responsible behavior.[9]
- Increased self-esteem and decision-making skills.[10]

Behaviorally based programs in particular (such as the *Reducing the Risk* curriculum) have been associated with increased use of contraceptives among some students and increased communication with parents among all participants.[11] When linked with the provision of school-based clinic services, sexuality education is associated with a reduction in unplanned adolescent pregnancies.[12, 13] Other studies have reported that students who have received sexuality education have fewer sexual partners, use condoms more consistently, and, when refusal skills are also addressed, engage less often in sexual intercourse.[14]

A recent review by the World Health Organization of nineteen studies on sexuality education programs reported that, contrary to some beliefs, no significant relationship exists between receiving formal sexuality education and initiating sexual activity; if anything, education results in postponement or reduction in the frequency of sexual activity and more effective use of contraception. Furthermore, two studies indicated that access to counseling and contraceptive services does not encourage earlier or increased sexual activity.[15] When paired with community-wide efforts, sexuality education has been associated with significant reductions in teenage pregnancy rates.[16]

While these findings are heartening—and helpful in responding to opponents—many desirable outcomes of sexuality education are not easily quantified. Consider, for example, the student who was pleased that she could learn about parenthood through a "mock" pregnancy (raising a chick from a fertilized egg) rather than by having a real baby! Or the teen who, after watching a teen theater skit on emotional abuse, found the courage to get out of a destructive relationship. Or the distraught gay teen who decided not to commit suicide, after calling the crisis hotline number given out in a sexuality class. These qualitative, often invisible impacts of sexuality education rarely garner the attention of evaluators but nevertheless offer much of the impetus for this work. The full value of comprehensive sexuality education may be realized only when learners face watershed experiences in their lives.

THE RATIONALE AND SUPPORT FOR COMPREHENSIVE SEXUALITY EDUCATION

Educators always have had compelling reasons for providing sexuality education to the young and old alike; today, there is a new sense of urgency to our work. As the twentieth century comes to a close, the AIDS pandemic continues to expand, disproportionately affecting gay men, adolescents, women, and people of color; unintended pregnancies and sexually transmitted diseases among teens and adults occur at an unacceptable rate; the reported incidence of child sexual abuse, sexual harassment, and relationship violence is ballooning; relationship disintegration (two out of three adult and three out of five adolescent marriages end in divorce)[17] is creating a new paradigm for the "family," with its own set of dilemmas and emotional consequences for children and parents.

The good news is that a majority of the American public strongly supports school-based sexuality and HIV education. Since 1943, public support for sexuality education has steadily increased: from 68 percent to more than 85 percent in 1988.[18, 19] Parents of school-aged children (about 30 percent of total adults in the country) are even more likely to endorse it.[20] When the topic is AIDS, the level of public support rises to as high as 95 percent. A majority also supports inclusion of "controversial" topics in sexuality education, such as contraception, abortion, and homosexuality, for children 12 years old and older,[21] and eight out of ten parents want their children to be taught about safer sex.[22] When given the opportunity to opt their children out of sexuality education, only about 1–3 percent do so.[23]

Over eighty mainstream organizations form a National Coalition to Support Sexuality Education, including the American Medical Association, American School Health Association, American Association of School Administrators, National School Boards, and several mainstream religious organizations.[24] Recently, the U.S. Conference of Mayors endorsed a resolution calling not only for comprehensive sexuality education, but for condom availability for students.[25]

Parents want to be the primary sexuality educators of their children, but they also appreciate the school playing a role. Most don't feel knowledgeable, comfortable, or skilled enough to teach about sexuality and HIV and fear they will do or say the wrong thing;[26] for whatever reason, fewer than 20 percent of parents take an active role in providing sexuality education.[27] They still want to be involved, however, whether as informal sexuality educators or as "sentinels" watching over the school-based program.

Children also want to be able to talk with their parents and cite them as one of their most influential sources of information;[28] however, some (especially adolescents) feel too uncomfortable to discuss many topics honestly and openly. In a telling recent survey, for example, 81 percent of parents reported believing that their teens were honest with them about sexuality, but only 22 percent of their teenage children said they actually were.[29] Additional barriers to parent-teen communication include embarrassment, poor communication in general, different values about sex and dating, and a desire to avoid conflict.[30]

Roughly half of 15–19-year-olds say that most young people do not have enough accurate information about sex and reproduction;[31] teachers, administrators, and students all agree that sexuality education should be part of the school curriculum.[32–34] Some adolescents want the schools to teach their parents about sexuality as well so they will better comprehend teenage sexuality.[35] Students also have thoughtful suggestions about the design of sexuality education programs (see box). As one writer has noted, perhaps educators should be less focused on what messages to *send* to young people, and more receptive to hearing what they want, need, and think will work with their peers.[36]

If We Listen to Students . . .

Here's what they recommend for their sexuality and HIV education programs:
- Use only those teachers who are knowledgeable, comfortable, open, honest, nonjudgmental, and able to facilitate discussion.
- Stop focusing exclusively on sexual "plumbing" (anatomy and physiology) and address topics that really interest us: STDs besides AIDS, emotional aspects of sexuality, relationships, life-styles, sexual practices, protecting yourself, personal safety, gender roles, and controversial topics like abortion and sexual orientation.
- Address both the positive and negative aspects of sexuality—not just "scare tactics."
- Don't moralize or judge students; it creates a negative, oppressive atmosphere.
- Take into account students' personal histories (such as sexual abuse) and recognize the realities of sexual pressure. Be aware that some people have been exploited sexually.
- Teach sexuality in coeducational classes to encourage open lines of communication and sharing of feelings.
- Replace outdated texts and films with current, realistic, nonmoralizing materials.
- Talk on the students' level—accept or use slang (not vulgarity) and share some personal experiences.
- Train more peer educators. Bring in peer guest speakers.
- Educate parents about sexuality and what takes place in sexuality education.
- Start sexuality and HIV education early—in elementary grades.
- Require comprehensive human sexuality before graduation from high school.

(SOURCES: Teen focus group conducted for the Office of the Superintendent of Public Instruction, Olympia, Washington [February 1993]; "Listen to the Young Speak Out on Liquor, Food, and Sex,"

PTA Today [February 1981]; Nancy Peterfreund and Karen Moe, "Seattle School District 1993 Teen Health Survey: Report on Findings" [March 1994].)

REALITIES IN TEACHING ABOUT SEXUALITY AND HIV

Effective teaching about sexuality and HIV is not easy, however, especially given the social and health realities our learners face today. Gone are the days when a health educator could feel successful by delivering a lecture, distributing a worksheet, and having students demonstrate what they had learned on a pencil-and-paper quiz. Much more is required for students to learn what they really need to remain safe, healthy, and happy in the modern world. Our students' life situations are getting more complex and dangerous; we need to use increasingly creative and stimulating teaching methods to accomplish our task.

Learners Are Diverse, with Diverse Needs

The nineteenth-century dream that America would become a "melting pot" in which its many subcultures would blend together has not been realized; modern society is really more like a "stew," in which we all share the pot but retain many distinct identities. Our communities are diverse—racially, ethnically, religiously, and politically—and will become only more so as we move into the next millennium. Current estimates project that by the year 2000, for example, one out of three elementary and secondary school students in the United States will be an ethnic "minority."[37]

Learners not only are culturally diverse but reflect differences with respect to their sexuality, relationships, and family structure as well. Within any classroom group, educators should anticipate having students with diverse characteristics and experiences:

- Many learners are sexually experienced (approximately 72 percent by the time they complete high school), some by choice and some not.[38]
- They practice monogamy, "serial monogamy," multiple concurrent partnerships, or celibacy.
- Roughly 10 percent are gay, lesbian, or bisexual.[39]
- Many have experienced family disruption through divorce or death, sexual exploitation, family or partner violence, unintended pregnancies, abortion, and sexually transmitted diseases.
- Though less often, students may be affected by HIV/AIDS, be transsexual or transgenderal, or have any number of genetic or hormonal challenges that may affect their sexuality.

Students now harken from every conceivable kind of family configuration: "traditional" nuclear, single parented, blended, extended, coparented, grandparented, foster parented, and same-gender parented. The "traditional" family of two married parents and their minor children living together is now the exception: as of 1992 only 26 percent of American families fit this model; fewer than 10 percent of families had a mom who did not work outside the home;[40, 41] and approximately 20 percent of American children live with only one parent, usually the mother.[42] Between the 1950s and mid-1980s, the proportion of 14-year-old females living with a single parent rose from 21 percent to 38 percent.[43]

Learners Face More Sexual Risks

Today's learners initiate sexual activity earlier, have more lifetime sexual partners, and face many more sexual risks than did their parents or grandparents. The United States is now the developed world's leader in many sexual problems, such as sexually transmitted diseases, HIV, rape, and child sexual abuse;[44] these problems are disproportionately reflected in the adolescent population.

The average age of first intercourse is 15.7 years for males and 16.2 for females;[45] among inner city youth, the average age of initiation is 12.5 years.[46] About 10 percent of 12-year-olds, and three-quarters of all young people aged 15 to 19, are having intercourse; 20 percent have four or more partners.[47, 48] The earlier they begin having sexual intercourse, the more likely they are to have multiple partners; if younger than 13, they are nine times more likely to have more partners than those who begin sexual activity at age 15 or 16.[49]

Few teens plan their first intercourse; 21 percent *never* use contraception, accounting for 75 percent of approximately one million teenage pregnancies per year, involving four out of ten girls before they turn 20.[50, 51] Sexually transmitted infection rates are increasing faster for teens than for young adults: from 1960 to 1988 the prevalence of gonorrhea among 15–19-year-olds increased 170 percent, more than quadruple the rate of increase among 20–24-year-olds. Two and a half million adolescents are infected with an STD annually, or one out of six, representing one-fifth of the national cases, increasing their chances for health problems such as ectopic pregnancies, infertility, pelvic inflammatory disease, and cervical cancer. Over one-fifth of people who develop AIDS are in their twenties and most likely were infected as adolescents;[52] 90 percent of HIV-positive teens do not know they are infected.[53]

Yet teens are reluctant to seek regular reproductive health care: sexually active girls wait an average of 11.5 months between initiating sexual intercourse and visiting a clinic.[54] Half of all teen pregnancies occur within six months of the first intercourse,[55] one-fifth within the first month.[56]

A recent survey on teen health risks, including sexual risk taking, sheds additional light on youth vulnerability.[57] Although nearly all students engage in some risk behaviors, starting at early ages, some groups of students are affected disportionately. Educators therefore must target prevention education on specific behaviors within specific groups.

Many students are engaging in risk behaviors by the eighth grade. Since students who drop out of school typically do so by the ninth grade, and stopping behaviors is much more difficult than preventing them in the first place, prevention education must obviously occur much earlier.[58–61]

All students are affected by others' behaviors—unwanted sexual pressures, harassment, and offers of illicit drugs.[62] For example, more than eight in ten public school students in grades eight to eleven say they have been subjected to unwelcome sexual comments or advances, usually from another student; six in ten admit to having been a perpetrator themselves.[63] Educators must provide universal education, including skill building (e.g., refusal skills).

Social Inequalities Affect Sexual Behaviors

Underlying many programs of sexuality and HIV education is an assumption that all individuals are able to choose their behaviors freely within the context of a coequal partnership, or that they are committed to maintaining their own good health. This assumption denies reality.

For example, an estimated 20–25 percent of girls and 15 percent of boys in the United States are sexually victimized before the age of eighteen; gay youth are even more at risk.[64] The power differential inherent in the sexual abuse dynamic lowers self-esteem and self-efficacy, associated with an increased incidence of premature pregnancy,[65] eating disorders, drug addiction, unsafe adult sex, and HIV infection for survivors.[66] Therefore, perhaps the best approach to preventing sexual abuse is to educate those who are more likely to grow up to be abusers— usually boys—in addition to teaching avoidance and reporting skills to their potential victims.[67]

Likewise, much AIDS prevention education is directed at women, admonishing them to limit their number of sexual partners, avoid risky behaviors, and have their partners use condoms.[68] Imagine a 120-pound woman telling her 190-pound drug-addicted, abusive partner that he must wear a condom! In some subcultures (e.g., Latino) women must not speak of sexual matters nor challenge their male partners' authority.[69] Perhaps AIDS prevention education for heterosexuals is more appropriately targeted to men, especially since condoms are a *male* prophylactic.

Most teenage mothers are impregnated by partners over the age of 20, not their age-mates, as is often assumed;[70] the younger the teen, the greater the age gap. On the average, teenage women have male partners three years older than they are;[71] 71 percent of married teenage women and 24 percent of married teenage men have spouses over the age of 20.[72] We recently witnessed a panel presentation by five 15-year-old mothers; all of their babies were fathered by men over 30! Yet many sexuality and HIV education programs presume that all or most teenage "dating" is happening between peers.

Socioeconomic inequities also play a role in early pregnancy, risk-taking behaviors of all kinds, and defeatist attitudes among some minorities. African-American males, for example, are less likely to believe that health prevention measures actually work or that they will survive their youth.[73] Similarly, "at-risk" youth (i.e., out-of-school, homeless, drug-using, or incarcerated) take unwarranted risks due to pessimism and low self-esteem. Lesbian, gay, or bisexual youth are more likely to engage in self-destructive behaviors[74, 75] and to be victimized by those who take advantage of their self-protective cloak of secrecy about being "different."[76] Some gay men engage in risky sexual behavior because of low self-esteem resulting from living in a society that degrades their sexual orientation.[77]

Media Influence on Sexual Attitudes and Behaviors

American adolescents watch six hours of television a day and view nearly 14,000 instances of sexual material each year. A scant one percent of these scenes make any reference to sexuality education, prophylaxis, or consequences such as sexually transmitted diseases or abortion.[78] Sexism, violence, and power inequities characterize heterosexual relationships; homosexual or bisexual people, if shown at all, are often negatively stereotyped. Nevertheless, teens rate television as their third most important source of information about sex (after peers and school), and half of them believe television relates a realistic picture of consequences.[79, 80] Many young people watch talk shows, in particular, to obtain information about sexuality—emotional aspects of relationships, sexual practices, diverse life-styles, and so on—not being provided by parents or school.[81]

Studies confirm that movies and music videos negatively affect attitudes about gender roles, rape, sexual attractiveness, and permissive sexual activity.[82] Most media, including magazines and advertisements, depict children and youth inappropriately sexualized beyond their years; images of sex and attractiveness are used to promote products to the young and old alike. Without the positive countermessages of comprehensive sexuality education, and lacking the skills to be critical consumers of media, youth develop distorted, dysfunctional views of sexuality, gender roles, and relationships.

Other Social Factors Affecting Youth Sexuality

Critics often blame sexuality education for "sexualizing" children earlier than in previous generations. In fact, many other social forces contribute to this phenomenon; comprehensive sexuality education provides one of the few counterbalances.

General improvements in health and nutrition cause young people to reach physical maturity much earlier than their predecessors; the gap between puberty and marriage age increased from an average of 7.2 years for women in 1890 to 11.8 years for women and 12.5 for men in 1988.[83] Faced with an extended adolescence and normal sexual desires, many youth don't wait until finishing their education or committing to a long-term, monogamous relationship before beginning sexual activity. In a culture that lacks any formal initiation into adulthood, the onset of sexual activity often provides a substitute.

Social norms, reinforced greatly by media messages, exacerbate peer pressure to "just do it" while the social stigma for sexual consequences (such as unintended pregnancy) no longer exists in most groups. Changes in family structure and parents' work patterns have resulted in a decline in adult supervision of youth; most students report having sex in their own homes, many in their parents' bedrooms.[84]

Both external and internal barriers interfere with the development and implementation of effective comprehensive sexuality and HIV education programs.

Adult discomfort and misperceptions about the nature of modern sexuality education play a significant role in preventing or limiting the development of effective programs. Adults are uncomfortable with adolescent sexuality in particular; consequently, they support programs based on their images of how they would *like* youth to be. Individual parents or community members frequently object to programs that address the real concerns of youth as being too "explicit" or "controversial." To paraphrase one educator's observation, the result is that "June and Ward Cleaver design sexuality education programs intended for Beavis and Butthead."

Teachers have more difficulty holding the attention of students today, in part because they must compete with students' experience of rapid-fire, colorful, "hip" media offerings. Educators cite student boredom and discipline problems as significant barriers to learning.[85] Aggravating the problem is the "saturation effect" of the same AIDS messages from many sources or annual duplicative lessons;[86] educators must use innovative, effective methods to captivate student interest.

Organized opposition is by far the greatest obstacle to effective sexuality education. Teachers and administrators alike cite minority opposition as their biggest concern in implementing programs, even in light of broad-based public support.[87] Sexuality and HIV education is a lightning rod for individuals, groups, and national organizations with broader agendas regarding public schools. Historically, such groups have succeeded in undermining or eliminating many sexuality education programs (see box). In Chapter 5, we discuss this issue in more detail and present some specific strategies for preventing and defusing opposition.

A Historical Perspective on Sexuality Education

Before the early 1900s, little attention was given to sex education of the young. Children were thought to be "asexual" and many believed that to bring up the subject of sex would invite experimentation, with emotional or physical consequences. As for adults, contracting a sexually transmitted disease or conceiving an out-of-wedlock pregnancy was evidence of moral failure, and doctors could refuse to treat such unfortunates.

In the early nineteenth century, several societal changes converged to launch the "social hygiene educational movement," primarily intended to reduce venereal disease. "Germs" were discovered to play a role in human illness, including sexually transmitted disease. Darwin's theory of evolution, espoused in the 1850s but not widely understood, was interpreted by social hygienists as both "a warning and a promise" in that humans are like their simian cousins in their beastly urges, but selective breeding (*eugenics*) could eliminate certain undesirable traits. Correct information about sex and heredity therefore was considered essential. Freud's assertion that sexuality begins at birth fostered a reassessment of the belief in the asexual nature of children and adolescents. As a result, schools added a new objective to the curriculum: "sublimation" of student sexual urges into more acceptable pursuits such as work, sports, music, or the arts. At the same time, the schools became involved in other topics previously considered to be the sole domain of the family: health and nutrition, child care, vocational training, and "temperance" education (i.e., substance-abuse prevention).

Since the early 1900s, the primary goal for sexuality education has been prevention of disease and dysfunction. However, its scope, character, and philosophy have widely fluctuated and evolved. During the early days of public school sex education, the main objectives were to uphold traditional sexual values, promote sexual restraint, and warn about the dangers of sex. In the mid-1940s, concern about STDs and marital problems of returning G.I.s reenergized sex education, which was broadened to address individual sexual adjustment within marriage. In the 1960s, soaring divorce rates, the women's movement, concern about teenage pregnancy, and a renewed interest in Progressive education provided the stimulus for a resurgence of sex education. Programs of this era included values clarification, promotion of tolerance for different sexual lifestyles, and more comprehensive coverage of topics. Eventually, intense organized opposition diluted or stopped many programs.

In the 1980s and 1990s, the AIDS pandemic has rekindled interest in sexuality and substance-abuse-prevention education as the only means of avoiding infection. The tone and character of sexuality and HIV education programs today vacillate between the antisex, moralistic, and prophylactic philosophy of the first half of the century and the sex-positive, pluralistic, and broader approach of programs in the second. Whether this latest upsurge in sexuality education also will succumb to backlash remains to be seen.

(SOURCES: Michael Imber, "Toward a Theory of Educational Origins: The Genesis of Sex Education," *Educational Theory*, Vol. 34, No. 3 [Summer 1984], 275–286; Lynn R. Penland, "Sex Education in 1900, 1940 and 1980: An Historical Sketch," *The Journal of School Health* [April 1981], 305–308; Lester A. Kirkendall, personal communication, 1986.)

Lack of training for teachers and administrators presents a significant internal problem. Fewer than half the states require specialized training for teachers of sexuality or substance-abuse education; most states accept a generic health or physical education certification. Consequently, preservice training institutions rarely address these topics adequately, and many new teachers feel completely unprepared to teach about sexuality or drug use, both of which are critical to HIV prevention education.[88-90] Even experienced health educators, competent in teaching reproductive anatomy and physiology, express lack of confidence in teaching about certain topics including STDs, sexual transmission of HIV, homosexuality, and abortion.[91]

Administrators would deal more easily with problems if they were better trained in creating and sustaining sexuality and HIV programs and handling controversy. Like teachers, many are uncomfortable both with the topic and with the tactics of opposition groups. Until institutions of higher learning address the needs of both preservice teachers and administrators, or school districts provide more inservice training, insufficient preparation will continue to negatively affect sexuality and HIV education. (We say more about teacher training needs in Chapter 5.)

Other internal barriers include lack of time, money, and current materials. Sexuality and HIV education must compete with many other subjects in an already crowded school curriculum; lack of sufficient instructional time is a serious concern. Many districts and states have no required health education curriculum within which to incorporate sexuality education; consequently, it frequently is grafted onto miscellaneous subjects, with an average of twelve hours total instruction per grade level[92]—what some consider to be the minimum just for HIV education.[93]

Few schools can afford the many available excellent curricula and other new resources. Students complain about outdated or insufficient materials, and teachers say having to create their own is a major deterrent. Some current HIV curricula are inadequate because they do not address topics such as homosexuality, diverse sexual behaviors, and sources of prophylactics.[94]

Support from higher authorities would make the task of implementing programs less daunting. Many states mandate HIV prevention education; however, few require *comprehensive* sexuality education or even revise their *existing* sexuality curricula. School board and state agency officials are often unwilling to risk backlash if they undertake a curriculum review process, a realistic but manageable scenario in most communities.

On the national level, health education is still trying to recover from the 1980s when policymakers were engaged in a sociopolitical struggle between "public health realists" and "moralizers."[95] Political leaders are still conspicuously reticent on the AIDS pandemic, promote and fund "abstinence only" and "revirginization" programs (despite questions about their effectiveness), and have canceled a planned national sexual behavior survey to verify the scope of the problem.[96]

Critics of sexuality education often query us, "Why is it, if schools have been offering sex education *[sic]* for so many years, we still have so many teen pregnancies, STDs, HIV, and relationship problems?"

First of all, fewer than 10 percent of students currently receive anything approximating *comprehensive* sexuality education,[97] and schools introduce many topics much later than needed. Parents aren't doing their part well enough, either; children report that parents are uncomfortable and wait too late to bring up sexuality issues with them. Starting education about sexual risk taking after sexual activity has begun is unlikely to affect established behaviors.[98]

What would the consequences be if other essential subjects were taught in a similar manner? What if math, for example, did not start until the fifth grade, was offered in a one-week unit (or in an assembly with a local mathematician), the boys and girls were separated for some topics (multiplication for one gender, division for the other), and some essential topics were excluded altogether (because "algebra would violate our children's math 'innocence' ")?

Complex, persistent social problems like unintended pregnancies, dysfunctional relationships, sexual abuse of children, and the HIV pandemic are complicated by broader changes occurring in society: the disintegration of families and communities, dwindling economic resources and educational opportunities, changing social norms, decline in the availability of social and health services, and persistently irresponsible media messages. These problems cannot be cured by education alone.

Part of the responsibility should be placed squarely on the shoulders of opponents who actively work against programs and restrict informed public discourse about sexuality education. They promulgate false dichotomies and simplistic slogans: "virgins" versus sexually experienced students, abstinence-only approaches versus "amoral, technocratic sex education," school versus parental rights, a return to the morals of an earlier time (1950s?) versus a "decadent society in which anything goes." They suggest that these are the only choices before us; such thinking makes for good newspaper copy, but poor health education policy.

The proper direction of sexuality and HIV education should be determined by information that is available about what is really needed and what really works, not by unfounded fears, ill-informed opinions, and unrealistic objectives. Today's problems are far too complex and learners too diverse for a "one size fits all" approach.

We believe that sexuality education, rather than contributing to sexual health problems (as some claim), has played a role in *reducing their rate of increase*. Considering the many barriers and historical opposition to sexuality education, to judge its potential effectiveness based on the limited documentation of its performance thus far is premature and wrong-headed—the equivalent of blaming a horse for losing the race when three of its legs were hobbled.

CHAPTER 2

Effective Sexuality and HIV Education: What Works and Why

If telling were the same as teaching, we'd all be so smart we could hardly stand it!

—R. Mager, *Developing Attitude toward Learning*, 1968

If effective teaching about sexuality and HIV prevention were the same as simply "telling" students about the dangers or even the joys of sex, community health educators and teachers would not have to worry as much as they do about students engaging in risky sexual behaviors or making poor relationship decisions. After all, educators have been diligently disseminating information on sexual topics for many years now, especially since the 1980s when AIDS education was recognized as the only weapon against the spread of HIV.

Increasing cognitive knowledge—an essential objective of sexuality education—has never been sufficient in affecting learner behavior, and health educators have long been held to a higher standard of behavioral outcomes than colleagues in other subject areas.[1] Until the recent advent of "outcome-based education," most teachers were content with simply increasing student cognitive knowledge; rarely were they concerned with facilitating affective or behavioral outcomes as well. Health and sexuality educators, on the other hand, always have sought to affect student behaviors related to substance use, smoking, nutrition, unintended pregnancy, sexual exploitation, HIV and STD, and many other concerns.

Some people believe if educators simply repeat messages of "Just say no!" often and emphatically enough, students will listen, learn, and behave accordingly. Researchers and educators now know that such "abstinence-only" approaches do not work with most learners: many do not heed messages from authority figures; different learners require different messages and approaches; and effective education demands more than preaching.

Our teachers tell us to 'just say no,' but who listens to their English teacher about whether or not to have sex?

(Student in a focus group, Olympia, Washington, February 1993.)

Now more than ever, sexuality and HIV educators must have an impact on learners that will carry over into their real lives. This means creating learning experiences that allow students to examine their sex-related attitudes, values, and current behaviors. It also means giving learners opportunities to develop and practice the *skills* they need to maintain healthy and personally satisfying sexual relationships. The ultimate goal for effective sexuality education is the development of sexually healthy people.

To us, "effective sexuality education" is what works best to meet the educational needs of learners. Learners have their own set of interests and expectations for sexuality education, such as wanting more information on certain topics, but may not be cognizant of everything they need to know. Educators also have objectives, dictated by their own professional and personal judgment and by school or organizational policies. Educators should help learners fulfill both sets of objectives—the learner's and the educator's—in order for the experience to be "effective."

Research reveals that sexuality education *can* have a positive impact on learners (see Chapter 1). That research, together with the authors' study of educational theory and philosophy, our experience teaching sexuality education, and extensive feedback received from our learners, gives us insight into what kind of sexuality education works best.

The remainder of this chapter outlines ten guiding principles for effective sexuality and HIV education, in the form of questions to ask when evaluating or designing an educational program, course, or workshop.

THE ELEMENTS OF EFFECTIVE SEXUALITY EDUCATION

Question 1: Does the program present a positive, accurate, and comprehensive view of human sexuality?

An effective sexuality program or workshop, first and foremost, promotes a sex-positive view of human sexuality: it treats sexuality as a potentially healthy, fulfilling aspect of human existence. A *comprehensive* program covers all relevant and essential topics, not just those considered noncontroversial.

Shame and guilt make poor bedfellows with expressive and healthy sexuality. Some people wrongly believe that promoting sex-negative messages and emphasizing the "dangers of sex" will discourage sexual activity among adolescents. To the contrary, research shows that feelings of shame, guilt, and discomfort with sexuality correlate with poor sexual decision making.[2–5] Also, negative feelings about sexuality (*erotophobia*) inhibit learning about sexuality;[6] similarly, extreme homophobia interferes with learning about HIV transmission and prevention.[7]

On the other hand, positive messages about sexuality foster safer behaviors. A study on contraceptive use found, for example, that participants who felt positive and comfortable about their sexuality were more likely to use contraception effectively.[8] Unfortunately, most programs fail to meet this primary criterion: for example, a recent review of HIV education curricula in the United States reveals that only three curricula in fifty states and two territories promoted a "positive" view of sexuality.[9]

Modern Western culture is saturated with negative messages about sexuality in general and about women in particular. Throughout Judeo-Christian history, as reflected in artistic, literary, and theological traditions, sexuality has been considered at best a "lesser" human attribute, at worst an evil one. Negative side effects of this cultural programming include personal discomfort with our bodies and feelings of guilt and shame, and public avoidance or suppression of discussion of sexual matters in education, research, the law, medicine, politics, and cultural activities. This cultural "conspiracy of silence" contributes to individual ignorance about sexuality and fosters unrealistic expectations in relationships, sexual dysfunction, and ill-informed sexual decision making.

Women, because of their obvious role in reproduction, have been equated throughout our history with matters of the "body" and denigrated in comparison with men, who are considered to be more "intellectual and spiritual."[10] Because of this general view, reinforced by some misogynist religious tenets, women carry a subtle burden of shame and blame, leading to sexual oppression on both the relationship and societal levels. Personal health consequences for women include sexual victimization, domestic violence and marital rape, and difficulty in contracepting successfully or practicing safer sex.[11, 12] Consequences on the societal level include limited career opportunities, unequal pay, sexual harassment, and inadequate attention to women's health concerns, to mention only a few.

Positive Messages about Sexuality and Gender

- Sexuality begins at birth (some say at conception)* and is neither evil nor "unclean."
- All parts of the human body are worthy of respect and care.
- Sexuality is a gift that can be explored, expressed, and treasured in many different ways.
- Men and women are different in some ways, but equally worthy of respect, love, and power.
- Loving relationships should be characterized by honesty, equality, individual integrity ("wholeness"), open communication, and shared responsibility.

*Mary Calderone, SIECUS co-founder, personal communication, 1985.

The underlying philosophy of a program affects not only the tone of its key messages but which topics are included, how topics are addressed, and, ultimately, how well educational needs are met. Students need to have accurate and complete information addressing their *real concerns and questions* and enabling them to make informed decisions about sexual behaviors and relationships. Peter Scales has noted that many sexuality education programs fail in this task: "Too many people . . . are still learning to spell epididymous *[sic]* and describe its 'primary function.' I still can't spell it, and it hasn't affected a single decision in my life." [13]

Comprehensive sexuality education includes topics that some adults would consider "controversial": varieties of sexual behaviors (including masturbation), safer sex practices (including proper use of a condom), sexual orientation, abortion, substance use and abuse, death and dying, and diverse values and life-styles. However, most sexuality education curricula avoid such topics.

Some "abstinence only" or "fear-based" curricula distort facts, leave out essential information, and exaggerate the risks of sexual activity and condom use to "scare" adolescents into remaining celibate until marriage (see box). Some focus on the failure rates and rare side effects of contraceptives but don't mention their protective effects for other health problems such as heart disease or address the comparative risks of childbearing. Most troubling, these curricula stress the impacts of sexually transmitted diseases but deliberately omit information on how to obtain prophylactics or treatment.

Common Characteristics of "Fear-Based" Curricula*

- Scare tactics to discourage premarital sexual behavior.
- Information about contraceptive methods usually omitted; if mentioned, failure rates are emphasized and overstated.
- Focus exclusively on the negative consequences of sexual behavior; students do not examine their own values about premarital sexual behavior.
- Medical misinformation given about abortion, STDs, HIV/AIDS, and sexual response.
- Sexual orientation not discussed, or homosexuality is described as an unhealthy "choice."
- Sexist bias evident in descriptions of anatomy, physiology, sexual response, and sexual behavior; stereotypical gender roles presented.
- People with disabilities omitted or reflected as nonsexual.
- Racist and classist comments in texts and stereotypes about various communities underscored.
- Religious bias evident and only one viewpoint on sexual behavior given.
- A limited number of family structures included; nontraditional families depicted as "troubled."

*These characteristics were gleaned from eleven curricula: Sex Respect by Coleen Mast; Facing Reality, by James Coughlin; Me, My World, My Future and Sexuality, Commitment and Family by Teen Aid; Family Accountability Communicating Teen Sexuality (FACTS) by Northwest Family Services; Learning about Myself and Others by Anne Nesbit; An Alternative National Curriculum on Responsibility (ANCHOR), and Families, Decision-Making and Human Development by Terrance Olson and Christopher Wallace; Responsible Sexual Values Program (RSVP) by April Thoms; The Art of Loving Well by Ronald Goldman and Nancy McLaren; Free Teens by Richard Panzer.

(SOURCE: Leslie Kantor, "Scared Chaste: Fear-Based Educational Curricula," SIECUS Report, Volume 21, Number 2 [December 1992/January 1993], 1–18.)

Lately, a movement to secure pledges of sexual abstinence from young people has been widely publicized.[14] While any strategy that encourages adolescent abstinence is commendable, the irony is, as Ira Reiss has noted, too often adolescent "vows of abstinence break far more easily than condoms."[15] Avoiding honest discussion about prophylaxis, and misrepresenting its effectiveness (as some would have sexuality educators do), leaves students with no protection if and when they do engage in sexual activity.

Many state-developed HIV education curricula stress abstinence and other such "noncontroversial" topics as dating and family issues to the exclusion of the other essential topics. For example, only three state curricula thoroughly address how to use a condom.[16] Teachers also report that they cannot or do not cover many topics crucial for students, e.g., birth control methods and where to obtain them.[17] See the box for reasons why one "controversial" topic should be included in the curriculum.

An Oft-Excluded Topic: Why We Should Teach about Sexual Orientation

- Because many students are either gay, lesbian, or bisexual themselves, or have parents or siblings who are (affecting as many as five to ten kids in every classroom).
- Because kids who believe they are gay, lesbian, or bisexual (or whose parents are) may harbor a lot of myths about themselves or their loved ones: that they will be gay just because a parent is, that gay people are child molesters, that survivors of sexual abuse will become gay, that all homosexuals will die of AIDS, or that gay people can never be happy in a relationship.
- Because schools have an obligation to support and enhance the self-esteem of all students, and to counteract stereotyping and prejudice that can lead to discrimination and violence against gays, lesbians, and bisexuals.
- Because many kids (straight or gay) have questions about sexual orientation, and schools are the most logical place for them to receive accurate, unbiased information.
- Because homophobia and heterosexism in schools and society place lesbian and gay youth at increased risk for emotional and physical risks, including social isolation, depression, substance abuse, and suicide, with suicide rates two to six times more than heterosexual youth.*

In reality, schools already are places in which children learn about sexual orientation—by student jokes and taunts of "fag" or "lezzy," and by heterosexism in the school curriculum and climate. Which values would we rather teach: that ignorance, intolerance, and hate are acceptable, or that we should respect and care about one another regardless of our differences?

*Ann Thompson Cook, "Who is Killing Whom?" *Respect All Youth Project*, Federation of Parents and Friends of Lesbians and Gays, Washington, D.C. Issue Paper 1, 1991.

(SOURCE: Adapted from Beth Reis, "Why Should the Public Schools Teach about Sexual Orientation," paper presented at the annual meeting of the Association for Sexuality Education and Training [ASSET], September 22, 1989. Copy available from ASSET [see Appendix C].)

Another glaring omission from most sexuality education programs is any discussion of sexual pleasure or intimacy. A truly sex-positive program acknowledges not only the potential risks of sex but the pleasurable aspects as well. To exclude these topics denies that desires for sexual release and for intimacy with another human being are powerful incentives for youth to become sexually active. Students need to know that, although these feelings are normal, not all sexual desires need be acted upon and that there are many safe ways to experience intimacy.

Other incidents of incomplete or distorted sexuality education occur in teaching about gender. Many curricula and educators overemphasize gender differences, avoid any discussion of female sexual desire, treat females largely as potential sexual victims and males as sexual aggressors, value female over male virginity, and place responsibility on the female for postponing sexual activity and handling contraception.[18-20] Some educators dismiss or downplay facts about biological differences to promulgate their own gender philosophy. Male perspectives may be overlooked, if not as a result of direct bias, then perhaps because of the traditional linkage of women with puberty and reproduction, the focus of many curricula.[21]

In such programs, students are denied an accurate, honest, and balanced perspective. How can we expect young people to trust adult messages that are tinged with half-truths and lies of omission, or to develop into well-adjusted sexual beings when they have been given primarily sex-negative, incomplete information about their sexuality? One of Joan's favorite poems ("Lies" by Yevgeny Yevtushenko) says that it is wrong to tell lies to the young; we believe it is wrong to deliberately misinform *anyone* about human sexuality, whatever the political rationale or supposedly good intentions.

Affirming, accurate, and comprehensive information about sexuality is consistent with democratic values in our society, essential to the development of critical thinking, and, ultimately, more effective with learners. Individuals who have correct, complete information about sexuality feel positive rather than shameful about their own sexuality, have realistic and fair expectations of partners, and are more likely to make good decisions and find sexual happiness in their lives.

A Personal Story: "If Only I Had Known . . ."

Evonne was doing a teacher training on sexuality content and methods. On this evening, the topic was sexual response differences in men and women.

Using graphs depicting the typical male and female sexual response patterns, she explained that men and women differ in the amount of time it takes to become aroused, reach orgasm, and return to an unaroused state. During her lecture, she noticed one of the teachers had tears in her eyes. She stopped to inquire.

The woman hesitated a moment and then answered, "I wish someone had given me this information a long time ago. It would have prevented a lot of grief and conflict in my marriage."

Question 2: Does the program respect and empower students?

When we use the word "empowerment" we mean three things: first, acknowledging and addressing the true needs, concerns, and realities of students; second, giving students the information and classroom experiences they need to become critical thinkers and responsible decision makers; and third, sharing responsibility and decision making power with students.

Some educational philosophers have suggested that if teachers truly want to develop democratic citizens, they should allow students to experience democracy in the classroom. Unfortunately, most classrooms are more reflective of benevolent dictatorships than democracies. Generally speaking, the person having the power and responsibility in the traditional classroom is the *educator,* who makes prior decisions about what's worth knowing, how it will be studied, and how learners will be evaluated. The flip side of this arrangement is that the teacher is usually held solely accountable for the quality of learning that occurs.

In the democratic sexuality education class or workshop, however, learners share not only in the decision-making process but also hold some of the responsibility for the quality of the learning experience. That is, they are asked what they need and want to learn; they assist in the planning and implementation of learning activities; they share responsibility for how well the group "works" together; and they cooperate in evaluating the experience and their own learning. (See Chapters 6 and 7 for more discussion of this approach.)

Fostering Student Empowerment in the Sexuality Education Classroom

- Ask students what they want to learn.
- Help students get to know one another.
- Develop ground rules *with* students (not *for* them).
- Promote respect for differences, open and constructive communications, support, and honesty.
- Promote cooperation rather than competition among students.
- Welcome spontaneity and appropriate humor.
- Help students develop skills and knowledge.
- Serve as a facilitator, guide, resource, and colearner.
- View the curriculum as flexible, depending on emerging student needs and current events.
- Involve students in planning and evaluating the program.

Involved in this way, students have the opportunity to make teachers aware of their real, current needs and concerns, rather than those projected for them. Such sexuality education is more relevant and useful to learners. Students also gain practice in accepting responsibility for their own actions, both within and outside the classroom. Furthermore, participatory sexuality education encourages students to think critically, an essential element of democratic citizenship sorely lacking in our society.[22]

Learners who feel respected and empowered in an educational experience also are more likely to take intellectual and emotional risks necessary for growth. In a learning environment that fosters respect, confidentiality, openness, collaboration, and mutual support, students feel more comfortable sharing and exploring their feelings, ideas, and concerns. In such a psychologically "safe" environment, students more easily gain knowledge, explore attitudes, and practice skills necessary for implementing good health decisions outside of the classroom.

How programs address issues of gender roles—and empower or disempower young men and women—is of particular concern. For example, the underlying message of some curricula (such as *Teen Aid* and *Sex Respect*) is that males are naturally sexual aggressors and females are their passive targets. This view places the primary burden for responsible sexual behavior on the female and negatively stereotypes males; it also denies the reality that young women, too, have sexual drives.

In a culture that actively promotes sexual expression by young people, both genders may feel pressure to become sexually active before they are ready. An empowering sexuality education program helps males and females examine such cultural messages and how they interfere with their potential for happiness. Gender-equitable education also recognizes that *both* genders are victimized by socialization into rigid gender roles.

Using trained "peer educators" is an especially effective method of empowering students. Peer educators are viewed as role models and deemed more credible than adults.[23, 24] (Please see Chapter 12 for more on peer education programs, including *teen theater.*)

Question 3: Does the program respect cultural and sexual pluralism and promote universal values?

Cultural pluralism, sexual pluralism, and *universal values* are fundamental but potentially conflicting concepts that educators must balance in teaching about sexuality.

Cultural pluralism is a philosophy that acknowledges and values the fact that our society is more like a "stew" than a "melting pot" in its demographic makeup; that is, our communities and our classroom groups consist of individuals from many racial, religious, and cultural backgrounds, with diverse beliefs, values, and practices.

Not only are our learners culturally pluralistic, they also are *sexually pluralistic.*[25] In other words, they differ in fundamental ways that impact their sexuality, that is, their gender, sexual orientation, sexual values and attitudes, sexual health, family configurations, personal history, sexual experience, and relationships. Such differences show up not only among groups but within individuals themselves as "overlays" of experience and origins, for example, an Asian/Hispanic, adopted, bisexual, HIV-positive woman who is married and child-free.

Whose Culture Is It, Anyway?

Educators should set a tone within the classroom that respects cultural and sexual diversity:

- **Use inclusive language (e.g., use "he or she" rather than "he," "partner" rather than "spouse," "caregivers" or "trusted adults" in addition to "parents").**
- **Use materials reflecting gender, racial, family, and relationship diversity.**
- **Invite guest speakers with a diversity of perspectives.**
- **Use culturally diverse visual materials.**
- **Design learning activities that are inclusive (e.g., don't assume that all learners are sexually active, or heterosexual, or intend to become married or to parent).**
- **Acknowledge the cultural and sexual pluralism represented in the group.**
- **Promote "interculturalism," that is, increased understanding and communication among cultures.**

Many sound reasons exist for respecting cultural and sexual pluralism in sexuality and HIV education. First, public schools should reflect the actual makeup of our society and schools, not what some imagine or wish it to be (see statistics on the American family in Chapter 1). Second, it is generally accepted that public school teachers should not promote a particular religion or political party; why, then, would we have the right to prescribe to students their sexual or relationship choices?[26]

Third, unless learners feel that their group or experience is specifically addressed and included in a learning experience, they are less likely to internalize important messages. Researchers have discovered, for example, that young girls do not relate to stories using the supposedly "generic" male pronoun.[27] Likewise, African-American or working-class gay men do not respond well to literature or educational programs targeted to white, affluent, and highly educated gay men.[28, 29]

HIV education, in particular, should be sensitive to cultural, relationship, lifestyle, and gender diversity within specific populations, for example, at-risk adolescents, people of color, substance abusers, homosexual men, heterosexually identified men who have sex with men, and women.[30] One example of a culturally appropriate program is the Jemmott curriculum, designed for urban black male adolescents, which effectively utilizes culturally specific videotapes, games, exercises, and black group leaders to engage the interest of this target population.[31]

A true democracy welcomes all voices, even when they conflict with each other on fundamental values. However, our society also holds some relatively universal values that may not be superseded by individual opinion. "Universal," in this case, does not mean that every person agrees. Most Americans believe, for example, it is wrong for an adult to have sexual contact with a child; however, some individuals reject and violate this premise. In such cases, society's universal value of protecting children from sexual exploitation overrules the "right" of an adult to act on his or her own values and impulses.

Also, America was founded on guiding principles that govern our interactions and establish basic human rights, even though not all (or even a majority) of our citizens always agree with them or are willing to extend such rights to everyone. These are "universal values": all individuals have dignity and worth and deserve equal and considerate treatment; each person is responsible for his or her own actions; everyone has the right to choose, practice, or reject religion; and everyone has the right to life, liberty, and the pursuit of happiness. Not everyone embraces these ideals, however; one telling study found that fewer than 40 percent of Americans support the full range of civil liberties reflected in the Bill of Rights. [32]

Universal Values about Sexuality, Family and Relationships

- **All children should be loved and cared for, preferably within a healthy, functional family.**
- **Parents should be the primary sexuality educators of their children.**
- **Schools and other institutions also should be involved in the sexuality education of youth.**
- **It is preferable for young adolescents to abstain from sexual intercourse.**
- **Sex is best and safest in loving, long-term, committed, monogamous relationships.**
- **It is wrong to coerce or force anyone into unwanted sexual contact or to knowingly transmit disease.**

Educators sometimes must perform a delicate balancing act to respect cultural and sexual pluralism and, at the same time, support universal values. Some educators, for example, agonize over how to reconcile gender equity ideals with cultural practices that subjugate women, for example, "female circumcision," which, in reality, is extensive genital mutilation intended to decrease female sexual pleasure and assure chastity.

Many educators also struggle with community norms that conflict with the universal value of respecting everyone's human dignity and civil rights. Sol Gordon points out, for example, that some communities hold racist values, but that does not give them the right to offer school curricula with a racist bias. [33] The same is true for sexist or homophobic community norms.

Opposing groups often express conflicting values about sexuality and gender. Witness, for example, the ongoing philosophical battles between such groups as Phyllis Schafly's Eagle Forum and the National Organization for Women (over women's proper place in society), the National Right-to-Life Committee and the National Abortion Rights Action League (over abortion), and the Aryan Nation versus Queer Nation (over equal rights for homosexuals).

What's more, teachers have a variety of personal and political values. For this reason, educators must be especially careful not to impose their own values on students, abusing their authority over them (see Chapter 5 for more on this subject). Educators should promote universal values while acknowledging and examining diverse cultural views on sexuality. We can be, as Sol Gordon says, "moral without being moralistic."[34] As public school and community educators, we have no responsible alternative.

Question 4: Does the program address a diversity of learning styles and abilities?

Students vary greatly in learning styles and abilities, which derive from complex interactions of physiological, psychological, environmental, and situational influences.[35] Different styles include a variety of preferences: for visual, auditory, tactile (feeling), or kinesthetic (movement) stimuli; for learning alone (independent), in peer groups (collaborative), or from an authority figure (dependent); for reflective or active involvement; for creative "right brain" or logical "left brain" activities; and so on.[36] Entire books have been written on this subject—one book alone lists thirty-two different possible learning styles! We highlight only some of the major categories of learning style differences in the boxed inserts; note the overlapping concepts between and among the models.

Learning Modalities: "Sensual" Ways of Perceiving Information

Learners may show a preference for using different senses to receive and process information:
- *Kinesthetic* ("muscle sense") or *psychomotor* (movement): learning by manipulating objects (such as by building clay models of the reproductive system) or moving through physical space (such as "milling" exercises).
- *Visual* (or *spatial*): learning by observing with one's own eyes (such as watching a film, reading, or watching someone perform a task) or manipulating objects in the "mind's eye."
- *Aural* (or *verbal*): learning by listening or speaking (which is another way of listening—to one's own voice).
- *Taste and smell:* the lesser senses are also used for learning.

Multiple Intelligences

At least seven distinct types of "intelligences" have been described; some are more highly developed in individuals than others:
- *Verbal/linguistic intelligence:* Related to written and spoken languages.
- *Logical/mathematical intelligence:* Often called "scientific thinking," deals with

deductive thinking and reasoning, numbers, and the recognition of abstract patterns.
- *Visual/spatial intelligence:* Relies on the sense of sight and the ability to visualize an object and create mental images.
- *Body/kinesthetic intelligence:* Relates to physical movement and knowings of the body, including the brain's motor cortex which controls bodily motion.
- *Musical/rhythmical intelligence:* Based on recognition of tonal patterns, including environmental sounds, and on sensitivity to rhythm and beats.
- *Interpersonal intelligence:* Operates primarily through person-to-person relationships and communication, and relies on all of the above intelligences.
- *Intrapersonal intelligence:* Relates to inner states of being, self-reflection, metacognition, and awareness of spiritual realities.

(SOURCE: David G. Lazear, "Multiple Intelligences and How We Nurture Them," *Cogitare*, Volume 4, Number 1 [Fall 1989].)

Social Interactions in Learning

Learners may prefer differing types of social interaction and primary sources of information in learning; these may vary, depending on the learning task:
- *Dependent:* Prefer to receive new information from an authority figure, such as the teacher or a guest speaker.
- *Independent:* Work better alone, e.g., doing independent research or individualized desk work.
- *Collaborative:* Inclined to work with a group of learners, e.g., doing small group tasks or group research projects.
- *Competitive:* Prefer to be a leader and in competition with other students for attention and grades.

(SOURCE: Barbara Fuhrmann and Anthony F. Grasha, *A Practical Handbook for College Teachers* [Boston: Little, Brown and Company, 1983].)

Learners also differ in their preference for active versus passive learning methods. Some learners prefer concrete experience or active experimentation, for example doing an analogous HIV "transmission" experiment. Others comprehend best through reflective observation and abstract conceptualization, that is, by listening to a guest speaker and making connections with the subject. (See Chapter 6 for a differentiation of methods that address active or passive learning preferences.)

In the past, researchers looked for a "one best method" of teaching that would work for all students. Today, educators know that the most effective approach is to utilize a *diversity* of methods, thereby increasing the chances that each student, regardless of preferred learning style, will be engaged by the learning experience.

Individual learners also have "overlays" of several learning styles—another reason for using diverse methods. Also, some students prefer different methods depending on the sexuality topic to be covered.[37] The more varied ways that teachers present the same concepts, the more likely each learner will learn, retain, and utilize them.

Traditional classroom methods (such as lecture and audiovisual presentations) favor learners who are authority dependent and who prefer audio/visual stimuli and passive learning. However, such passive methods are not as effective with learners as those requiring more active involvement, such as role play, demonstrations, and student projects.

Edgar Dale's "Cone of Experience and Learning"[38] asserts that, in general, learners retain . . .

- Only 10 percent of what they read.
- 20 percent of what they hear (e.g., audiotape, lecture).
- 30 percent of what they see (still photos).
- 50 percent of what they hear and see (video, observing a demonstration, seeing something on location).
- 70 percent of what they say (participating in a discussion, giving a talk).
- 90 percent of what they say and do (doing a dramatic presentation, simulation, firsthand experience).

Gender differences play a role in learning style preferences. According to modern theorists, female students exhibit different stages of intellectual development than males,[39] have distinct perceptual styles,[40] and even use language uniquely.[41,42] Female students are at a disadvantage in traditional classroom environments, where males find the presentation methods and competitive learning process more to their liking.[43]

Females also suffer discrimination in schools in the form of male-centered and biased curriculum materials, less interaction with the teacher, lower academic expectations, and sexual harassment.[44,45] Such experiences perpetuate rigid gender roles and limit personal and academic achievement for females. They have no place in the sexuality education classroom.

Research also shows that, although females generally are more verbal than males, when both genders are in a group, males interrupt females more often, regardless of the age of group members. This behavior silences women, even when discussion is regarding a topic about which females are knowledgeable and in which they have a lot of personal investment.[46,47]

Learning Activity: "Balancing the Gender Scales"

Seat learners in two circles facing inward, with girls in the inner circle and boys in the outer circle (a fishbowl—see Chapter 10).

Have the girls talk with each other for 20 minutes or so (depending on age of the learners) about their experiences of being female, without any interruptions from boys. Instruct the boys to remain silent, observe, and take notes about what the girls say. (Do not participate in the discussion yourself, but enforce ground rules if necessary.)

Processing: Return to large group setting and discuss the *process*, not the content, of the experience.

Ask the girls to address . . .
- What it was like to talk without being interrupted.
- What it was like to have the boys listening.
- How they felt talking with just girls.
- What they learned from the experience.

Have the boys discuss . . .
- How it felt to be silenced, to be expected to listen, and take notes on what girls were saying.
- How they coped with it.
- What body language they used.
- Whether they were able to concentrate.
- What they learned from the experience.

Discussion. Make connections between what they experienced and what research reveals about female and male communication.

Follow-up possibilities
1. Continue discussion in small, same-gender groups, in which boys and girls talk about the experience of being their gender. Have groups share the highlights of their discussions with the large group.
2. Finish with a focus writing exercise (see Chapter 8) on the above activities.
3. Follow with an activity focused on an aspect of male experience.

Our task as sexuality educators would be overwhelming if we attempted to accommodate every learning preference within the context of every learning experience. Yet, if we truly want to be effective with our students, we should be aware of learning-style differences and routinely incorporate a wide variety of methods within our teaching. (See Part II for further discussion of diverse methods for teaching about all sexuality education topics.)

Contraception from Many Angles

Use diverse methods to appeal to a variety of learning styles and preferences when teaching about contraception:
- Watch a short video on how contraceptive methods work *(auditory* and *visual).*
- Pass around examples of various birth control methods *(visual, tactile, active).*
- Display posters with contraceptive messages *(visual).*
- Have students cut up magazines and make a collage of media messages that promote sexual activity *(tactile, visual, active).*

- Let students fill condoms with water to demonstrate capacity and strength *(tactile, experimental, active)*.
- Have students work in small groups to design a physical analogy to barrier methods using their bodies *(collaborative, kinesthetic, reflective)*.
- Give options for doing solo or small group research on methods *(independent or collaborative)*.
- Invite a clinic nurse to speak to the class *(dependent, auditory, visual, reflective)*.
- Have students visit a family planning clinic or local drugstore to price contraceptives *(concrete experience, active)*.
- Have students write about how it would feel if they had a contraceptive failure *(reflective, active)*.
- Have students create and act out a role play about discussing contraceptive options with a partner *(active, collaborative, interpersonal)*.

Question 5: Does the program address all three learning domains?

Changing risky behaviors and reinforcing healthy behaviors are primary objectives of most sexuality and HIV education programs. In the past, many educators falsely assumed that learners would alter behaviors or develop important skills simply by virtue of their increased knowledge. We now know, however, that students require much more than "the facts" to help them become truly competent in sexual and health decision making.[48]

Human behavior is the result of a complex interaction of physiology, knowledge, attitudes, beliefs, behaviors, and skills. If sexuality and HIV education programs are to have an impact on student behavior, they must be designed to address all three learning domains: i.e., the *cognitive* ("thinking") domain, in which facts and concepts are considered; the *affective* ("feeling") domain, where feelings, attitudes, values, and beliefs are examined; and the *behavioral* ("acting") domain, in which psychomotor and other skills are addressed.

In other words, knowledge is *necessary* but not *sufficient* in facilitating behavior change. Even when programs address both knowledge and attitudes, but not skills, they have little or no effect on learner behaviors.[49] On the other hand, some programs focused primarily on skill building (e.g., the *Reducing the Risk* curriculum), with little emphasis on content, have yielded significant cognitive growth.[50] However, overemphasis on any single domain, to the exclusion of the other two, will not facilitate the comprehensive understanding that should be the goal in sexuality education.

Within each of the learning domains, some approaches are more effective than others. In the cognitive domain, a concept-building approach is more effective than fact accumulation; in the affective domain, facilitating examination of learners' own values and attitudes is superior to the "preaching" of prescribed values; and in the behavioral domain, actual or role-played practice works better than observing others in learning and retaining new skills and behaviors. (See Chapters 4 and 6 for more discussion on teaching within each of the learning domains; see

Chapters 8–12 for teaching methods categorized by domain and for examples of activities in each.)

Question 6: Is the program interdisciplinary and integrated "across the curriculum"?

The topic of human sexuality is interdisciplinary in nature. In order to fully comprehend the broad topic and many of its subtopics, one must draw upon many disciplines, including biology, psychology, sociology, political science, home economics, women's studies, and history. A comprehensive understanding of HIV/AIDS, for example, requires familiarity with the etiology and epidemiology of the disease (biology), its impact on the individual (psychology) and groups in our society (sociology), the politics of combatting the disease (political science), and our culture's previous experience with epidemics (history). In addition, HIV/AIDS touches upon a number of professional fields, including medicine, social and health services, health education, corrections, and the ministry.

The most effective programs in sexuality or HIV education incorporate many disciplinary perspectives rather than focusing on one: (1) by offering a separate, interdisciplinary course or workshop on sexuality; (2) by integrating sexuality education into a comprehensive, interdisciplinary health education course or program; or (3) by "infusing" sexuality and HIV education "across the curriculum," that is, within several subject areas.

The latter method, most applicable to school settings, involves separating the topic of sexuality or HIV education into various disciplinary components and inserting them at relevant places within the regular curriculum. A related example for the elementary level is "Primarily Health," an integrated, whole language-based health education curriculum for grades K–3 (published by the Comprehensive Health Education Foundation; see Appendix D for contact information). On the secondary level, subtopics within HIV/AIDS education can be broached within biology, psychology, sociology, history, and even English and mathematics classes (see box).

Integrating sexuality and HIV lessons across the curriculum, and linking them with comprehensive health education rather than offering isolated, out-of-context lessons or elective courses, is preferable for several reasons. First, an infusion approach ultimately reaches more students, whereas many may miss the "one-shot" lesson in a required health class or not sign up for an elective course on sexuality or health. Second, learning about sexuality within a context of health education acknowledges and reinforces many shared concepts within sexuality and health education topics—for example, abstinence, responsibility, self-care, and health. (See boxed insert, "Shared Concepts in Prevention Topics," in Chapter 4.)

Third, an infusion approach dignifies human sexuality as one of many essential subjects within the regular school curriculum rather than as a "special" or optional subject of study. Finally, many more teachers will be involved, enriching sexuality education with their diverse disciplinary perspectives and expertise.

Integrating HIV Education
Across the Curriculum

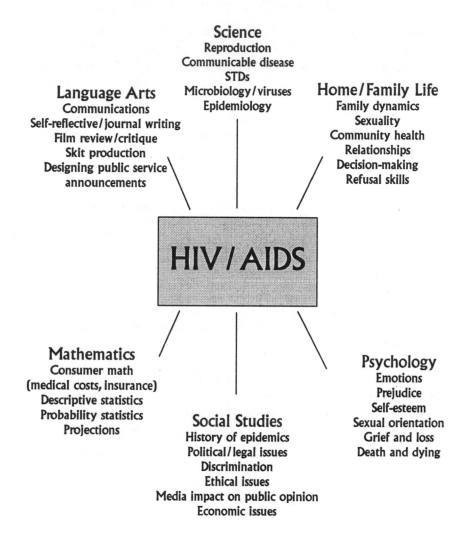

Science
Reproduction
Communicable disease
STDs
Microbiology / viruses
Epidemiology

Language Arts
Communications
Self-reflective / journal writing
Film review / critique
Skit production
Designing public service
announcements

Home / Family Life
Family dynamics
Sexuality
Community health
Relationships
Decision-making
Refusal skills

HIV / AIDS

Mathematics
Consumer math
(medical costs, insurance)
Descriptive statistics
Probability statistics
Projections

Social Studies
History of epidemics
Political / legal issues
Discrimination
Ethical issues
Media impact on public opinion
Economic issues

Psychology
Emotions
Prejudice
Self-esteem
Sexual orientation
Grief and loss
Death and dying

Of course, the ultimate success of the infusion approach depends a great deal on having numerous teachers who are well trained and comfortable in teaching sexuality topics. They also must be able to collaborate with one another to plan a coherent program. Unfortunately, most schools are structured so that teachers work solo within "self-contained" classrooms or, in secondary settings, are segregated into subject-area departments. Neither situation fosters the teacher communication necessary for collaborative, cross-disciplinary work.

Consequently, many attempts at infusion in school-based programs result in spotty, poorly conceived, monoperspective, or overlapping coverage of sexuality topics. The same is often true in colleges, where several different departments offer competing sexuality "overview" courses, each with its own disciplinary focus and bias.[51]

Current school reform is changing departmentalized curricula in schools and colleges, however. Many schools are creating interdisciplinary studies programs, in which a topic is taught in an integrated, coordinated fashion by a team of teachers from complementary disciplines. Sexuality education, because of its multidisciplinary nature, may be on the cutting edge of this trend.

Integrating Sexuality Education in Elementary Language Arts

Effective communication is a key goal of effective sexuality education—a goal shared with language arts programs.

Why not, then, teach the concepts and values of sexuality by employing such methodologies as reading books, writing poetry, talking with others—in short, by building upon the components of language arts programs? Reading books about relationships, talking with one another about feelings, and writing or drawing pictures of families are all of keen interest to elementary age children and help them develop their ability to communicate (language arts) while teaching important concepts in sexuality education.

Children learn about themselves as sexual beings long before they enter schools. Those life lessons of cooperation, love, uniqueness, responsibility, and belonging are taught through daily interactions in families and communities. Viewing sexuality as a part of life allows us to teach elementary sexuality education without concern or trepidation.

Sexuality education in elementary schools must acknowledge humans as beings who do not survive without touch. Often educators teach topics such as HIV/AIDS and child abuse prevention to elementary-aged students without giving them the opportunity to learn to identify and describe their feelings, explore family relationships and responsibilities, initiate or participate in friendships, or learn skills and attitudes for getting along with classmates. How can students be expected to learn to enjoy a life of mutually respectful, loving relationships when we teach them only the dangers of sex? They must be given a framework on which to hang such information and skills.

Elementary sexuality education can be integrated within the existing language arts program to emphasize important life lessons of communication, cooperation, responsibility, belonging, problem solving, and negotiation.

(SOURCE: Roxanne-Hood Lyons, 1994.)

Question 7: Is the curriculum comprehensive in scope, age-and experientially-appropriate, and logically sequential?

We advocate teaching to identified student needs and interests, rather than relying too heavily on prepackaged curricula. However, many teachers prefer (or are required) to use a published curriculum, even if only as a supplement. Highlighted throughout this book are several good curricula and resource guides, including *Reducing the Risk* (ETR Associates), *When I'm Grown* and *Life Planning Education* (Advocates for Youth), *Values and Choices* (The Search Institute), *F.L.A.S.H* (Seattle/King County Deptartment of Public Health), and *New Methods for Puberty Education, Teaching Safer Sex, Streetwise to Sex-Wise,* and *Positive Images* (The Center for Family Life Education, Planned Parenthood of Greater Northern New Jersey). (See Appendix D for complete titles and sources.)

We also suggest some important criteria with which to choose and evaluate published curricula yourself. Presented thus far in this chapter are several general principles for effective sexuality and HIV education programs, each of which is equally applicable to evaluating effective curricula, that is, they should promote universal values, be positive in tone, accurate, comprehensive, culturally pluralistic, interdisciplinary, and geared to different learning styles and all three learning domains. In addition, curricula should be age and experientially appropriate and logically sequential—that is, content should be addressed at the appropriate developmental time and in a logically consistent order.

Effective curricula take into account differences that exist, in general, between age groups and provide appropriate content and learning activities for each developmental stage. Whether evaluating curricula or designing lessons of your own, you may find it useful to know student developmental differences with respect to sexuality knowledge and attitudes (see box).

Developmental Differences in Sexuality Education Students

Grades K–3: Students are likely . . .
- To be egocentric, that is, they view the world from their own perspective, making little distinction between their own points of view and those of others.
- To develop some independence from parents and gradually orient toward peers.
- To be curious about external body parts.
- To be highly competitive and capable of unkindness to each other.
- To understand information in terms of their own experiences.
- To perceive cause and effect in terms of mere happenstance.
- To trust the information given to them by authority figures.
- Not to understand the sexual terms and events they discuss.

Grades 4–5: Students are likely to be . . .
- In different stages of prepuberty and early puberty.
- Becoming aware of sexual feelings and desires—either in themselves or in others—and be confused about them.
- Increasingly sensitive to peer pressure.
- Capable of concern for others.
- Exploring [gender] roles.
- Interested in learning about sexuality and human relationships.

- Able to discuss human sexuality.
- Still confused between what really is and what might be possible.
- Able to internalize rules and know what is right or wrong according to those rules.
- Able to perceive only linear, unidirectional, cause-effect relationships.
- Interested in discrete lists of causes and "noncauses" of illnesses.
- Interested in internal body parts; perceiving the body as a collection of discrete parts.
- Focused on concrete aspects of body parts, such as size, color and shape.

Grades 6–9: Students are likely to be . . .
- Engaged in a search for identity (including sexual [orientation] identity).
- Asking "Who am I?" and "Am I normal?"
- Very centered on self.
- Influenced by peer attitudes.
- Concerned about and experimenting with relationships between boys and girls.
- Confused about the range of heterosexual and homosexual feelings many of them will have experienced.
- Worried about the changes in their bodies.
- Interested in internal body functioning and able to view the body as an integrated system.
- Able to understand that behavior has consequences, but may not believe that the consequences could happen to them.
- Fearful of asking questions about sex that might make them appear uninformed.
- Beginning to understand complex relationships between multiple causes and multiple effects with regard to illness; that is, to understand the concept of "interaction."
Beginning to understand the notion of prevention.

Grades 10–12: Students are likely to be . . .
- Still struggling for a sense of personal identity, especially those students who are confused about their sexual [orientation] identities.
- Thinking that they "know it all."
- Seeking greater independence from parents.
- Still heavily influenced by peers, but open to information provided by trusted adults.
- Near the end of this period, beginning to think about establishing more permanent relationships.
- Experiencing a sense of denial about their vulnerability to AIDS and other dangers.
- Sexually active.

(SOURCE: Reprinted from *Criteria for Evaluating an AIDS Curriculum*, with permission from the National Coalition of Advocates for Students, Boston, revised 1992. Bracketed notes are ours.)

Selection of an appropriate curriculum also should take into account the sexual experience of learners. For example, *Postponing Sexual Involvement* is designed for middle school students and successfully promotes a norm of delaying sexual intercourse for abstinent students; however, the program does not affect frequency of intercourse nor use of contraceptives among students already sexually active. *Reducing the Risk* and the Schinke-Blythe-Gilchrist curriculum, on the other hand, are designed for high school students and effectively emphasize norms of avoiding unprotected intercourse, either through abstinence or the use of prophylaxis;[52] use of these curricula would be inappropriate for younger, sexually abstinent students.

In addition to being comprehensive in scope and appropriately staged, good sexuality education curricula should be logically *sequential,* that is, presenting and gradually building upon key concepts, facts, and skills appropriate to each developmental level. Individual topic threads should be woven throughout the curriculum so they logically build upon student knowledge and skills gained from earlier levels. An example of an appropriately sequenced content thread on reproductive anatomy and physiology is given in the boxed insert.

Teaching about Reproductive Anatomy and Physiology, Grades K–12

Level 1 (middle childhood) messages
- Each body part has a correct name and a specific function.
- A person's genitals, reproductive organs, and genes determine whether the person is male or female.
- Boys and men have a penis, scrotum, and testicles.
- Girls and women have a vulva, clitoris, vagina, uterus, and ovaries.
- Both girls and boys have body parts that feel good when touched.

Level 2 (preadolescence) messages
- The maturation of external and internal reproductive organs occurs during puberty.
- At puberty, boys begin to ejaculate and girls begin to menstruate.

Level 3 (early adolescence) messages
- The sexual response system differs from the reproductive system.
- Some of the reproductive organs provide pleasure as well as reproductive capability.

Level 4 (adolescence) messages
- Sexual differentiation occurs early in prenatal development.
- Chromosomes determine whether a developing fetus will be male or female.
- For both [genders], hormones influence growth and development as well as sexual and reproductive function.
- A woman's ability to reproduce ceases after menopause; a man can usually reproduce throughout his life.

- **Both men and women can experience sexual pleasure throughout their [lives].**
- **Most people enjoy giving and receiving pleasure.**

(SOURCE: *Guidelines for Comprehensive Sexuality Education: Kindergarten–12th Grade* [SIECUS National Guidelines Task Force, 1991].)

In Appendix A, we have included an overview of criteria to use when evaluating sexuality and HIV education programs that was developed by the Association for Sexuality Education and Training (ASSET). This organization of Pacific Northwest sexuality educators provides, upon request, their "Curriculum and Materials Review Packet," which includes the criteria, advice on setting up and working with a curriculum review committee, and forms to use when conducting a review.

Question 8: Is the program supported and reinforced by the family, peers, religious groups, clinics, and local media?

The family is the first and most powerful influence on a learner's sexual knowledge, attitudes, values, and comfort level with sexuality. Then peers become another important source of information—and misinformation—and a touchstone for sexual attitudes. Religious teachings provide a moral framework for young people as they explore sexual life-styles and relationships. Various community agencies, such as health clinics and schools, provide factual information, resources, and opportunities to reflect upon sexuality issues and behaviors. The media send out persistent but mixed messages about sexuality and gender that strongly influence students.

Each of these groups teaches about sexuality, whether explicitly or implicitly, intentionally or unintentionally. Sometimes unspoken messages are the most powerful. Even when various sources conflict in their messages and cause some confusion, more information about sexuality is better than less; people rarely make *worse* decisions by having *more* information. Students use their intellect and own value perspectives to sort out which messages are relevant and useful to them and which are not. The most effective teaching about sexuality, however, occurs when the many different possible sources of information for learners actively cooperate to provide explicit, coherent, comprehensive, and coordinated messages about sexuality and HIV.

Many examples exist of effective collaboration among the many sources of sexuality education: after-school programs for parents and their children; school and community-based programs utilizing trained peers; schools cooperating with local health clinics to offer comprehensive health services, including contraceptives, to students; churches and other religious groups inviting community health educators to conduct workshops; school and community-based educators coordinating efforts to improve delivery of services and reinforce messages; and local media campaigns developed to supplement and reinforce educational programs.

Research indicates that collaborative programs are more effective than those more limited in scope. The best example to date happened in the small community of Denmark, South Carolina, in which parents, churches, schools, the media, and other community organizations collaborated to implement a skill-based program and to reinforce each other's messages: teachers and administrators received graduate level training in sexuality education; parents, clergy, and community leaders attended workshops; peer counselors were trained; a Teen Life Center was created to provide contraceptive counseling and services at the school; a media campaign was started; and a K–12 sexuality education curriculum was implemented. Within several years, teenage pregnancy rates in the county dropped by more than *50 percent,* while rates in three demographically similar counties (with no such program) *increased.*[53] A subsequent evaluation of the program found that when key elements of the program were dropped—for example, the provision of contraceptive services by the Teen Life Center and the resignation of the school nurse—the pregnancy rate climbed again.[54]

In another program, teenage pregnancy rates were reduced by 36 percent (compared with a 15 percent rise in a control group) when parents, clergy, school staff, and local media were all giving out the same messages: "Wait to have intercourse," but "If you don't, protect yourself."[55]

School and Parent Collaboration: One Educator's Story

A mother and her two adolescents were attending a four-week family series on sexuality education. The mother reported that the most important part of the program for her was the ride home. Once she was in such a deep conversation with her children that she drove around the block ten times so they could finish.

(SOURCE: Anne Terrell, Education Director, Planned Parenthood of Tompkins County, New York.)

The supposed natural friction or competition between parents, communities, and schools is a dangerous myth. As noted in Chapter 1, the vast majority of adults support public school involvement in sexuality education. Parental involvement minimizes objections and excusals and increases parent-child communication.[56] In reality, all adults have an investment in working together, on many levels and with many different voices, to help young people comprehend and navigate the complexities of human sexuality and relationships.

Question 9: Are the teachers willing, comfortable, and well trained?

The teacher, authorities in this field agree, is the *single* most important factor in the effectiveness of a sexuality education program. Attributes of the ideal sexuality educator include good skills and personal qualities as a teacher, in-depth knowledge of sexuality content and methods, and, especially, comfort with sexuality (see box).

Desirable Qualities of the Sexuality or HIV Educator

- A broad base of knowledge in human sexuality content and issues as a foundation for teaching.
- General comfort with sexuality, and healthy attitudes toward his or her own sexuality.
- Genuine enthusiasm for and comfort with teaching about sexuality or HIV.
- Respect and trust of learners and an appreciation of the diversity of attitudes, values, feelings, personal attributes, and experiences within a group of learners.
- An ability to work effectively with other professionals, parents, and community members.
- Skills in teaching methodology, including the ability to create a supportive atmosphere, facilitate discussion, maintain confidentiality, and design and offer a wide variety of learning activities.
- Ability to empathize and communicate well with learners.
- Flexibility and nonauthoritarian style.
- Clarity about his or her own values and the impact they may have on teaching about sexuality or HIV.
- The ability to recognize his or her own strengths and limitations, e.g., knowing when to ask for help.

Studies consistently reveal that many teachers feel unprepared for teaching about sexuality or HIV. In the late 1970s, practicing teachers, when asked to evaluate their preservice training, named three subject areas they were "completely unprepared to teach": sexuality education, substance abuse, and ecology. In one study, 70 percent of elementary teachers reported they would teach sexuality education only if required to do so.[57–59] Most teachers felt that training should include "sensitivity training" to help them increase their comfort level with sexuality.[60]

More recent research indicates that many teachers still feel inadequately prepared: one-third say they need more information on all topics they teach, and more than half specify a need for more training on STDs, sexual transmission of HIV, homosexuality, and abortion in particular.[61] A recent review of catalog course descriptions reveals that although some colleges offer content courses on sexuality, few offer methods courses and even some health education courses don't address sexuality or HIV.[62]

Even teachers who are well informed, skilled, and enthusiastic about teaching about sexuality often feel a lack of support from their community, administrators, or colleagues. Nonetheless, students say they would rather learn about sexuality education from their regular classroom teacher than from guest specialists.[63] If the trend toward teaching sexuality "across the curriculum" continues, many more teachers who never expected to teach about sexuality or HIV will be asked to do so. Already many teachers have been pressed into the task, out of necessity, whether they felt ready or not, which is unfair both to teachers and their students.

Teacher training institutions have been slow to respond to this need. In 1983, a study of 777 teacher preparation institutions declared that they had "no more clearly defined what preparation for sex(uality) education is today than they (had) in the 1960s."[64] Most training is obtained via inservice education, which is rarely of sufficient length or depth.[65] Current studies are finding little improvement in this situation.[66]

Clearly, changes should occur at three levels to redress this critical training need: (1) state education agencies should set certification and training standards for teachers of sexuality education; (2) training institutions should require sexuality content and methods courses for all preservice teachers; and (3) school districts should provide adequate opportunities for "remedial" training to inservice teachers. (We address the teacher training issue further in Chapter 5.)

Question 10: Does the program promote lifelong learning?

Some sort of education about sex is inevitable. . . . Teachers and parents act as though the time and circumstance under which a child receives sex education were determined entirely by them. Instead of keeping children "innocent," the net result of this attitude is to leave their entire education to inaccurate and pernicious sources.

(Lester Kirkendall, *Sex Education and Human Relations,* 1950)

Learning about sexuality is an ongoing process that begins at birth—when adults first hold and interact with a child—and continues throughout life. As individuals grow and their circumstances, relationships, needs, and perspectives change, so do their needs for information. Furthermore, the body of human sexuality knowledge is vast, complex, and constantly expanding, not narrow and static, as some believe.

Learner needs for education about sexuality, therefore, can never be quenched by completing a single workshop or course at one point in time. Truly effective sexuality education consists of many opportunities for learning about sexuality, in many different contexts, and at many different levels. Some learning will occur in formal settings, such as classrooms; much of it, however, will happen outside the classroom within the real lives of learners.

The most effective formal sexuality education fosters development of skills and knowledge that serve learners as they continue to face choices and situations in the "real" world: skills in communication, assertiveness, and critical thinking; knowledge of community resources, such as clinics, information hotlines, libraries, and other educational opportunities; and the skills and comfort level to utilize these resources.

Finally, educators should acknowledge explicitly that everyone should expect learning about sexuality to continue throughout life.

In this chapter, we have outlined ten guiding principles for planning, implementing and evaluating effective sexuality and HIV education programs. Although no one program will meet all these ideals fully, use them as "lenses" through which to evaluate your work in sexuality and HIV education.

CHAPTER 3

Creating a Productive Learning Environment

We never educate directly, but indirectly by means of the environment. Whether we permit chance environments to do the work, or whether we design environments for the purpose makes a great difference.
—John Dewey, *Democracy and Education*

In 1916, Dewey noted that most American classrooms center attention on the information giver (teacher), with few opportunities for peer dialogue, collaboration, or experiential learning. He warned that, in this type of environment, students are unlikely to learn about democracy, because they do not have the opportunity to *practice* skills and attitudes needed for responsible citizenship. Unfortunately, Dewey's observation still holds true for many American classrooms and has much relevance for the sexuality education classroom in particular.

The best environment for effective teaching about sexuality is similar to that required for producing democratic citizens. Some writers have even suggested that the environment found in the best sexuality education classroom also fosters citizenship skills.[1] Learning about the sensitive and personally relevant subject of human sexuality thrives best in an atmosphere that promotes cooperation and dialogue with peers, contemplation of one's values and attitudes, and practice of new and old skills. In this kind of classroom, the teacher relinquishes the traditional "authority" role in favor of a more student-centered approach. (See strategies for facilitating a learner-centered environment in Chapter 7.)

"Learning environment" consists of much more than just physical surroundings. Many social, cultural, and psychological factors also contribute to the overall learning climate: the makeup of the group, the philosophy of the teacher, the learner's relationship to the teacher and peers, and any psychological "baggage" that learners bring to the experience. Comfort with sexuality, both teachers' and students', plays an especially powerful role in teaching and learning about sexuality.

As was addressed in Chapter 2, the extent to which students feel empowered is another critical element of successful teaching about sexuality. Students in traditional learning environments have little input into what is learned or the teaching methods used. However, the effectiveness of sexuality and HIV education is enhanced when it directly addresses identified learner needs and when learners are actively involved in designing their own learning experiences.

Physical features of the sexuality education classroom also influence the psychological climate and learning outcomes. Some researchers estimate that the physical environment *alone* is responsible for at least 25 percent of learning that takes place.[2] Consciously designing physical space to be congruent rather than in conflict with teaching objectives enhances learning.

In this chapter, we discuss the attributes of a psychologically safe and productive classroom—especially learner empowerment and comfort with sexuality—and present strategies for accomplishing them. We also address characteristics of the physical environment that can facilitate or hinder learning.

The Role of Sexuality Comfort in Learning about Sexuality

Most learners come to the sexuality education classroom naturally curious and motivated to learn. At the same time, they may feel shy, giddy, or reluctant to participate because of their discomfort with sexuality. Some (especially males) pretend to know more than they do, as a way of obscuring their discomfort and lack of knowledge. Learners who have suffered traumatic sexual experiences (e.g., sexual abuse or assault) may have to overcome intense emotional dissonance to learn about sexuality.

As learners begin a sexuality workshop or class, they also may expect their teacher to feel awkward and embarrassed about sexuality. They may anticipate expressions of teacher discomfort—blushing or getting flustered—that would make the learning experience unpleasant or more uncomfortable for them, too. These concerns may interfere with learning unless teachers take steps to counteract them. Until students feel it is "safe" and comfortable to talk about sexuality, they are unlikely to fully engage in the experience or learn what they need to know.

Recent research has documented a strong relationship between one's comfort with sexuality, attitudes about sexuality, and sexual knowledge.[3] Evonne found that individuals with a high comfort level with sexuality also have higher levels of knowledge and tend to be more tolerant in their attitudes. Similarly, as students gain more knowledge about sexuality, they also experience an increase in comfort and changes in acceptance of sexual values and life-styles of others.

Some people worry that increasing student comfort with sexuality will lead to increased sexual activity and its concomitant health risks. Quite the contrary, research has shown that increasing one's comfort with sexuality has several positive behavioral outcomes such as better communication with partners, more effective use of contraceptives and more appropriate sexual choices.[4] While students with higher sexuality comfort report increases in their tolerance for others' behaviors and beliefs, their own sexual standards and behaviors remain constant.[5] Besides, many learners already feel "comfortable" enough to engage in sexual activity; what they lack is comfort and skills to utilize protective behaviors, such as refusals or prophylaxis.[6]

Statistically speaking, positive correlations among sexuality comfort, knowledge, and attitudes do not mean that any one of these *causes* the others to happen.

However, we believe a causative relationship does exist between increasing sexuality comfort and affecting sexual knowledge and attitudes; we base this claim on long-term observation of learners in sexuality classes, and their self-reports about the role of comfort in their ability to learn.

In other words, we believe that learners who feel at ease in the sexuality classroom are *more likely to learn* and to change their attitudes about sexuality, two essential components of behavior change (see Chapter 4). Also, students who feel comfortable with sexuality may be more likely to *retain* knowledge gains and attitude changes, which often are only temporary in sexuality education programs.[7, 8]

A critical first objective of a sexuality educator, therefore, should be to create a classroom environment that fosters increased comfort with sexuality. Student comfort operates on four levels in sexuality education: with the teacher, with fellow students, with the topic, and, finally, with what will happen in the class.

The Educator's Role in Learner Comfort

Teacher comfort with sexuality establishes an overall tone for learning, either restricting or enhancing the extent to which students feel comfortable.[9] Educators communicate in many subtle ways their own feelings about teaching about sexuality: by physical demeanor, by what is said or not said, by topics covered or not covered, and by reactions to what students say and do in class.

Sensing their teacher's feelings, students respond in kind, being more or less likely to ask questions or to risk making themselves vulnerable by participating in activities. As one student said to an apparently comfortable teacher, "I appreciate your matter-of-fact, down to earth style. I think we try to copy your comfort level!" Lessons covered hastily by an embarrassed educator, on the other hand, reinforce learners' own feelings of discomfort and embarrassment, provide unclarified information about sexuality, and frustrate learners' needs to discuss and comprehend sexuality issues.

In recent focus groups, teenagers shared their opinion of the HIV/AIDS education in their schools. The general consensus: "It was lousy." What's more, they singled out teacher discomfort as the greatest deterrent to their asking questions or getting them answered directly and honestly.[10] One teen elaborated: "It was so obvious that the *last thing* our teacher wanted to do was teach us a unit on AIDS. Her basic attitude was 'Look—I am required to cover this stuff for one hour, so let's get it over with.' Then, at the end of the hour, she asked if we had any questions. Did she honestly think anyone would *dare* to ask a question when she was so uncomfortable with the topic? Besides, we didn't trust her not to tell our parents every single thing we said to her."

Demonstrating your comfort and competence early in a learning experience is a critical first step in establishing credibility and will prevent problems later on. Learners want to know that you are comfortable and knowledgeable about the topics to be covered, and that you are skilled as a teacher, open-minded, and respectful of their personal beliefs and life-styles. Be explicit about your background, expertise, and philosophy for teaching sexuality education. In the boxed insert are additional strategies for establishing your credibility and launching a good class.

Ten Ways to Get Off to a Good Start

1. Share your credentials for teaching sexuality education.
2. Tell students why you think it is important for everyone to learn about sexuality.
3. Demonstrate your comfort with hearing sexual slang, translating it into correct terminology.
4. Demonstrate, if possible, that you cannot be shocked easily by student revelations or comments.
5. Don't avoid certain topics or issues.
6. Express your anticipation of and sensitivity to student discomfort with sexuality or with certain topics.
7. Promise to maintain student confidentiality (except for revelations you cannot keep confidential, e.g., disclosures about sexual abuse or harassment).
8. Tell students what you hope to accomplish in the class.
9. Be explicit about your philosophy of education and how you view your role in the class.
10. Let students know what you expect of them and how they will be evaluated.

Educator credibility in the sexuality education classroom is easily perishable. Learners are quick to spot a hypocritical teacher in any topic area, but their "radar" seems especially well tuned for those teaching sexuality education. Perhaps this is because of the unusually sensitive nature of the topic or the high amount of their personal investment. Whatever the reason, sexuality educators face extraordinary expectations to fulfill their promises, practice their stated philosophy, and maintain a psychologically safe environment.

Educator Introduction as a Process

Self-introduction should be a deliberate and ongoing process:
- If you are a classroom teacher, your students will have hearsay information about you before they enter the classroom. Try to augment that reputation in a positive fashion. Be deliberate about the concrete facts you reveal about yourself throughout the term of your working relationship with them.
- If you are a community educator, guest speaker, or trainer, consider what you will say about your credentials. Keep your self-introduction brief by giving those pieces of information most relevant to the situation and likely to impress the group.
- Be honest and straightforward; never represent yourself as someone you

aren't. For example, sexuality educators doing parenting education are often asked if they are parents; if you aren't, confront this issue head-on so it cannot be used against you.

- If there is time in your agenda and if appropriate, introduce yourself during participant introductions.
- Give pieces of information about yourself throughout the session. At the beginning, learners often are most focused on their own comfort and inclusion needs; they are more likely to hear information about you that relates to a specific topic during the agenda.

Educators lose credibility in a hurry when they express respect for diversity but then make comments biased against particular groups or points of view, or chastise students who disagree, or tell sexual jokes (most of which derive their humor by denigrating others). Consistency in what you *say* and *do* in class, in terms of language and behaviors toward students, does much to enhance your credibility.

Some students distrust a teacher who is too open about personal values or experiences, or who "preaches" to students about certain sexuality topics and issues. Obviously, teachers are not "value-free"; you bring your own set of beliefs and prejudices to the classroom. If you feel strongly about a certain topic, try to remain neutral as much as possible when teaching about it; otherwise, students who disagree with you may feel alienated, reducing your credibility and approachability for those students.

On the other hand, students benefit from occasional reminders that teachers are sometimes uncomfortable or emotional about certain topics, and that you have experienced your own formative life experiences (see Chapter 5 for cautions regarding personal disclosures).

Ways to Maintain Your Credibility

- Keep your promises.
- Teach without "preaching."
- Acknowledge your own embarrassment when it happens.
- Know and admit your own limitations as a sexuality educator (e.g., "I don't know much about that topic").
- Demonstrate that you genuinely care about your learners both as people and as learners.
- Don't tell jokes that are inappropriate or offensive (most are).
- Don't be judgmental about learner beliefs or choices.
- Avoid bias in your language.
- Act consistently with your stated philosophy of education.

Strategies for developing and maintaining credibility need not be addressed explicitly in lock-step fashion, but can be useful as a mental checklist while planning units or workshops. Incorporating them consciously into presentations and lessons lays important groundwork for creating an environment in which students feel more comfortable learning about sexuality.

Developing Student Comfort with One Another

> I feel really comfortable in this class, both with you and the other students.
> I usually have trouble speaking in front of people I don't know very well,
> but I already feel at ease speaking in class. That is a great feeling!
>
> (Note from a student)

Just as the teacher-student relationship is extremely important to effective sexuality education, so are the relationships between and among the students in a group. Participants in a sexuality class need to feel confident not only that they can trust and depend on their instructor, but that they can count on their colearners as well to be supportive, nonjudgmental, and compassionate.

Learners may know one another in a different context (such as another class), but a sexuality education class involves more personal risk for them. Some who would be active participants in a math or history class might be less forthcoming asking questions about sexuality (especially if it is related to personal experience); simply posing a question implies some knowledge of the topic. Consequently, more so than in other classes or contexts, students want to know what they can expect from their classmates.

Two main processes foster a sense of mutual support and psychological safety within a group: (1) establishing and maintaining ground rules; and (2) helping students get to know one another.

The Use of Ground Rules in Sexuality Education

Ground rules are a set of agreements, or explicit group norms, about how a group will operate to protect both individual and group rights. They vary depending on group needs and the developmental age of the learners, but typically they address the following issues and concerns:

Confidentiality. Group members should agree that nothing that occurs or is said by an individual will be revealed outside of the session. Advise learners that on rare occasions the educator may have to break this ground rule if required by law or special circumstances.

Right to "pass". Because of the sensitive, personally challenging nature of some activities and discussions, every person has the right to pass on any activity.

Avoiding generalizations and making "I" statements. Learners should avoid making sweeping statements about groups or issues: for example, "All women (or all men) are . . ." Encourage students to accept ownership of their opinions by beginning statements with "I" rather than "you," "they," or "those people."

Openness and sharing of personal experience. Being honest and open is desirable in a sexuality class; however, caution students not to reveal so much that they make themselves or others feel uncomfortable or vulnerable.

Privacy. Respect and protect each person's right to privacy.

Encouraging full participation. Ask students to share responsibility for involving everyone in class activities and discussion by monitoring their own participation and encouraging others to make contributions.

Integrity of every contribution. Encourage students to pose any questions they have even if they seem ill-informed (e.g., the "no question is dumb" ground rule).

Acknowledgment and acceptance of feelings. Remind students that at times some people, including the educator, feel uncomfortable, which is O.K.

Respecting and appreciating differences. Students will disagree, but they should not judge or show disrespect to others. Diversity of opinion should be valued.

Ground rules define limits for the group. First of all, they establish the rights of individuals to hold their own opinions, to express them in ways that do not infringe on other's rights, and to participate fully in the learning experience. Second, they establish for the students that the intended nature of the group is educational, not therapeutic. In other words, students should not share intimate details about their lives, nor expect the group to help them resolve personal problems. Otherwise, both the group and the teacher may find themselves confronted with issues they are not skilled or willing to handle.

Classes in any topic area benefit by having ground rules; sexuality education classes *require* them. Because of the personally sensitive topics and diverse value perspectives within a sexuality education class, emotions sometimes run high, and personal boundaries are more easily violated. Ground rules increase "psychological safety" in the group, help prevent group process problems, and defuse interpersonal conflicts.

A Case Study: The Importance of Ground Rules

A couple of years ago there was a sexuality class that really flopped. On the very first day they were talking about flirting and come-ons. A student—I'll call him "Rob"—announced that he already knew how to handle a come-on.

He said, "Girls don't come on to guys unless they're sluts, so they deserve what they get. And if a guy ever tried anything, I'd punch the faggot out."

After class, two people came up to the teacher and asked to be excused for the rest of the unit. They each sat down in private and had long talks with the teacher.

It turned out that one student ("Jenny") had been raped by her boss the week before. She felt as if Rob was blaming her . . . saying it's your own fault if you get raped. Of course, it isn't; but it's easy to feel that way when it's you. She couldn't stand to be in class with Rob.

The second student (I'll call him "Michael") was furious at Rob's name-calling.

Michael's father was gay and he wasn't going to stick around while people called his father names. "Faggot," of course, is a put-down, just like racial and religious slurs.

In fairness, you have to understand that Rob had no idea that Jenny had recently been raped or that Michael's father was gay. It never occurred to him that anyone would be offended by his remarks. He needed a little education. He needed to learn that there are ways to express your opinion without demeaning other people . . . and he needed to realize that you never know the life experiences of most of the people around you.

(Source: Beth Reis, M.S., *9/10 FLASH* [Seattle: Seattle–King County Department of Public Health, 1988], 2–3; reprinted with permission from Family Planning/STD Program, Seattle–King County Department of Public Health.)

Developing ground rules as a group can be accomplished in a variety of ways (see Chapter 7) but should be done early in the learning experience. They can be posted or distributed to all students.

When facilitating ground rule development, the teacher may have some items s/he especially wants to see included in the list (e.g., "limit side-talking"). Learners will generate most essential guidelines, however, if given the opportunity; also, they feel greater ownership and respect for ground rules they create themselves. If they overlook an essential guideline, simply suggest its inclusion.

Establishing ground rules early on makes it easier to handle offenses when they occur. Rather than singling out and embarrassing a student by creating a ground rule at the time of an inappropriate behavior, address violations by reminding the whole group of a relevant ground rule previously established. For instance, if a student (Ami) expresses disapproval of another student's (Lee) opinion, you can note, "Let me remind *everyone* of our ground rule about respecting individual opinions and perspectives. Lee has a right to his own opinion. So, Ami, what is *your* opinion on that issue?" Stated in this way, the reminder gently corrects Ami while reinforcing the ground rule.

Helping Students Get to Know One Another

> I thought the exercise we did helped "break the ice" so we can communicate better with each other. Most of us felt uncomfortable at first and that felt somehow reassuring.
>
> (Student in a sexuality class)

Students develop trust and increased personal investment in the group as they get to know one another and learn it is safe (assuming group members actually are worthy of their trust). Giving students opportunities to become better acquainted enhances their sense of psychological safety and increases their willingness to cooperate with one another.

Learners can easily maintain anonymity in a group (especially if the group is large) unless the teacher actively works to involve them. Students may share other classes and school activities, for example, without ever having had an open, honest conversation with one another about who they really are and what they really care about. Adult learners, in particular, are adept at maintaining psychological distance from a group, even when the topic is sexuality.

Learner introductions accomplish several tasks at once: (1) familiarize everyone (including you) with student names; (2) reveal something interesting and unique about each individual (which helps you and others to remember names); and (3) begin the assessment of needs and interests (e.g., by asking, "Why are you taking this class?"). Many different strategies are used to accomplish introductions (see inserts).

"Getting to Know You"

Ask each person to tell the group his or her first name and one of the following activities:

1. Say why s/he is taking the class or workshop and what s/he hopes to learn (the standard introduction method).
2. Add a descriptive adjective to his or her first name, beginning with the first letter of the first name (e.g., "Eclectic Evonne," "Joyful Joan"). This device helps in memorizing names especially if, at the end of the introductions, you ask several volunteers to take turns recalling all the names and adjectives.
3. Say something about him or herself; the next person does the same, after repeating the first person's introduction; the third repeats the pattern; and so on until the whole group has been introduced.
4. Tell the group briefly about someone s/he considers a role model or personal hero and why.
5. Have students answer five questions about themselves (e.g., favorite color, food, recreational activity, one thing they want to learn) on a sheet of paper and tape it on their chests; then circulate ("mill") in the large group, silently reading other students' answers; then find one other person whose answers raised interest and have a conversation. Repeat the process several times, or have pairs join with other pairs.

One caution here about doing introductions in sexuality education classes. You may be tempted to introject sexuality content immediately (e.g., "Share how you got your early information about sexuality"); however, such questions may be intimidating or may elicit negative stories that create an undesirable tone in the first moments of class. A wiser course is to progress gradually from relatively innocuous questions to ones that have some sexuality content, allowing learner comfort to build and a positive tone to be established.

After completing introductions, use additional strategies to enhance student familiarity, such as small group discussions and activities, class interviews of individuals, large group discussions, and guest panels with an "open chair" for students. See Part II for a description of these and other methods.

Using humor in introductions makes them fun as well as informative; it also assures students that you welcome laughter, helps you connect with learners, and may relieve some students' apprehension about participating. The "Blatant Lies" strategy (see box) evokes predictable laughter.

"Blatant Lies"

1. Have students think of two "facts" about themselves (one or both of which can be a "blatant lie").
2. Share the facts in pairs, having partners guess which of the statements are false or true.
3. Have individuals introduce their partners and share their "facts"; have the group make guesses as to their veracity.

(NOTE: This exercise can take considerable time and is not recommended for use with large groups.)

(SOURCE: Kelly Riggle-Hower, at the Northwest Institute for Community Health Educators.)

Some people believe that precious instructional time is wasted in conducting activities, such as introductions, that are not obviously content related. On the contrary, spending the time necessary to build a supportive group is an investment that pays off when students feel more comfortable studying sexuality in that group and in taking risks that enhance learning.

Educators who lead "one-shot" learning experiences also should take a few minutes to do introductions, either individually or via a quick group poll (see box). Even if the group has a shared history and individuals supposedly know one another, thought-provoking introductions elicit new information and provide you with information about the group at the same time.

Quick Introductions in a One-Time Experience

If you are a workshop leader or guest speaker, use one of the following alternatives to do introductions:
- When the group is small (fewer than ten), ask for a thirty-second introduction from each participant.
- Distribute a brief survey to participants prior to the session, and then poll their responses, for example, "how many of you teach at the elementary level?").
- Conduct a brief verbal poll by asking participants to stand if their response is

"yes," for example, "How many of you are taking this class because (1) you want to, (2) your advisor signed you up, (3) a friend encouraged you, or (4) you need the credit?"

- If the group is large, conduct introductions in small clusters, starting with pairs and working up to several pairs together. Circulate among the groups, listening to participant responses; then, in the large group, solicit examples of interesting information gleaned.

Developing Student Comfort with the Topic

Learners typically begin sexuality education with some apprehension and discomfort, which the teacher can help them overcome. First of all, educators serve as role models, demonstrating comfort through physical behaviors and attitudes and appropriate, facile use of sexuality-related language. Second, educators can implement strategies specifically intended to increase learner comfort with sexuality.

Educator use of language about sexuality and gender plays an especially important role in fostering learner comfort. Language provides a valuable "window" into a culture and into those who are products of that culture. The language of Western culture reveals general discomfort with sexuality, as well as misogyny and heterosexism, in the slang and euphemisms used to describe sexual anatomy, in sexual jokes, and in gender-biased language.

Most children (and adults) were taught to describe their genital areas and body functions euphemistically (e.g., "down there," "wee wee"), later substituting whatever slang was used by peers. Even adults rarely know or feel comfortable using correct sexual terminology. Learners often worry they will use incorrect words or say something considered offensive to others, which prevents them from asking important questions or contributing ideas. Teachers can help learners increase competence in using sexuality-related language (see box).

Building a Common Vocabulary in Sexuality Education

Use a variety of vocabulary-building and clarifying processes:
- Model and encourage the use of correct terminology rather than euphemisms. Make the link between medical and colloquial terms. Remember, it takes time for learners to learn a new vocabulary.
- Make lists of correct terminology with learners; post them or have them available as handouts and use for reference in future lessons.
- Discuss how slang is often sexist, racist, heterosexist, or homophobic; talk about how slang sometimes hurts people and violates ground rules you have established.
- Translate student slang into correct terminology; remember, students may use offensive terms to test you, or it may be that they simply know no other words to use.

- **Do not allow the use of terms, comments, or jokes that are derogatory of race, religion, nationality, gender, sexual orientation, age, or disability; discuss why it is important not to use them.**
- **Provide a "question box" for anonymous questions, which you can translate into appropriate language. (See Chapter 9 for a complete description of the process for handling anonymous questions.)**

Gender bias in language is inappropriate in sexuality education, if not technically incorrect. The "generic" male pronoun to refer to both genders, for example, is rapidly disappearing from our public discourse, in part because research has revealed that females feel excluded by it.[11] Sexuality and HIV educators should use gender-inclusive language (i.e., "he or she," "her or his," "they," "one") even if it sounds cumbersome or violates traditional rules of grammar; encourage learners to do likewise.

Educator modeling of "sexually pluralistic" language also helps learners develop inclusive, respectful language. Using the word "partner," for example, to refer to a person in a relationship acknowledges the existence of unmarried couples, as opposed to "spouse," which refers only to a legally married (i.e., heterosexual) person. Another example is "person living with HIV" rather than "AIDS victim" or "AIDS patient," to respect those who consider themselves living with a disease rather than being a victim.

The language of sexuality and gender is often highly politicized. For example, some individuals, depending on their beliefs, use either "pro-choice" or "pro-abortion" to describe those who favor legalized abortion, and "anti-choice" or "pro-life" to describe those who oppose it. The objective approach for the sexuality educator when dealing with this topic is to use terminology that reflects the preference of the group described (i.e., "pro-choice" for one and "pro-life" for the other), not revealing one's own bias. Other politically loaded words in this field include "feminist," "men's rights advocate," "traditional" or "family values," "fundamentalist," "secular humanist," "essentialist" or "social constructionist," and "queer."

Double entendres (words with double meanings, one of which may be considered indelicate or risqué) can be an occasional annoyance or source of unexpected humor in the sexuality education classroom. Educators and learners alike can be blind-sided by unintentional use of a word or phrase that has a sexual double meaning. When such distractions occur, the educator should simply acknowledge the humor and perhaps use it as a "teachable moment" about the role of sexual euphemisms in our culture before returning to the original topic (see boxed insert).

Saying More Than You Meant to Say

One of our favorite stories about being side-tracked by a *double entendre* came from our colleague, the late Mary Lee Tatum, a widely respected junior high school sexuality educator in Falls Church, Virginia. Mary Lee was demonstrating the proper use of a condom by stretching it over two of her extended fingers when a student asked, "Why do condoms fail sometimes?"

She responded, picking at the condom with the fingernails of her other hand, "Well, sometimes they get a little 'prick' in them." The students, who had immediately gleaned the *double entendre* ("prick"), were falling out of their chairs laughing before it occurred to Mary Lee what she had said.

It's easier to talk about sex when it's O.K. to laugh.

(Student in a sexuality class)

Appropriate humor in the sexuality classroom, whether unintentional or deliberate, can enhance comfort level and learning. Laughter provides an outlet for the emotional tension that builds up when talking about serious and personally loaded subjects. However, humor that is offensive or belittling has the opposite effect—most sexual jokes, for example, are not appropriate, since they frequently play on prejudice and intolerance. [12]

Spontaneous Humor in the Classroom

I decided to videotape one of my presentations on sexual anatomy and physiology to high school students so I could improve my technique. Upon reviewing the videotape, I made a very interesting observation: every time I had said the word "erection," I also had unconsciously raised my index finger in an erect position. Although I had observed students giggling during this portion of my presentation, I had been unaware until viewing the videotape that my own body language was the source of the humor!

(SOURCE: Story told by Kelly Riggle-Hower, community educator, Seattle)

Sexuality *is* a serious subject, but educators also need to accept that funny things *will* happen in class and it should be O.K. to laugh. How you deal with spontaneous humor in the classroom demonstrates your comfort level with sexuality and with students and, in turn, makes them feel more at ease. If you frown and express disapproval, for example, you not only squelch the students' natural response, but communicate that perhaps sexuality is too solemn a subject to laugh about. On the other hand, by accepting student laughter (and joining in, if so moved) you communicate the subtle message that humor is a desirable feature of healthy intimate relationships.

Some students, however, use joking behavior to mask serious questions and concerns; therefore, even when treating a humorous comment as such, be conscious of what else the student might be trying to communicate. If you have reason to believe the comment or joke veils a concern deserving follow-up, pursue it with the student individually after the session.

Today's class made clear to me my ignorance and uncomfortableness about not only my own sexuality but male and female anatomy and the sexual organs. I was very anxious at the beginning of the class; however, the drawing exercise we did made me feel more at ease with my own feelings. I expect to be embarrassed in the future but know I will not be alone. Talking about sexuality and listening to others inspires me to gain more knowledge and challenges me to participate.

(Student in a college sexuality class)

Activities specifically designed to increase comfort with sexuality language and topics help to lower anxiety. As learners participate, each successive experience becomes less intimidating. Lessening of discomfort occurs naturally over the course of a learning experience about sexuality, but consciously designed activities work more quickly, mitigating this barrier to learning.

Examples of desensitizing activities include opportunities to practice correct terminology, having a guest speaker talk about living with HIV/AIDS, seeing a video or slide presentation with accurate images of sexual anatomy, and practicing the correct application of a condom on a substitute "phallus," such as a banana. In the *Reducing the Risk* curriculum, students complete a homework assignment to visit a local drugstore and locate and describe contraceptives, helping them overcome the discomfort typically associated with obtaining condoms. [13]

Learning Activity: "Draw the Body Parts"

Divide students into gender-mixed groups, give them markers and six-foot lengths of newsprint, and tell them to draw and label the primary and secondary sex characteristics (both internal and external) of life-sized images of the male and female. Reassure students that artistic ability is unimportant and you do not expect them to have much correct knowledge of sexual anatomy—you are just interested in seeing what they already know.

Have each group post their two drawings and describe to the large group how they have labeled the parts. Don't make any corrections at that time. Just thank each group for sharing their drawings.

Discussion. Solicit from each group information about the *process* that occurred in their group as drawings were produced:
- Who did the drawing? (Male or female)
- Were different artists chosen depending on which gender was being drawn? Who took a leadership role in each case?
- Which sex characteristics were drawn first? Last?
- Which gender drew the genitalia in each drawing?
- Why?

Discuss how they felt while doing this activity:
- How many people felt uncomfortable at first?
- Did participating in this exercise increase or decrease your comfort?
- Why was there so much laughter? (There always is!)

- Were you surprised by how much you already knew?
- How did you feel about this activity overall?

(NOTE: Although this exercise can be used to assess student knowledge or launch a lecture/discussion on sexual anatomy, and physiology, its primary purpose is to develop comfort.)

Comfort with sexuality topics increases as students gain more knowledge and competence. For example, as students learn about condoms, use correct terminology to discuss issues related to them, and practice communication and other practical skills, their comfort and ability to utilize condoms appropriately increases.

Students often hold negative attitudes not only about certain sexuality topics, behaviors, and language but also about certain groups, for example, homosexual people. Extreme homophobia interferes with learning about AIDS or sexual diversity;[14] conversely, extremely positive attitudes toward gays and lesbians result in *more* learning.[15] Exercises specifically designed for decreasing homophobia are described in the box and in Part II ("Gender Orientation and Society"—see index of activities in Appendix D). Reading personal accounts and having guest panels are also effective methods.

A Fantasy Exercise: "Heterosexuals in an Alien World"

Prior instructions. Lead a relaxation exercise prior to the fantasy, then invite students to close their eyes and listen. For this fantasy exercise, all students should operate as though they were heterosexual in orientation.

Fantasy. Imagine, if you will, that it is a year sometime in the distant future on the planet Earth. We have survived the age of AIDS, but not without significant loss of life and radical effects on our society. Heterosexuals, who were disinclined initially to believe the extent of the threat or to alter their behaviors accordingly to avoid contracting the virus, have seen their numbers dwindle drastically. Homosexuals, initially hard-hit by the virus, responded rapidly and effeively to educational efforts to prevent contracting the disease, and have seen their numbers restabilize and, over the years, even grow to outnumber heterosexuals.

Advances in technology have separated the procreative function from sexual relations, via in vitro fertilization and successful incubation of infants, leading to a predominance of artificially conceived and incubated humans. As a result of these and other monumental changes, homosexuality has regained its early historical status as the highest form of love, and heterosexuals (many of whom still reproduce through natural means) now represent an oppressed and defiled minority, derogatorily referred to as "breeders." Religious teachings have been reinterpreted to cast aspersions on the heterosexual orientation as "unnatural and immoral." Legalized discrimination and acts of hatred and violence toward heterosexuals have become commonplace.

Task instructions. In small groups, brainstorm strategies that you, as heterosexuals, can use to deal with this oppression. How will you continue to function as

persons who are heterosexual and still survive in this society? Select a recorder to report your strategies to the large group.

(NOTE: This exercise serves two purposes: (1) to increase empathy for homosexual, bisexual, and transgenderal people; and (2) to evoke generation of survival strategies reminiscent of those currently used by oppressed sexual minorities, e.g., hiding one's true orientation, joining forces with others, organizing, lobbying, demonstrating, litigating, publishing literature, sponsoring pride events, creating separate communities and "friendly" businesses, etc.)

(SOURCE: Activity designed by Evonne Hedgepeth, inspired by Brian McNaught, author of *On Being Gay* and *Gay Issues in the Workplace*.)

Developing Comfort with What Will Happen in Class

Learners typically begin sexuality and HIV education with preconceived notions about what will happen—some positive, some negative, many unrealistic. In fact, many don't know *what* to expect and fear they will be embarrassed or asked to do something that violates their personal boundaries. Such trepidations are alleviated by telling learners what will happen in class.

First of all, establish and enforce ground rules to create a level of trust by outlining the boundaries for participant behavior; then learners won't have to worry they will be verbally attacked for expressing an unpopular opinion. Post an agenda for each session to alert learners to your plans and foster their cooperation in accomplishing them. If any of your planned activities involve risk taking (such as an anonymous survey), tell learners what you expect of them and how their input will be used; if a planned video has a potentially upsetting segment (such as a birth scene or depiction of a rape), give learners prior warning and offer the option of leaving during the showing. Finally, provide a "safety net" for individuals who prefer not to participate in activities by occasionally reiterating their right to pass.

Other Factors in Student Comfort

Teachers increase learners' comfort by guaranteeing their privacy as much as possible. As you try to make sexuality education relevant, you may be tempted to ask personal questions, for example, whether students have ever had experiences related to the topic. Surveys about life experience, family configuration, sexual orientation, or gender role identity are useful tools to demonstrate diversity and illustrate key concepts; however, such information should be obtained in ways that protect individual identities. In many states, it is illegal to pose such questions to schoolchildren, even anonymously; check with the district for its current policy.

Students can be asked, "What are the *different types* of families that exist?" rather than "What kind of family do *you* have?" Students then may contribute answers without revealing anything about their own situations. Also, except where prohibited, surveys can be collected without names, or assigned for individual consideration only.

Some debate exists over whether students, particularly younger ones, are more comfortable learning about sexuality in a same-gender group. Some educators and parents claim gender segregation is necessary to prevent embarrassment and preserve "mystery"; others believe that separating males and females only fosters misunderstanding and ignorance about the other gender.[16, 17] We believe the desire to separate children for sexuality education says more about adult discomfort than what is effective or comfortable for students.

First of all, students do not agree they should be segregated for all sexuality-related content, although they may value separate sessions occasionally or for certain topics. Second, both boys and girls need to learn about the feelings, experiences, developmental issues, and perspectives of the other gender. Third, most students—indeed, most people—feel some initial discomfort talking about sexuality in a mixed-gender group; if it were advisable to separate younger students, then why not older ones (or adults, for that matter)?

All students need to conquer their discomfort with sexuality to become more competent discussing sexual matters in relationships. Communication and trust-building exercises between genders can be used to develop that competence. Separating the genders only reinforces the notion that men and women will never bridge their differences to communicate effectively.

On the other hand, separating the genders on occasion gives each gender the opportunity to discuss mutual concerns and information they might not feel comfortable sharing in a mixed group. Girls, especially, may benefit from having such experiences. However, these sessions should be integrated into the regular, coeducational program.

Group size also greatly affects learner comfort. Some learners feel more comfortable in a large group, which provides some anonymity; others prefer small groups in which they can get to know and trust other participants. (We address ideal group size later in this chapter, under physical environments. Also see Chapter 7 for consideration of large and small group facilitation processes.)

EMPOWERING STUDENTS IN SEXUALITY EDUCATION

Many strategies for developing comfort in the sexuality education classroom also empower students; for example, helping students get to know each other, establishing ground rules, and deliberately enhancing student comfort with desensitizing activities.

Making education relevant to needs and interests is an essential element in learner empowerment; teachers should ask learners what they need and want to learn. Learners are, after all, the best authorities on their own needs, interests, and preferences for content and learning methods. Also, because education takes place within *specific* contexts with *specific* groups of people, assessment should be done for each learning group, not surmised from general population surveys or projections about target groups.[18] Learner assessment allows you to ascertain the saliency of certain topics in a planned curriculum and to make connections with what learners already know.

Some specific methods of determining student needs include brainstorming topics as a group (see Chapter 12), conducting a needs survey (Chapter 9), having a group discussion (Chapter 10), giving pretests of knowledge and attitudes

(Chapter 13), doing a conceptual or topic "webbing" (or "mind-mapping") exercise with the large group (Chapter 6), or asking students to write you notes on an ongoing basis (Chapter 13).

Informal assessment happens before and during the sexuality unit or workshop as you observe, listen to, and work with learners. *Formal assessment* tools, such as webbing, pretests or interest surveys, reveal additional information (see Chapter 6). Ongoing assessment during the learning experience, such as asking for student feedback, can be used to adapt the planned curriculum to emerging student needs and interests.

Engaging learners as co-planners and co-evaluators of sexuality and HIV education programs is another way of empowering them. This notion may seem radical to some, but most educators now recognize the wisdom of including students on program-planning and advisory committees. Also, once learning groups are formed, all learners can be consulted to identify and prioritize the topics to study.

One method of accomplishing this is to have the group brainstorm all possible topics within a subject and then ask each student to list his or her top ten preferences. In an ongoing class, do this survey before the unit begins; in a one-time experience, either survey the participants ahead of time (if feasible) or ask them in the first few minutes of the session to identify their most pressing questions or concerns. You then can adapt your plan accordingly, as feasible.

Brainstorming and surveying topics accomplish several objectives simultaneously: (1) they reveal existing learner knowledge about the subject (by their ability to discern subtopics); (2) they demonstrate how much there is to know about the subject; (3) if webbing is used, it demonstrates relationships among subtopics; and (4) they reveal to you which topics should be covered as a large group or in individual or small group projects.

Students also can be polled for ideas about specific learning activities, projects, materials, or other resources for the class. Often learners, if asked, suggest creative activities or valuable resources such as guest speakers. Evonne once asked her high school students if they knew of any additional resources for their American history class—one student's family owned one of the few existing copies of the Zapruder film of the Kennedy assassination and another asked if her grandfather, an American survivor of the Pearl Harbor bombing, could be a guest speaker.

Asking students to contribute their own ideas for the class has two benefits: (1) increased student investment in and ownership of what happens; and (2) an expansion of your own stock of ideas for teaching the class. Ultimately, the educator is responsible for what happens—the students' role in planning is, at best, supplementary. However, involving students in planning the program, to whatever extent possible, empowers students and enriches a program.

> Competition is the worst possible arrangement as far as relationship is concerned.
> (Alfie Kohn, *No Contest: The Case against Competition*, 1992)

Traditional schooling in this country was built on an ethic of individual achievement and advancement over one's peers. Conventional methods of teaching and evaluation reflect this underlying philosophy, which does not prevail in other cultures or even within all subgroups in this culture. [19]

Research has shown that, in general, competition does not facilitate learning; nor does it serve learners in many other important ways. Competitive learning environments pit learners against one another, fostering peer distrust, envy, and lack of empathy. [20] Competitive methods also exacerbate fear of failure, which can be a barrier to learning and is especially intense and detrimental for female students. [21]

Cooperative learning, by contrast, fosters greater cognitive achievement than either competitive or individual learning experiences, no matter what the subject, age level of the students, or nature of the learning task. [22, 23] Cooperative learning experiences also have a number of significant *affective* and *behavioral* outcomes relevant to sexuality education: collaborative work is more likely to increase learners' feelings of self-worth and competence, to increase their understanding and sensitivity for people who are different, and to improve communication and interpersonal relationship skills. [24]

Today, many educators utilize cooperative learning methods and have replaced competitive testing and grading with individualized "outcome-based" assessments and narrative evaluations. These reforms will positively affect all subject areas eventually but have always been crucial to effective sexuality education. Small group work, as noted above, facilitates group building and increases student comfort. Collaborative projects allow two or more individuals to explore topics of interest that the class as a whole will not study. Fostering noncompetitive attitudes in a sexuality class also reinforces respect for cultural pluralism—that is, when people work toward a common goal, rather than competing for resources and attention, their personal differences seem to matter less.

Productive collaborative work requires good communication, a valuable skill that directly transfers to maintaining effective relationships outside of the classroom. Finally, learners benefit from learning how to cooperate with others (including partners) to solve problems and plan their lives together, rather than feeling they must stand alone.

For more information on practical strategies in cooperative education, such as forming effective groups and grading, see *Learning Together and Alone: Cooperative, Competitive and Individualistic Learning* by Johnson and Johnson. [25]

Students also should play a role in evaluating sexuality education programs. If you want to know whether a product is good or not, should you ask the company that made it, or the consumer? Similarly, learners have unique perspectives on their own learning, which, in conjunction with your observations, provide a more accurate evaluation than your view alone. Students should evaluate the learning experience on three levels: (1) their own performance in the class; (2) the program in general; and (3) your performance as educator. (See Chapter 13 for evaluation strategies for each of these three categories.)

As logical as this approach to evaluation sounds, many educators overlook it as a basic strategy for empowering students. Expecting learners to evaluate their own performance puts much of the responsibility for learning where it belongs—with the learner. If they know from the beginning that they will be asked to give an accurate report of their growth and participation in class, they take learning activities more seriously. Initially students who are accustomed to a competitive grading system are inclined to represent their work in the most favorable light; however, with time, practice, and instruction in the value of honest self-evaluation, students eventually produce meaningful reports.

Students also should give their opinion of the class in general, that is, what activities were especially helpful, how effective was group process, which resources were most valuable? Finally, students should evaluate you, providing vital information that will improve your teaching (see Chapter 13). If you truly value feedback from students and take it into account as you continue to teach sexuality or HIV education, you give power not only to your current students but to those with whom you work in the future.

MAKING THE MOST OF THE PHYSICAL ENVIRONMENT

The physical climate in the classroom—that is, group size, room arrangement, temperature, and other features—can work for you or against you in the job of facilitating learning. This is especially important to effective sexuality and HIV education.

Total group size, for example, is a major factor in how quickly a group will develop intimacy and cohesion. In our experience, between twelve and eighteen is the ideal group size for teaching sexuality education—it is large enough to provide some anonymity, yet small enough that individuals get to know each other quickly and can contribute frequently to group discussion. The National Coalition of Advocates for Students recommends in its *Criteria for Evaluating an AIDS Curriculum* that student groups for HIV education not exceed twenty.[26]

Most educators, however, are expected to work with much larger groups, rarely having the option of smaller educator-learner ratios for sexuality or HIV sessions. One feasible alternative, then, is to break larger groups into smaller units (e.g., dyads or triads) for discussion and activities; some small groups may even be ongoing for certain tasks.

> I like the fact that we break up into smaller groups. It seems easier to talk about things then.
>
> (Student in a sexuality class)

Placement of learners in a space greatly affects group interactions. The traditional classroom configuration of successive rows of chairs facing the teacher, called a "sociofugal" arrangement (literally, "fleeing the social"), is intended to *restrict* interactions among students. This arrangement interferes with two important objectives of the sexuality education class: to increase discussion and to utilize the group as a legitimate source of ideas and information. Such objectives are better accomplished when students are arrayed in a circular or semicircular pattern, or "sociopetal" arrangement ("seeking the social").[27]

Terry Beresford recalls doing a training workshop as a community health educator in an abandoned chapel on the top floor of an inner city building formerly used as a hospital for infectious diseases, with the pews nailed to the floor. "We improvised and coped," she says, "but talk about overcoming obstacles to the development of a happy and learning-conducive ambience!"

Your location in relation to learners also subtly affects group process and communicates much about your role, your attitude toward learners, and your comfort with the topic. Standing in a central location and with more freedom of movement than the students automatically infers a higher status for the educator.[28] Since a key objective of effective sexuality education is to empower learners, occasionally remove yourself from center stage and encourage discussion within the group to teach learners to value each other as important resources. Occasionally sit among the students during a discussion; your physical location will communicate that you have temporarily relinquished your authority role in favor of facilitation and that you truly value their contributions to discussion. (See Chapter 7 for further discussion of effective group facilitation.)

The best room structure allows flexibility in moving furniture and students quickly into various configurations appropriate to the learning task: circular or semicircular for presentations and large group discussions; clusters of small groups or pairs for group tasks; and single desks with plenty of space between them for individualized tasks, such as reflective writing or drawing.

Learners also have personal preferences for their location in the room, and their proximity to you and other learners; you should try to accommodate these desires as much as possible. For example, a learner's choice to sit distant from the teacher (or the group) may indicate their distrust of the group or previous abuse by an authority figure; learner preference for closeness may reflect a desire for inclusion or attention. Ideally, learners should be able to shift easily between "a state of separateness and a state of togetherness" according to their changing desires and comfort level during the learning experience.[29]

Community health educators and other guest speakers face exceptional challenges in managing effective physical environments. Typically, they have no opportunity to examine the space until shortly before the session; furthermore, guest educators may have limited authority or ability to make necessary alterations. Whenever possible, ask ahead of time for a desirable room arrangement, or arrive early enough to make last-minute changes. Also, solicit learner assistance in creating a conducive learning environment, during one-shot or ongoing classes, reinforcing the notion that students share responsibility with you for the success of the learning experience.

Another aspect of the classroom physical environment deserves special mention. In Chapter 2, we discussed the importance of culturally pluralistic teaching. If your classroom is filled with books and posters showing images of mainstream, white, middle-class, heterosexual, normally abled kids in "Leave It to Beaver" families, what is communicated to students whose experience does not fit these images?[30] Even if your group is homogeneous in makeup, diverse images remind students that our society is not.

Approximately 80 percent of human communication occurs through nonverbal cues;[31] therefore, how you present yourself, arrange your classroom, and choose material resources speaks volumes to students about your philosophy in teaching sexuality education.

In this chapter, we have discussed aspects of establishing a psychological and physical climate to foster learning in the sexuality and HIV classroom. Just as a plant grows best if started in good soil with lots of nutrients, our learners thrive in environments that are psychologically safe and personally empowering.

Plants require more than a starter medium in order to grow, however; they also need sunlight, water, and further feedings. Similarly, educational growth requires a healthy dose of intellectual challenge, which at times may even feel uncomfortable to learners. In the next chapter, we examine theoretical underpinnings of effective sexuality education and ways of stimulating students to learn and grow.

CHAPTER 4

Theory and Research for Teaching about Sexuality and HIV

In November of 1991, Earvin "Magic" Johnson, basketball superstar, announced he had contracted the HIV virus. The public response was electrifying; the news spread to every street corner, family room, and school yard of the United States almost instantaneously. Political leaders made their first official statements on the subject. Thousands of individuals who previously had denied their own risk were suddenly instilled with a burning "need to know" about HIV infection. Health clinics and hotlines were overwhelmed with a dramatic increase in requests for HIV tests and information, and many people reduced risk-taking behavior. [1, 2]

"If it could happen to Magic, maybe it could happen to me," they worried. Many people, for the first time, felt vulnerable. With the Johnson announcement, the American public experienced a "sea change" [3] in heterosexual awareness of the threat of HIV infection. In particular, the disclosure resonated with many people of color who had not identified with other celebrities infected with the virus, most of them white, gay, or infected by nonsexual means (e.g., blood transfusions and drug use). [4]

The general public was not ignorant of AIDS prior to Johnson's revelation; to the contrary, heterosexuals and people of color, along with everyone else, had been exposed to relentless "AIDS 101" information through assorted media. Most people knew how the virus was contracted, that it was deadly, and how to avoid it. Yet many in America did not comprehend their own risk for HIV infection. Health officials and educators were puzzled and dismayed by research showing that, despite widespread general knowledge about HIV/AIDS, many individuals remained oblivious to their own risk and failed to make changes in their behavior to protect themselves and others from infection. [5–8]

Why, then, was a solitary event so effective in changing behavior when other means of educating the public over several years had failed? Obviously, the piling on of facts was not working. Was it simply the right time for the message? Was there something special about the event, or the messenger? Or had the accumulation of facts simply reached critical mass?

Ask educational theorists and you might hear various explanations for the phenomenon. Perhaps Johnson's revelation had caused many individuals who viewed him as a role model to *personalize* their own risk for the first time. Or perhaps evidence of the *susceptibility* of an apparently healthy athlete convinced others to contemplate their own. Or maybe the event had *disequilibrated* people, facilitating a conceptual leap in their understanding.

These concepts are essential elements of several prevailing theories that inform and guide modern health education practice. The theories are called by many different names—social learning theory, cognitive behavioral theory, social influence theory, Piagetian theory, "stages of change" theory—but they share some basic tenets useful to the practicing sexuality educator.

Current research on sexuality and HIV education confirms that sexuality and HIV education that is well grounded in educational theory greatly enhances learning.[9] Unfortunately, none of us has the luxury of sitting back and waiting for a serendipitous event such as a popular athlete's disclosure of his HIV status to create "a need to know" in our learners. Educators have to know how to spark that motivation artificially in a classroom setting, and then capitalize on it with the most effective teaching methods.

Another compelling reason why sexuality educators should use only the most powerful, theory-based methods is that we typically are given so little time. Both teachers and administrators cite inadequate instructional time as one of the greatest obstacles to the implementation of effective sexuality education.[10] However, research confirms our own experience that the amount of time spent in sexuality education is not nearly as important as the *quality* of the experience.[11, 12] Theory-based teaching helps sexuality educators make the most of the time spent with learners.

The modern sexuality educator, therefore, should be conversant in the theory and research that underpins modern sexuality education. In this chapter, we briefly review a few relevant theories, synthesize their common elements, and present their implications for teaching about sexuality and HIV/AIDS. Our intention is not to provide comprehensive or in-depth coverage of all theory and research relevant to sexuality education; that task would require several chapters. However, we trust this overview will provide the experienced educator with a thought-provoking review and novice educators with an inspiration to study further.

TEACHERS DON'T "TEACH"—OUR STUDENTS "LEARN"

> I don't understand why my students did so poorly on the last test. I covered that material with them for a whole month!
>
> (Anonymous teacher)

How often have you heard someone say that educators "teach" concepts or skills or attitudes—almost as if we open up students' heads and pour knowledge in? Or, that if we simply "cover" a body of material in a course or workshop, learners will learn it?

Educators do not really "teach" facts, concepts, or skills, but students do learn them with our assistance. We are helpful bystanders (coaches, if you will) in a process that happens *within* the learner. Yes, we can stimulate that process, encourage and support it, but no one can guarantee that learning *will* happen. Ultimately, it is the learner who makes sense of the experience, incorporates all or part of it into his or her existing mental "schemes," or rejects it altogether.

Recognizing how learning truly happens makes it easier to avoid the trap of thinking or acting as if we, rather than the learners, are the most important players in the learning process. Otherwise, we may overuse teaching techniques we do especially well (at the expense of what works best with learners) or accept more responsibility (or credit) than is merited. Effective sexuality and HIV education should be driven by how students *learn*, rather than how teachers prefer to *teach*.

Some educators delineate three domains of learning: *cognitive, affective,* and *behavioral.* Actually, such distinctions are arbitrary, since real-life learning involves much overlap among these categories. Nonetheless, they serve as useful constructs with which to analyze teaching behaviors. We asserted in Chapter 2 that the most successful teaching about sexuality addresses all three domains, that is, teachers should assist students in learning new facts and comprehending key concepts underlying them (cognitive domain), in examining their feelings, attitudes, beliefs, and values (affective domain), and learning and practicing health-positive skills and behaviors (behavioral domain).

Many educators and curricula mistakenly focus on providing students with "facts" through lectures, videos, and worksheets, requiring only cognitive processing. Their faulty assumption is that if one simply exposes students to enough random, disjointed ideas, eventually the information will "take" and student behaviors will be affected accordingly. The typical result, unfortunately, is the acquisition of isolated facts, unlikely to be retained or used once learners complete the obligatory test at the end of the unit.

Several educational philosophers have decried this "filling up the vessel" approach to education. Alfred North Whitehead *(The Aims of Education)* called it "passive reception" of "inert" ideas, disconnected not only from student experience but also from each other. Paulo Freire *(Pedagogy of the Oppressed)* termed it the "banking system" of education, advocating instead education that requires students to "problematize" (think critically) about subject matter. John Dewey *(Experience and Education)* argued that students act intelligently only as a result of education that has personal and social meaning.

Approaching teaching today as if making an "investment for the student's future," not addressing current concerns and needs, is a bankrupt notion. Whitehead summarized it best:

> The mind is never passive; it is a perpetual activity, delicate, receptive, responsive to stimulus. *You cannot postpone its life until you have sharpened it.* Whatever interest attaches to your subject-matter must be evoked *here and now*; whatever powers you are strengthening in the pupil, must be exercised here and now; whatever possibilities

of mental life your teaching should impart, must be exhibited here and now. That is the golden rule of education, and a very difficult rule to follow.

(Whitehead, *The Aims of Education*, p. 18; emphasis is ours)

FOUR GENERATIONS OF SEXUALITY EDUCATION PROGRAMS

Sexuality education of the 1960s and early 1970s was based largely on the banking model of education. Since then, sexuality education in the United States has evolved through three more "generations."[13]

Sexuality educators of the *first generation* believed if they simply provided correct information to students about pregnancy, sexually transmitted diseases, and prophylactics, students would abstain from unprotected sexual activity. Evaluation of programs of this generation, however, indicates that although student knowledge increases, risk-taking behaviors continue unabated.

The *second generation* of sexuality education placed greater emphasis on values clarification and skill building, especially communication and decision-making skills. Teachers and programs of this generation gave out facts but also gave students opportunities to "clarify" values and improve skills in communicating values to partners. The anticipated result of these programs, that students will avoid risk-taking behaviors, has not been borne out by research. Learners do become more cognizant of their own values, and more tolerant of those of others, but they do not exhibit behavior change.[14]

Third-generation curricula and programs were developed in reaction and opposition to the first two. Criticizing second generation sexuality education programs as "value-free" or morally relativistic, curricula were developed (e.g., *Teen Aid* and *Sex Respect*) with a specific moral message about sexual activity before marriage: "Just say no!" Designers of such curricula believe that teaching students about prophylaxis gives out a "double message," in actuality promoting sexual behavior. Some of these curricula use scare tactics and misinformation to dissuade students from taking risks. Research-based evaluations of third-generation curricula have been significantly flawed, but do report significant changes in student attitudes about premarital intercourse.[15] However, recent analysis has shown that these curricula, like their predecessors, have no significant impact on actual behavior.[16]

An emerging *fourth generation* of curricula builds upon the successes and failures of the previous three, as well as upon several theories about behavior change. Examples of fourth-generation curricula are *Postponing Sexual Involvement (PSI), Reducing the Risk (RTR),* and an unnamed curriculum by Schinke and Gilchrist.[17] Like some third-generation curricula, these programs have underlying value messages ("norms"): that adolescents should delay the onset of sexual activity and abstinence is best (PSI and RTR) but if teens still decide to be active, they should practice safer sex behaviors (RTR). Fourth-generation curricula and programs are founded upon several theories of behavior change, including social learning theory, social inoculation theory, and cognitive behavioral theory (addressed later in this chapter).

Some fourth-generation curricula have been rigorously evaluated, revealing significant impacts on behavior. Both *PSI* and *RTR* have been shown to foster delay in initiating sexual intercourse, and *RTR* also increased use of contraceptives by sexually active youth. [18]

Apparently, curricula and programs with a strong, valid theory base are more likely to affect behavior. Many first-generation sexuality education programs fail to take into account educational theory related to any of the three learning domains, neglecting the affective or behavioral domains altogether and relying upon ineffective teaching methods for the cognitive domain, that is, using "telling" as the main method. Later generations of curricula address other domains, but don't always use effective methods for cognitive growth. In the next section, we examine a well-known theory of cognitive development and apply it to effective teaching in sexuality and HIV education.

PIAGETIAN THEORY APPLIED TO SEXUALITY AND HIV EDUCATION

Piaget described mental life as consisting of a system of mental *schemes* with which humans use existing knowledge and comprehend new information. [19] Piaget did not speak of these schemes in a physical sense; however, imagine a network of brain neurons and synapses, much like a three-dimensional puzzle. The mental schemes of children are few and simple; as children grow into able adults and learn new information and concepts, their interlocking schemes become more numerous and complex.

Sexuality educators often see evidence of this construct. Each individual comes to a learning experience with his or her unique way of viewing sexuality, health, and relationships. These learner schemes reflect infinite variety, a function of diverse experiences, developmental levels, and abilities: a sexually experienced student has an entirely different set of schemes than one who is inexperienced; a student living with herpes likely has different schemes about achieving sexual intimacy than s/he had before infection; a woman who has terminated a pregnancy probably feels differently about abortion than someone who has never faced that decision.

When presented with new information, a person's schemes may be affected in one of several ways. If compatible with the learner's current set of schemes, the information is simply added on by means of a mental process Piaget called *assimilation*. Using the three-dimensional puzzle as an analogy, this would be like simply adding a new piece without changing the puzzle's essential structure. For example, if a student in sexuality education already has a strong foundation of knowledge about HIV and is simply told about a new drug that shows promise, s/he can easily assimilate the new information within existing schemes.

If, on the other hand, the new information cannot be assimilated because of limitations in existing schemes, two things can happen: (1) the information can be rejected (i.e., no learning), or (2) the schemes must be transfigured to allow incorporation of the new information, a process Piaget called *accommodation*. Using the puzzle analogy again, the structure must be altered so the new piece will fit.

Consider, for example, the female student whose schemes include a belief that all men are potential rapists. After hearing a male guest speaker who actively works to end sexual violence, she may have to readjust *(accommodate)* her schemes—her beliefs—in order to make them fit with the learning experience. Of course, she also may reject the guest speaker's example as exceptional, keeping her original beliefs more or less intact.

So imagine, if you will, the process of learning as a dynamic one in which mental schemes grow, change, and become more elaborate as the learner is exposed to many discrete and interrelated pieces of new information.

Another key concept in Piaget's theory, illustrated in the above learning situation, is *disequilibration* ("dis/ e qui li bra' tion"). For this aspect of his theory, Piaget apparently borrowed from Freud, who hypothesized that the human organism has a basic desire to maintain equilibrium (or static balance) in its physical and psychological states.

According to Freud, disequilibrium is an uncomfortable state (e.g., hunger, cold, fear, loneliness) that humans naturally seek to avoid. The effort to redress these physical or psychological needs, thereby regaining a state of equilibrium, drives much of human behavior.

Piaget applied the notion of equilibrium to cognitive growth, asserting that humans are more likely to learn when the quiet state of their mental schemes is disturbed by the introduction of new facts, ideas, concepts, or realities. The cognitively "disequilibrated" person, then, is motivated to assimilate or accommodate new information in order to return to the more comfortable state of cognitive equilibrium; in other words, s/he is infused with a "need to know." In the above example, the female student is disequilibrated by being confronted with a man who does not fit her stereotype, perhaps motivating her to learn more—or she might just work harder to find evidence to confirm her belief.

Other examples of potentially disequilibrating learning experiences abound: viewing an emotionally stirring video or theater production; listening to an HIV-positive guest speaker; participating in a values clarification exercise; interacting with peers; visiting a health clinic or purchasing a condom for the first time; assessing one's own comfort level with sexuality, and so on. Of course, none of these experiences is guaranteed to disequilibrate all students; conversely, *any* learning experience has the potential to disequilibrate. Even the introduction of a single fact—for example, that sperm can live up to seven days—could spark disequilibration.

Consequently, the most effective sexuality educator presents learners with situations or information that cause disequilibration, thereby creating a "need to know" that, in turn, increases the likelihood that learning will happen. In other words, disequilibration forces an opening in the learner's mental schemes, so that new knowledge can enter. This way of thinking about teaching and learning is quite different from the notion of pouring in "X" amount of information until the learner gets full!

Another useful construct from Piaget's theory is that there are two fundamentally different kinds of knowledge or "ways of knowing": *figurative* and *operative*.[20] *Fig-*

urative knowing refers to basic sensual processing of information regarding the "present, static configuration of a thing":[21] the ability to read a letter or word and recognize its symbolism for something else, for example, illustrates figurative knowing. In Bloom's taxonomy, figurative knowing is low on the hierarchy (being able to recall, list, identify, define, and distinguish facts about a topic).[22]

Operative knowing is more sophisticated, requiring an ability to "operate upon" other knowledge acquired figuratively, that is, being able to compare and contrast, synthesize, analyze, extrapolate from and evaluate facts, observations, and definitions about a topic.

To understand the distinction between these two ways of knowing, consider what happens when you try to read a book while sleepy or distracted. You may be able to process only the words as separate, figurative symbols—for example, "the," "possibilities," "are," "exciting"—without comprehending how they *operate* together to make meaning—that is, "The possibilities are exciting!"

Health educators frequently observe figurative versus operative knowing in sexuality education: the learner who can correctly label the parts of the male reproductive system but doesn't understand how they work together to deliver sperm out of the body; the clinic patron who comprehends different effectiveness rates of various contraceptive methods (figurative knowing) but does not understand how they work (operative) nor which method would be best for her and her partner; or students who can list ten reasons for postponing sexual involvement (figurative knowledge) but don't have the skills to remain abstinent (operative knowledge).

Both kinds of knowledge—figurative and operative—are essential to learning about sexuality. Unfortunately, many educators emphasize figurative knowing over operative knowing for several reasons: (1) they may be most comfortable and experienced in using teaching methods that lead to figurative knowledge (e.g., lecture); (2) they face opposition by people who do not want children to have operative knowledge about sexuality; and (3) figurative knowledge is easier to measure on an "objective" test. Some teachers are satisfied if their students, after being presented with some definitions, facts, and observations about a topic, can regurgitate them relatively unadulterated for a test. The fact that the students have gained little or no comprehension of the underlying operative principles, relationships, or applications of a topic may escape the teacher's attention or concern.

The focus on figurative learning is exacerbated by pressure upon sexuality educators to "document" learner achievement—something more easily addressed by quantitative tests of figurative knowledge than qualitative assessments of operative knowledge. Accumulated data on figurative knowledge is simplistic and obtained at the expense of more meaningful learning; educators do learners a disservice by succumbing to this pressure in the name of "accountability."

> Let the main ideas which are introduced into a child's education be few and important, and let them be thrown into every combination possible.
> (Alfred North Whitehead, *The Aims of Education*)

Another way individuals learn, according to Piaget, is by building upon their understanding of basic *concepts* acquired while experiencing their world as young children. During early development, humans gain first a "sensorimotor" understanding (using perceptual and motor senses) and, later, a cognitive understanding of basic concepts such as length, horizontality, rotation, conservation, and categorization of objects. These essential concepts provide a foundation for understanding more complex concepts with which individuals grapple as they develop and learn.

Concepts may be visualized as the linchpins in the mental schemes of an individual. Imagine a person's mental schemes as a construction of old-fashioned wooden Tinker Toys: figurative knowledge is represented by the colored sticks of many lengths and concepts by the many-holed wheels connecting the sticks—that is, facts—together.

Students come to a learning experience with their own preexisting constructions of concepts and facts. For example, most students already have an understanding of basic concepts such as family, love, attachment, pleasure, sacrifice, commitment, pain, difference, growth, change, disease, and loss, gained through earlier experiences and studies. Your challenge, then, is to help learners link new and more advanced information to the existing conceptual framework, building upon and broadening them and, occasionally, introducing new concepts.

Again, teachers do not "teach concepts"; rather, concepts exist only within the learner. All that you can do is assess a learner's current understandings and then provide learning experiences that are likely to lead to conceptual growth.

CONCEPTUALLY BASED SEXUALITY AND HEALTH EDUCATION

How can a teacher help students build on conceptual knowledge in sexuality and health education? With a class of fifth graders, for example, you could build upon the students' understanding of the concept of *change* to help them understand puberty as a time of change—some of it positive, some negative, just like most changes in our lives! Make connections between the feelings associated with the changes during puberty and other changes in their lives—moving, changing schools, gaining a new sibling or parent figure, and so forth. Help them see that change is a natural part of life.

Similarly, most students at this age have experienced a loss of some kind— perhaps a pet, a treasured possession, or even a friend or family member. Help students relate their own "loss" experiences to those that HIV-positive individuals face: loss of health, jobs, recreational activities, financial security, friends, family, and their lives as they have known them. Ask students to reflect on how they felt when they suffered loss, to help them empathize with HIV-positive individuals.

Many learning activities in sexuality and HIV education are conceptually based. Activities in HIV and STD prevention curricula, for example, can demonstrate the concept of "transmission." In one such activity, students sit or stand in a circle facing each other, rolling out a ball of colored yarn as the teacher describes risky behaviors that hypothetically occurred between individuals. By the end of the exercise, an elaborate web of connections among the students has been constructed with the yarn, visually demonstrating how a real STD transmission network might develop.

In a similar exercise, two key concepts—transmission and abstinence—are illuminated at once. A few students are secretly designated to be "carriers" of several STDs and then all students in the group are asked to mill about, shaking hands with one person, then another, then another, each time writing down that person's name. At the end of the exercise, the teacher discloses the names of students who initially were "infected" and asks each person who shook their hands to stand up. Then anyone who shook hands with any of those standing also stands up. By the end of the exercise, most or all of the students will be standing (some of them having been "infected" with more than one STD), except for the one individual who was instructed to "abstain" (not shake hands) and another who "used protection properly." The *Reducing the Risk* curriculum uses a similar exercise to illustrate the statistical risk for pregnancy and the concept of abstinence.[23]

Conceptually based learning activities are more effective than conventional approaches to learning for several reasons. First, activities such as the ones described above involve everyone and are more personally engaging than a lecture or video. Second, such activities disequilibrate students, in part because of curiosity about the purpose of the exercise and its relationship to the topic. Third, once those connections are made, the activity builds upon previous understandings of a concept.

Conceptually based teaching also directly focuses learners' attention on key ideas within content, rather than assuming they will be able to discern them from a collection of facts. This approach allows the teacher to organize the curriculum around shared core concepts within health topics (see boxed inserts) and to maximize learning in the limited time typically devoted to health education.

Once learners apply a previously understood concept to a new topic (e.g., "transmission" to HIV/AIDS), the next steps are (1) to elaborate on the topic with additional factual information or experiences *(elaboration),* and (2) to reinforce or "harden" the new learning *(crystallization).* Using the puzzle analogy again, think of elaboration as the addition of new pieces, attached to a particular concept or cluster of facts. Then the crystallization process equates to gluing that section of the puzzle to stabilize it, but only *temporarily* since schemes are never permanently fixed; humans are continually disequilibrated with new information, and their schemes are altered, throughout life. However, some individuals' schemes are more hardened and less amenable to new learning than others.

Ways to facilitate the process of elaboration include any of the methods described in Part II. Crystallization of knowledge occurs naturally as a result of elaboration, but more so if students are given opportunities to reinforce and apply their new knowledge, such as documenting their work in a portfolio, writing about it in a journal, or using a new skill.

Discerning which concepts and facts are the most essential is a critical factor in successful teaching in the cognitive domain. In Chapter 6 we offer a tool for identifying key concepts and topics in sexuality and HIV education. Also presented is a planning model that involves first assessing learner comprehension of essential concepts and then planning conceptually based lessons to disequilibrate learners.

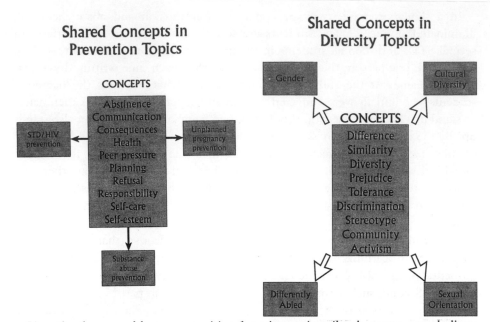

Shared Concepts in Prevention Topics

CONCEPTS

Abstinence
Communication
Consequences
Health
Peer pressure
Planning
Refusal
Responsibility
Self-care
Self-esteem

STD/HIV prevention

Unplanned pregnancy prevention

Substance abuse prevention

Shared Concepts in Diversity Topics

Gender

Cultural Diversity

CONCEPTS

Difference
Similarity
Diversity
Prejudice
Tolerance
Discrimination
Stereotype
Community
Activism

Differently Abled

Sexual Orientation

Piaget's theory addresses cognitive learning primarily; however, we believe many Piagetian tenets apply as well to teaching in the affective and behavioral domains. For example, a learner's mental schemes could be said to include attitudes, beliefs, and values (affective) as well as facts and concepts. The ability to name a behavioral skill necessary to healthy behavior (e.g., "just say no") is only *figurative* knowledge, whereas knowing how to use it is *operative. Disequilibration,* or challenging one's current way of thinking, definitely plays a role in attitude change and, ultimately, in behavioral change (see the next section). And new skills could be said to be *crystallized* through practice.

SOCIAL LEARNING THEORIES APPLIED TO SEXUALITY AND HIV EDUCATION

As important as it is to *know* health risks and prevention strategies, cognitive knowledge alone is not sufficient to influence behavior. Students may have a cognitive understanding of contraception, they may know about HIV/AIDS and behaviors that put them at risk, and they may grasp concepts essential to healthy living; but they won't necessarily act in accordance with their knowledge if they do not personalize their risk, believe in their ability to act, feel supported by peers, or have necessary skills to act on their intentions. Many sexuality education programs overemphasize cognitive learning and fail to address the equally important affective and behavioral aspects of becoming and staying sexually healthy.

Inadequacy of skills for negotiating with a partner, for example, constitutes a major obstacle to practicing healthy sexual behaviors. A 1990 study of HIV/AIDS knowledge, attitudes, and behaviors among young adults revealed that most of the subjects had appropriate, accurate, and useful knowledge about HIV, particularly about risky behaviors.[24] Yet most did not personalize risk, and even if they did, were unable to talk to partners about the use of barriers. Attitudes such as denial, low self-esteem, depression, suicidality, internalized homophobia, and attitudes about condom use also play a role in blocking healthy behaviors.[25]

Fourth-generation curricula are based primarily on *social learning theory,* which recognizes that learning occurs not merely within the learner but also in a particular social context. Learning is an interactive process between the learner and his or her environment; learners are influenced by cues from their environment (including the actions of others), by their own expectancies about outcomes, and by beliefs about their own ability to act.

Several overlapping theories are categorized under the umbrella term "social learning theory": social cognitive theory (also called social learning theory); cognitive behavioral theory; social inoculation theory; and social influence theory. In the following section, we summarize each theory briefly and then discuss some of their shared concepts and how they inform effective teaching in sexuality and HIV education.

Social cognitive theory posits that maintaining healthy behaviors (such as avoiding unprotected sex) is affected by (1) an understanding of what must be done to avoid sex or to use protection *(knowledge);* (2) one's belief in the anticipated benefit of delaying sex or using protection *(motivation);* (3) belief that particular skills or methods of protection will be effective *(outcome expectancy);* and (4) belief that s/he can effectively use these skills or methods of protection *(self-efficacy).*[26] Another important principle of social cognitive theory is that people learn by observing the behaviors of others and the consequences they experience from those behaviors.

Cognitive behavioral theory postulates that in order to resist pressures to have sex, a person must (1) personalize the information *(personalization);* (2) master *skills* to avoid unprotected intercourse; and (3) believe in his/her ability to use these skills *(self-efficacy).* Obviously, much overlap exists between cognitive behavioral theory and social cognitive theory.

Social inoculation theory suggests that individuals can be "immunized," so to speak, to resist future peer pressure to engage in risky behaviors by practicing ahead of time what to do in such situations *(behavior rehearsal).* Much as an inoculation works to help the immune system recognize and attack invading germs, individuals can learn to recognize and resist forms of peer pressure by practicing refusal skills in role plays and other such simulation exercises.

Social influence theory emphasizes the role of *social norms* in influencing individual behavior: if an individual perceives that certain behaviors are acceptable within his or her peer group, s/he is more willing to engage in them. If the social "norms" can be changed, presumably so can individual behaviors.

As you already may have noted, these theories have many concepts in common:

- *Personalization.* Do learners believe the information is relevant to them personally?
- *Susceptibility.* Do they believe themselves to be vulnerable (to HIV, unplanned pregnancy, STDs, etc.)?

- *Efficacy.* Do they believe in the effectiveness of a particular behavior or object (i.e., safer sex behaviors or latex products)?
- *Self-efficacy.* Do they believe in their own ability to enact the behaviors necessary to stay healthy (or well adjusted in their relationships)?
- *Social norms.* Do they perceive social support for their beliefs and behaviors?
- *Skills.* Do they have the skills to act on their beliefs, attitudes, and perceptions?

These concepts are the essential building blocks for designing learning activities intended to affect, enhance, and/or change learner behaviors. Here we describe how these concepts apply to sexual health concerns and how each can be addressed in effective sexuality/HIV education.

Personalization

Educators often speak of the importance of personal *relevance* of education to learners. Why? Because if learners see relevance in the material and believe it holds meaning for them personally, they may be more likely to learn and retain the information.

In sexuality and HIV education, more so than in other subjects, personal relevance is a requirement. First of all, students *expect* sexuality education to be personally meaningful; when it is not relevant or realistic, students may reject it wholesale. Recently, a college student said to us, "I'd like to take another class from Ms. Davis [not her real name] because I'm interested in gender studies, but I can't stand the fact that she is stuck in the 1970s. A lot of changes have happened in the dynamics between men and women since then."

Second, the topic of human sexuality is, by its very nature, personal. Consequently, many students reject abstract or theoretical material that is not connected with real-life issues.

As noted in Chapter 2, students are more likely to personalize from learning activities in which they see something of themselves, for example, in the people depicted, in the situations they are likely to encounter or have already experienced, and even in the group leader. Therefore, materials that present and discuss a diversity of images, relationships, and sexual behaviors help each learner relate more easily to a topic. Likewise, a teacher who reflects the cultural, gender, or sexual orientation of a homogeneous class may be more likely to be perceived by some as more credible (e.g., a gay man teaching gay men). Adolescents, especially, benefit from having peer educators with whom they identify and communicate more easily than with adults.[27] Learners in "special populations" benefit from programs tailored to address their unique needs and realities (see box). Activities depicting situations learners are likely to encounter are more personalizable than outdated or unrealistic scenarios.

By contrast, a role play addressing the dilemma of a young woman deciding whether or not to "let" a guy kiss her at the end of a first date denies the realities of modern adolescent relationships, and would be laughable to most students.

Using "abstinence only" approaches with *genitally active students* is like closing the barn door after the horse is already out; while the value of abstinence should be emphasized with all students, education about safer sex behaviors is more likely to address the needs of these students. [28]

- *Female students* may benefit from occasional segregated sessions so they can discuss, without interruption or competition from males, concerns unique to them. [29]
- Many *"at-risk" youth* (runaway, homeless, troubled or incarcerated, gang-affiliated, etc.) distrust authority figures and value approaches using peer leadership and high student involvement in planning. Their unusually high risk for substance abuse, prostitution, and risky sexual behaviors, which correlate with unplanned pregnancy, HIV, and STDs, also must be addressed. [30]
- Some *substance abusers* respond better to HIV prevention messages from peers, who have "been there," than from authority figures. [31]
- *Mentally and physically challenged individuals* may require basic information about privacy and social behaviors, and acknowledgment that they are sexual. [32, 33]
- Many *deaf students,* because they can't hear the ubiquitous media information about HIV (and some of them have difficulty reading English) require basic "AIDS 101" information that most hearing individuals already have. [34]
- In general, *African-American men* are less likely than white men to believe that health interventions actually work *(efficacy)* and are more pessimistic about their own health in general. They may respond more readily to reality-based, affective education that instills hope rather than reinforces fear and despair. [35] Many urban black learners may respond more readily to education using African-American music, videos, art, films, stories, and other nonwritten materials. [36]
- Teenage pregnancy prevention programs for *African-American women* should acknowledge that some young women desire to become pregnant for socioeconomic reasons and out of concern about the high mortality rate of their male peers. [37]
- *Mexican-American adolescents* may hold traditional attitudes about sex, maintaining a strong double standard regarding responsibility for virginity and contraception. [38]
- Some *Native American students* may benefit from a teaching approach that recognizes their need to reconcile conflicting demands of two cultures and that utilizes traditional practices such as storytelling and rituals (e.g., using a "talking stick" for group discussion). [39, 40]

NOTE: Maria Natera offers the following caution when generalizing about cultural groups: "The dividing line between cultural sensitivity and negative stereotyping is sometimes difficult to detect. While members of a group share cultural characteristics, each individual should also be seen as an individual with unique skills, needs and interests." [41] Dr. Natera's caution applies as well to stereotyping based on gender or sexual orientation.

Recognizing and addressing student diversity in teaching about sexuality and HIV is only part of the personalization equation. Developing activities that help students see relevance in topics they think are not important and helping them make connections with their own lives are also important. For example, an activity in the *Reducing the Risk* curriculum asks students to imagine what they would do if told they were HIV-positive. Most adolescents do not think of themselves as susceptible to HIV; yet this exercise forces them to "personalize" the experience of being HIV infected and consider its likely impact on their lives. Another example is an exercise that Evonne has used with high school students to help them personalize the likely consequences of an unintended pregnancy (see box).

Learning Activity—The "Chick Project": Personalizing an Unintended Pregnancy

I created "The Chick Project" to give high school students an opportunity to observe the growth and development of a fetus and, at the same time, to personalize the experience of becoming pregnant.

After all the students had agreed to participate in the project, I presented each (including males) with a fertilized Araucana* chicken egg and said "Congratulations! You're pregnant!"

Each egg was marked with its "parent's" name, and we developed a rotation schedule for turning the eggs every four hours (except at night). A dozen or so students wanted less responsibility, so they shared their rotation schedule as a group; a few wanted more responsibility and worked as a smaller team; one student, glad the project was providing her an opportunity to try out parenthood "without freaking out (her) parents," built her own incubator and took sole responsibility for her chick.

Although all had agreed to do the project, most students expressed reluctance to follow through when actually confronted with the responsibility of a "pregnancy." So we discussed the analogy with real pregnancies—even a "planned" pregnancy can evoke feelings of regret or ambivalence. Some students wanted to be released from the project, but I gave them only two options: *adoption* (only after the hatching of their chick) or *abortion* (cracking his/her own egg open into a toilet and flushing it). Notably, none of these students elected abortion, although one seriously considered it only to be convinced by peers to "carry the pregnancy" and let them adopt the "baby."

Most students took the project very seriously, some becoming emotionally attached to their eggs and very excited during the "births." However, the thrill of being new parents wore off when students had to feed the chicks and clean soiled cages every day!

Throughout the project we discussed many parallels between our simulation and real life pregnancy and parenting. For example, students who had taken less responsibility for the turning of the eggs felt less attachment to their hatched chicks. Several students whose chicks did not hatch (including the "parent" who had considered abortion) expressed feelings of grief and guilt.

Overall, the "Chick Project" was an amazing success, effective beyond my wildest expectations. Frankly, I was surprised that streetwise adolescents would be so invested in an activity I had half-expected them to consider silly. Perhaps the activity tapped an important need in them to create a new life and experience parenting in a safe, nonpermanent way. In any case, they learned that once a conception has occurred, none of their options is easy and whatever they choose may change their lives forever.

*Araucana ("Easter Egg") chickens were used because they have colorful individual markings by which they can be identified after hatching.

(SOURCE: Evonne Hedgepeth, The Open High School, 1976)

If students cannot relate information (e.g., about unintended pregnancy) to their own lives, they may be less likely to believe themselves to be susceptible or be less motivated to use health-positive behaviors. In Part II we highlight many other activities that sexuality educators can use to help learners personalize information.

Susceptibility

Many learners deny their susceptibility to health consequences, especially adolescents, who are notorious for believing themselves immortal, whether hitch-hiking, jumping off a bridge into shallow water, riding a motorcycle without a helmet, or having unprotected genital sex. Teenagers doubt or deny their susceptibility to sexual consequences, in particular, for a number of reasons: failure to recognize the possible outcomes of risky behaviors; not understanding the relationship between sex and disease or pregnancy; ambivalence about pregnancy; and denial based on discomfort, shame, guilt, or lack of experience with consequences.[42]

Adults, too, deny their susceptibility to the consequences of sexual behaviors. A case in point is the denial by many heterosexuals of their own risk for HIV. In one study of college students, most said they recognized the severity of AIDS, but believed their own risk was very low.[43] One college-aged author asserts what she believes is the general perception among her peers: being heterosexual and contracting HIV is "about as likely as having a piano fall on your head."[44] Contrast this belief with reality: heterosexual transmission is estimated to account for 71 percent of AIDS cases worldwide, and in this country, women represent the fastest-growing category.[45]

Other studies reveal the role that a belief in one's own susceptibility plays in risk taking. Young gay men, for example, are more likely to engage in unprotected anal intercourse than older gay men, who have watched many of their friends die of AIDS-related complications.[46-48] One study found that the extent to which one holds an image of someone in the final stages of AIDS serves as a powerful inducement to safer sex practices.[49]

Individuals in committed relationships are more likely to forgo protection, perhaps because they believe they are no longer susceptible.[50] Moreover, *both* partners must perceive that they are at risk before risk reduction behavior will occur.[51]

On the other hand, very young learners may fear HIV infection and other tragedies, for themselves or those they love, even when the risk is in fact very low.[52] With these students, the educator must counter learners' exaggerated perceptions of susceptibility with realistic appraisals.

Teaching about susceptibility means using learning activities that help students assess their true risk. Two such activities, in the *Teaching Safer Sex* curriculum,[53] utilize information sheets that describe levels of risk of various sexual behaviors and worksheets that help students analyze their relative risk. Students consider the question, "How does one increase the probability of avoiding or acquiring an STD through wise or unwise behaviors?" In addition to individual and small group work, these activities also employ large group discussion, continuum exercises, case history analysis, and a self-test to understand personal susceptibility. Another effective method is using guest speakers, demographically similar to learners, who have experienced negative sexual consequences of risky behaviors, for example, HIV-positive adolescents.

In Part II we present several methods that can increase learner awareness of susceptibility; see the index of learning activities in Appendix D for reference to specific activities.

Efficacy

Even if learners believe themselves susceptible to health or relationship consequences, they still may not trust the effectiveness *(efficacy)* of certain behaviors or products recommended to lower their risk. A large percentage of adults (from 30 to 50 percent) believe, for example, that condoms are less effective in preventing STD or HIV infection than studies indicate they really are.[54, 55] Some learners lack confidence that changing one's own behaviors (e.g., exercising improved communication skills) truly can have a positive impact on a relationship.

Students gain confidence in the efficacy of behaviors and technology in a variety of ways. They learn skills by observing others performing them successfully (such as refusal tactics in teen theater scenarios or videos), by self-practice in role plays, or by experiential learning exercises (such as simulation of correct condom use). They are more likely to believe in the efficacy of safer sex behaviors and prophylaxis if both the messenger and the message are perceived to be credible.

Learning Activity: Contraceptive Counseling Role Play

Evonne designed the following activity to help high school students comprehend both the *efficacy* of contraceptives and a person's *self-efficacy* in using them.

Preparation. Have students review information (via fact sheets, pamphlets, clinic visits, etc.) on various contraceptive methods to become familiar with effectiveness rates, methods of use, cost, and so forth.

Role play. Ask several students (ones who will be comfortable and competent) to play the following roles:

John and Josephine are a married couple, with three children and precarious family finances; for health reasons Josephine cannot risk another pregnancy yet they are morally opposed to the IUD and to abortion, which they believe result in the killing of a developing baby. They would not object to other contraceptive methods, which must be effective.

Sharon is a third-year college student who has infrequent sexual encounters with different partners, sometimes under the influence of drugs or alcohol. She definitely wants to avoid pregnancy, but hates the pill because she thinks it makes her gain weight. She doesn't feel comfortable asking her partners to wear condoms.

Kathryn is a single mom, on welfare; she definitely does not want more children; she is in a long-term relationship, but is not sure her partner is faithful to her. She is uncomfortable touching her own genitalia.

The volunteers play the role of counselees in a family planning clinic (or other counseling setting) considering their contraceptive options. They are instructed to stay true to character; for example, Kathryn, who is uncomfortable touching herself, should reject the diaphragm as a method. The remainder of the students serve as "counselors," helping the clients make decisions about birth control.

This activity helps students apply their figurative knowledge about contraceptives (i.e., make it "operative") and to understand that the effectiveness of a method is a function both of the method's general effectiveness rate ("efficacy") and an individual's (or couple's) self-efficacy in using the method.

Students today are caught in the middle of a political controversy that undermines their trust in condom efficacy. Some opposition groups are engaged in a disinformation campaign about condom effectiveness and safer sex practices, in an attempt to discourage any sexual activity outside of monogamous, lawful marriage. Recent studies on condoms, however, provide compelling evidence that latex condoms, *if used consistently and correctly,* are 96 percent effective in preventing pregnancy[56] and up to 99 percent effective in preventing HIV infection.[57] In a recent study of heterosexual partners (one of whom was infected with HIV), there were *zero* incidences of HIV transmission among couples who used condoms consistently for about 15,000 episodes of vaginal and anal intercourse, compared with a 4.8 percent infection rate per year for couples who used condoms inconsistently.[58]

Opponents of condom education often cite lower effectiveness rates obtained in studies of couples who used condoms inconsistently for pregnancy prevention. More subtly, they focus on *failure* rates, rather than on the significantly high effectiveness rates.

Admittedly, condoms do not provide 100 percent protection; neither, however, do seat belts (40–55 percent effective), helmets (85 percent), vaccinations, smoke detectors, or, for that matter, abstinence (74 percent effective when used as a method for preventing pregnancy).[59, 60] At issue here is *relative* risk versus absolute protection; most people use seat belts and helmets, obtain vaccinations, and install smoke detectors despite some risk of failure. Among nonabstinent individuals, the choice is between *safer sex* and *very dangerous* sex; to assume that young people will eschew genital activity if adults simply deny them easy access to latex products and information about correct usage is both unrealistic and irresponsible. Furthermore, the job of sexuality education requires providing learners with skills and knowledge they might need both now and in the future.

Self-Efficacy

A person develops self-efficacy by gathering information from four main sources: (1) personal experience performing a behavior successfully; (2) vicarious experience observing others successfully performing the behavior; (3) encouragement from others that they are capable of performing the behavior; and (4) internal physiological states.[61]

Self-efficacy is a key concept in developing and maintaining healthy sexual behaviors and relationships. Students may have a low sense of sexual or relationship self-efficacy for a variety of reasons. Females suffer from lower self-efficacy than males in general due to internal locus of control issues.[62] Women who have experienced sexual abuse or rape have lowered self-efficacy and are at increased risk for unintended pregnancy or HIV infection.[63, 64] Girls who first had sexual intercourse at age 14 or younger are at much higher risk for a plethora of problems—multiple partners, STDs, unintended early pregnancies, substance abuse, less discrimination in choosing partners[65–67]—likely due to decreased self-efficacy. Gay, lesbian, or bisexual youth may have less self-efficacy than other adolescents due to low self-esteem.[68]

Self-efficacy is enhanced through several mechanisms: opportunities to observe and practice skills such as assertiveness, effective communication, condom use, and negotiation of safer sex; exposure to positive role models and social norms; improving self-esteem through long-term positive feedback; and learning constructive ways to relieve states of anxiety or desire. Many of these methods are easily incorporated into school-based and community-based sexuality education. Educators especially should help students address their discomfort with sexuality, which negatively affects self-efficacy.

On the other hand, some discomfort or anxiety may be necessary to influence behavior change. Studies have found that a *moderate* level of anxiety, such as fear of contracting HIV, actually is helpful in motivating individuals to change behavior (too little anxiety does not provide an impetus to change, and too much can immobilize the person).[69] These findings lend further credence to Piaget's notion of disequilibration as a necessary antecedent to learning.

Social Norms

Social norms are expected modes of acting and behaving by virtue of membership in a certain social group in order to gain or maintain approval or status. Perceived norms significantly affect the willingness of an individual to initiate and continue health-positive behaviors.

Social norms are difficult to change, but sexuality and HIV education can have an impact. A compelling example is the *Postponing Sexual Involvement* curriculum, which has successfully influenced student norms using peer educators both to present a structured educational program and to serve as positive role models (see Chapter 12). The program utilizes peer educators representing a cross section of students and provides learning activities relying heavily on role play (see Chapter 11) to reinforce the norm of postponing sexual involvement.[70]

Teen theater is another effective way to positively affect social norms (see Chapter 12). Dramatic presentations and improvisations based on realistic scenarios captivate student interest and are more believable when presented by peers. Student theater is most effective when it utilizes open-ended role plays and actively involves the audience in problem solving or solicits reactions to the scenes and characters.

Studies with gay men have shown the impact of changing social norms on sexual behaviors. In one key study, popular opinion leaders among gay men in an urban setting were trained to deliver risk-reduction messages and give personal endorsements of safer sex to their social network. Men exposed to these messages reported a significant drop in risky behaviors, an increase in condom use, and a reduction in the number of sexual contacts.[71] Changing group norms also influences contraceptive behavior among heterosexuals.[72]

Public media campaigns also affect norms. The "Keep It Up, Seattle" advertising campaign, for example, encourages gay men to avoid risky behaviors.[73] Likewise, some communities have instituted advertising campaigns promoting abstinence and safer sex to reduce teenage pregnancy and HIV infection. Announcements of HIV status by celebrities such as Magic Johnson and Arthur Ashe also affect group norms on a wide scale.

Peer support is critical to *maintaining* health-positive behaviors. For example, studies have shown that gay men are more likely to "relapse" into risky behavior when they perceive that peer support for safer behavior is minimal.[74] Continued support from sexual partners also is essential.[75] School-based programs promoting positive social norms may require "booster shots" in the form of follow-up sessions in successive years.[76]

Perceptions of social norms, especially among adolescents, are as influential on behavior as actual norms.[77] For example, one study revealed that teens who perceived that their peers were using condoms were five times more likely to do so themselves.[78] The impact of perceived norms appears to be even more marked among high-risk youth.[79] Teens often have distorted notions of what is acceptable and prevalent among their peers, based on others' exaggerations about sexual exploits and their own lack of experience and knowledge.

The implications of this concept for sexuality and HIV education are twofold: (1) communities, parents, and schools should coordinate efforts to introduce and support health-positive norms; and (2) educators should use learning activities to help learners, especially adolescents, align perceived norms—that is, "everyone is doing it"—with reality.

Skills

The last key concept common to proven learning theories is *skills*—the ability to act on knowledge and beliefs, to apply information relevant to particular situations, and to utilize social support. Several categories of skills are necessary to healthy sexuality and relationships:

- *Interpersonal:* Communication (discussing, sharing, listening, and expressing feelings, needs, values, and beliefs), problem solving, negotiating, setting limits, self-protection (from assault or abuse), and parenting skills.
- *Intrapersonal:* Values clarification, self-esteem, analyzing situations, decision-making, "self-talk" (see Chapter 11).
- *Resource-related:* Locating information, reading, knowing, and using community resources including clinics and other health care providers, counselors, clergy, teachers, and other school staff.
- *Technology-related:* Using prophylaxis (condom, contraceptive pill, diaphragm), personal hygiene products, and other health-related technology.

Many learners lack essential skills for dealing with potential sexual risks or relationship issues. One study found, for example, that approximately 40 percent of heterosexuals were unable to communicate about safer sex behaviors with a potential sexual partner.[80] Communication abilities in adolescent couples also influence whether or how well they use contraception.[81]

Skill development requires that learners first observe and then practice a skill many times. Many educators are unwilling or unable to commit the time necessary for skill development in sexuality and HIV education, are uncomfortable facilitating role play or other such skill-building methods, or are restricted from using such methods. However, the payoff in terms of meaningful and useful student learning is well worth the investment. Several curricula provide excellent skill-building activities, including those listed in Appendix E; also see Chapter 11 for a review of behavioral methods and description of specific activities.

BEHAVIOR CHANGE THEORY

Sexual behavior is probably the most intensely private domain in our society. Therefore, sexuality and HIV educators must operate on an assumption that learners will make their own sensible and satisfying decisions about all areas of sexuality (1) if they have access to information they can understand, (2) if they have access to appropriate services, (3) if their specific sexual values are taken seriously by those assisting the decision-making process, and (4) if they have the self-efficacy, motivation, and skills needed to act upon their decisions.

This *learner-centered* approach underlies effective sexuality education; it also is reflected in the Transtheoretical Model (TTM) of change developed by Prochaska, DiClemente, and others.[82–85] Although many behavior change models exist, we focus on TTM because interventions based on this model have been thoroughly researched and shown to be effective in several behavioral areas: drug and alcohol abuse, weight loss, smoking cessation, and, most recently, HIV risk taking.[86] Interventions based on TTM generally have been used for one-on-one counseling and education; however, the model also is applicable to group education because of several key concepts shared with social learning theory: *personalization, suscepti-bility, efficacy, self-efficacy, social norms,* and *skills.*

Visualize for a moment how a counselor or adviser usually thinks about someone who "needs" to make a behavior change. They might recommend to the client a list of logical, linear steps needed to reach a goal, whether it be losing twenty pounds, stopping smoking, or practicing risk-free sex. Unfortunately, typical human behavior is rarely so logical or linear: most individuals don't follow all prescribed steps in order, or they stop before reaching the goal, or they relapse into former behaviors. Or some people may never act; having skills doesn't necessarily mean one will use them or change behavior. In all these cases, individuals may be left with a perception of total failure—an "all or nothing" approach.

The TTM model hypothesizes that behavior change happens in a cycle or spiral of stages or steps leading to a specific goal or endpoint, whether it involves adopting a positive behavior (e.g., using birth control) or stopping a risky one (e.g., not engaging in acts that risk HIV infection). Many people who want or need to change do not reach their goal on the first attempt, but must go through the cycle a number of times before the behavior change becomes permanent.

TTM also recognizes that individuals begin such a process with different prior experiences, levels of personalization, motivations, self-efficacy, learning styles, and feelings of ambivalence. People assisting the change process, therefore, must identify interventions that will work with the individual in their current stage and then help him or her take incremental steps toward the goal.

TTM outlines five stages of change: *precontemplation, contemplation, prepara-tion, action,* and *maintenance.* Each person who needs to make a behavior change must move successfully through all five stages, no matter how briefly. At each stage, the individual displays characteristic attitudes and requires stage-appropriate intervention methods by the educator.

Precontemplation. In this stage, the learner may be surprised or resistant to hearing that a particular behavior is a problem, likely has no intention of changing in the near future, may be unable even to imagine changing, or may feel hopeless about his/her ability to make change. The impetus for change comes not from the individual, but from others. The educator's task with learners in this stage is to increase understanding—to raise consciousness—of risks and problems associated with the current behavior (personalization and susceptibility) by using disequilibrating methods (e.g., peer education, simulations, real-life homework, probability analysis exercises, etc.) and to give relevant information.

Contemplation. The learner becomes aware that a problem exists; s/he seriously considers change and is beginning to be receptive to feedback and information. At this point, the learner is still thinking, not doing, and exhibits a high level of ambivalence regarding change. S/he is typically indecisive, unable to appraise the pros and cons of change realistically. The educator's challenges with individuals in this stage are (1) to help learners become aware of and express feelings about their risks and their self-image, and (2) to utilize activities to tip the pro/con balance in a direction favorable to change. Use values clarification exercises and introspective methods (such as focus writing, journal writing, anonymous questionnaires, case studies, etc.) to increase awareness of feelings and understanding of self during change. Use discussion and small group methods (e.g., analysis of information) to reveal to the individual the positive reasons to change along with the risks of not changing. Also, strengthen self-efficacy by giving positive feedback and referrals to resources (e.g., counseling).

Preparation. In this stage, intention begins to affect behavior. The learner sees that personal change is possible and begins taking some steps to make it happen. S/he feels "ready for action." The educator should work to increase the learner's faith in the efficacy of the behavior or product (i.e., condoms) and to improve skills in using it. Extensive practice methods (with positive feedback for use of skills) such as role play, rehearsal, and self-talk are valuable. Use "real-life" methods, such as visits to clinics, or volunteering for a group providing support to people living with HIV. Help learners develop a change plan that is self-generated, limits obstacles, won't make the situation worse, and will work. Use introspective methods (e.g., journal writing), self-tests, and other methods to help learners clarify values, examine their own commitment, and implement plans.

Action. During this stage, the individual is actively carrying out change, for example, using condoms during each sexual interaction for at least six months. The educator's task now is to support the person in taking small steps toward the goal and to reinforce *self-efficacy.* Make sure the learner has information about resources—clinics, counselors, telephone "hotlines," and the like. Endorse appropriate *social norms* (e.g., with peer education) and help learners identify and develop their sources of social support.

Maintenance. The individual in this stage is sustaining a change and avoiding relapse when confronted with "triggers." The educator's task is to help the learner recognize these triggers and practice *skills* for resisting a return to former behaviors. Also continue to reinforce appropriate *social norms* and provide positive feedback for positive behaviors.

Educators will recognize various stages of change among any group of learners, reflected in individual attitudes about behaviors; however, it usually is not feasible to identify or teach to each learner's current stage. Even if the individuals' stages are recognizable, sexuality educators cannot guide learners through all stages, from precontemplation to maintenance, with typically short-term learning experiences. But they can, by following the principles of effective sexuality education and utilizing a wide variety of methods, help all learners take some steps toward a positive goal; in this way, educators can be catalysts for change.

FUTURE DIRECTIONS: A FIFTH GENERATION OF SEXUALITY EDUCATION PROGRAMS?

Historically, sexuality education has been *reactive* to identified social problems, that is, narrowly focused on prevention of negative sexual consequences such as unintended pregnancy, HIV, STDs, substance abuse, and sexual abuse or exploitation.

Comprehensive, positive, *proactive* sexuality education, by contrast, addresses all needs of the developing sexual person: learning about love, desire, intimacy, friendship, and commitment; enhancing self-esteem; improving relationship skills (beyond those for prophylaxis only); clarifying one's values; examining gender roles and stereotypes; recognizing and appreciating diversity; developing skills in life planning, problem solving, parenting, and healthy living; becoming a critical consumer of media messages; exploring spiritual aspects of sexuality; and achieving personal success and happiness, within or without a sexual relationship.

The existing body of research and theory on teaching and learning about sexuality gives educators some clues for designing effective, proactive programs. While social learning theory recently has provided a valuable theoretical framework for programs to affect specific learner behaviors, it does not speak to the broader and equally important objectives of comprehensive sexuality education. Other theories—Piagetian and TTM, for example—provide some useful guiding principles as well.

Our hope is that the practice of sexuality education soon will evolve to a new level that integrates many diverse theory- and research-based approaches for teaching to all domains and all perspectives of comprehensive sexuality education.

CHAPTER 5

Meeting Special Challenges in Sexuality Education

> My most challenging experience as a sexuality educator was when a parent accused me of "raping" his son because I had shown the class a film on puberty.[1]

> I felt betrayed in a public meeting when my principal didn't stick up for me and the sexuality education program—I knew she would have for any other school program.

> I thought my heart would break when a student, who I suspected was being sexually molested by her father, asked me if I would be her Dad instead.

> A student asked me if I was gay, and I struggled with whether I should answer truthfully or not.

> (Comments from sexuality and HIV educators)

Teaching is a demanding and exhilarating job no matter what the topic. Teaching about sexuality and HIV, however, presents unique problems and rewards even for the experienced classroom teacher or community health educator.

In this chapter, we discuss ten special challenges in teaching about sexuality and HIV. Our list is not all-inclusive; we selected issues that many sexuality educators report as concerns and that we have encountered in our own work. We also suggest strategies for preventing or dealing with problems when they arise.

RESPONDING TO COMMUNITY REACTIONS

By far the biggest concern of community and school sexuality educators is lack of support from their community or administrators. Sexuality educators cite fear of opposition as their single greatest obstacle; they are especially concerned about organized opposition and lack of preventive action by supporters.[2] One survey found that one in four teachers believed parents do not support sexuality education, one in three thought their principals were nervous about possible controversy, and one in five believed their administrators would not support them.[3] These perceptions persist despite consistent evidence of widespread community support (see Chapter 1) and stated support by administrators.[4]

Historically, educators have allowed a vocal minority to have an inordinate say in the development of sexuality education programs, resulting in a general "chilling effect" on program scope and effectiveness.[5] In recent years, organized opposition to sexuality and HIV education has become increasingly sophisticated, well financed and politically powerful, effectively gutting or eliminating many successful programs across the country.[6, 7]

In Chapter 1 we mentioned the Denmark, South Carolina, community that experienced a 50 percent reduction in teenage pregnancies after implementing a community-wide, collaborative program. Several years into the program, when significant opposition to the school curriculum and the provision of contraceptive services to students led to termination of the Teen Life Center's contraceptive services, pregnancy rates returned almost to their preprogram rates.[8] In Alabama, several "pro-family" groups mounted a successful campaign to remove all ten of the state's health textbooks from the approved list, leaving the state with no text for HIV/AIDS education.[9] In another community, organized opposition led to the removal of a K–3 sexuality education curriculum because it *named the genitals.*[10]

Key national groups that oppose school-based comprehensive sexuality education include the American Center for Law and Justice, the Christian Coalition, Focus on the Family, Citizens for Excellence in Education, Concerned Women of America, Traditional Values Coalition, and the Eagle Forum, to name just a few. Tactics often used by such groups include distributing misinformation about sexuality/HIV education programs, appealing to emotionalism, making false accusations, intimidating school board members and teachers, and busing members to school board meetings outside their own district to challenge programs.

To keep opposition in perspective and reinforce and capitalize on existing community support for your program, educators can be proactive by using three key strategies: *prevention, defusion,* and *self-care.*[11]

Preventing Problems in the First Place

The first key to developing and maintaining community support for successful sexuality or HIV education programs is *prevention* of opposition. Many problems can be preempted by establishing an advisory committee that reflects many community constituencies: parents, health services representatives, business people, clergy, elected officials, informal leaders, teachers, administrators, and students.

Most importantly, identify your allies, be sure a few are included on the advisory committee, and work to build a network of support before problems develop. Parents of school-aged children represent, on the average, only 30 percent of the adults nationwide;[12] therefore, educators need to draw upon a larger base of support by involving concerned community members who are not parents. Include representatives of any groups from which you anticipate active opposition, so that their concerns are addressed from inside rather than outside the process. These individuals should be few in number, capable of rational dialogue and collaboration, and unlikely to engage in obstructionism. In any case, the committee's decision-making process should be majority vote, not consensus, since the latter is often difficult to achieve in such circumstances.

Other practical strategies for establishing a successful program are listed in the box. Several useful resource guides for creating and maintaining programs are available through *SIECUS* (listed in Appendix C).

Guidelines for Starting a Successful Program

- Engage in broad-based planning involving parents and representing many points of view.
- Establish a small advisory committee.
- Develop a statement of shared values for sexuality/HIV education.
- Adopt realistic goals.
- Be willing to compromise, but within limits.
- Provide training for teachers, administrators, and school board members.
- Have a student excusal option for parents who do not want their children to attend.
- Know the opposition and their concerns.
- Be politically active.

(SOURCE: Peter Scales and Martha R. Roper, "Challenges to Sexuality Education in the Schools," in *The Sexuality Education Challenge: Promoting Health Sexuality in Young People* [Santa Cruz, Calif.: ETR Associates, 1994], 69–90.)

Defusing Problems When They Occur

Even supporters occasionally have concerns about specific aspects of a sexuality or HIV program; if unaddressed, these concerns can undermine a program. Thus, communication with parents and the advisory committee must be kept open once a program is up and running. When a question or concern is raised, follow the same guidelines you would use for handling parental or community complaints about any other topic (see box). Your standard approach should not be altered because of the subject matter; nor should whole programs be abandoned or substantially changed because of the concerns of one or a handful of parents.

Dealing with One-on-One Confrontations

When confronted by individuals opposed to your school or clinic program, follow these basic rules:

Rule 1. Be pleasant. Be firm. Stay focused. Don't get sidetracked or emotional yourself, even if they are being emotional or irrational. Stay neutral.

Rule 2. Acknowledge their concerns. Let them know you hear them and that you respect their right to comment on the program.

Rule 3. Remember the true facts about the program or topic. (They may have been given false information, so give them facts and then ask them what they think.)

Rule 4. If they make outrageous statements, repeat them so they hear how they sound: (e.g., "You're asking me why I should care that people are dying of AIDS?")

Rule 5. Remind them that ALL children or clients are deserving of dignity and respect and a safe school or clinic environment.

If in a public school setting:

Rule 6. Remind them that you are a *public school educator* with a responsibility to serve ALL children, not just their children, and

Rule 7. That the mission of *public education* is to teach children how to live peacefully in an increasingly diverse society.

Rule 8. Let them know that, although they may hold an opinion different from yours or from the school/clinic, public policy must reflect universal values, not your or their personal beliefs.

(SOURCE: Adapted by Katie Meyer and Deanne Larsell from a handout, "How to Deal with the Opposition," by Virginia Uribe.)

Responding to parents of students in your program is quite different from dealing with a group without the same legitimacy. Often the most dedicated opponents of sexuality education programs have no school-aged children, or none enrolled in the targeted school. One sexuality educator told us about a small group of parents who successfully undermined her program even though their own children were being home-schooled!

Long lived, successful programs can be threatened when an existing curriculum comes up for review, providing opportunities for the opposition to mount new challenges. This scenario occurred in the 1980s in many school districts around the country when HIV/AIDS components were added to existing sexuality education curricula.

In the 1970s, many excellent sexuality education programs succumbed to attacks by organized groups, in part because administrators were unaccustomed to dealing with opponents' strident, sometimes threatening tactics. Today, many educators are standing their ground in defense of health education programs, emboldened by legislative mandates and a compelling interest in providing sexuality education as the only means of preventing AIDS.

A charge often leveled against sexuality education is that it promotes "secular humanism." Opponents use this diversionary tactic to put teachers and administrators on the defensive, by suggesting they are engaging in "religious instruction" that violates the separation of church and state, or that they are "anti-Christian." Information about secular humanism in the following box can help you respond to this unfounded allegation.

A Few Words about "Secular Humanism"

The most vocal and dedicated opponents of sexuality education are religious fundamentalists who believe that sexuality educators are promoting "secular humanism" in schools. Indeed, some of the most effective teaching methods used by sexuality educators, such as role play and values clarification activities, are defined as hallmarks of "humanistic education." However, neither sexuality educators nor opponents are generally aware of the philosophical foundation of such methods or their remote relationship to the humanist movement.

In essence, humanism refers to a faith in the ability of humans to solve their own problems, with or without divine guidance. A "humanist" is defined as an individual who has a "strong interest in or concern for human welfare, values and dignity."[13] The humanist movement emerged during the Renaissance, largely in response to centuries of dogmatic thinking and corruption of church leaders who had restricted religious, political, and social discourse during the Middle Ages. This philosophical shift facilitated modern scientific and cultural progress and was reflected in both religious and secular domains.

Humanistic educational philosophy is a modern development with only distant ties to the broader humanism movement in that it acknowledges the conscious role of the individual in human learning. Representing one of the three major schools of thought in psychology and education, humanistic philosophy asserts that humans learn not exclusively as the result of either environmental (Skinner) or biological (Freud) factors but by virtue of their own conscious mediation of the two. The role of divine guidance in human activities is neither addressed nor dismissed by humanistic educational philosophy.

Therefore, humanistically oriented teachers assume that learners make choices about their behaviors based not only on their beliefs but also on their ability to *reason*. This assumption forms the foundation of health education, but threatens some individuals who feel that both children and adults should accept without question the teachings of religious or other authority figures (i.e., parents). To such opponents, the true evil of humanistic education lies not in its content but in its facilitation of "inquiry, analysis, skepticism, judgement and dissent."[14]

Sexuality education is not the only topic area vulnerable to charges of promoting "secular" humanism; social studies, biology, and any other topics in which humanistic methods are used and critical thinking fostered also are subject to such criticism. However, sexuality education classes are often targeted both because of the use of humanistic teaching methods and the controversial nature of the topic.

Educators and opponents alike often overreact to charges of "secular humanism" because neither group generally recognizes its true meaning. Humanism simply refers to a respect for human dignity and the worthiness of addressing human problems. As a broad philosophy, it thrives in almost all religious and secular settings of the modern world.

Courts have ruled consistently in favor of public school-based sexuality education, refusing to support charges that sexuality education violates religious freedom, equal protection under the law, the right to privacy, or parental rights. Furthermore, they have ruled that teaching about sexuality and HIV is a justifiable public health measure. The Supreme Court, among others, has upheld the public school's right to inculcate community values, select teaching materials, and require student attendance at sexuality education classes (even without an excusal option).[15] As one judicial opinion stated, "If the course is necessary to the education of one child, it is equally necessary to the education of all students."[16]

Self-Care in Crisis Situations

Becoming embroiled in a long-term, impassioned conflict with individuals or organized groups can take a toll on an educator already doing stressful work. If this happens to you, both your physical and psychological health necessitate that you keep matters in perspective and not get overwhelmed.

Self-care strategies include typical stress management techniques—good nutrition, rest, exercise, or whatever else reduces stress for you. Conferring with fellow sexuality educators and taking time out from the conflict can help. Most importantly, remove yourself from center stage whenever possible, calling upon others (administrators, colleagues, supportive parents, and clergy) to advocate for the program in your place.

In summary, developing and maintaining community support for sexuality education programs means following these basic guidelines: start slow, involve the community, keep communications open, don't overreact to challenges, activate those who support you, and take the long-term view. Compromise may be required in order to initiate a program or keep it; being too rigid or far-reaching can make your program more vulnerable to challenges.

If significant opposition does develop, keep matters in perspective. Remember that the opposition represents a small minority, even if they are louder than most. Their wishes should not overrule the right of the majority to have their children receive comprehensive and *effective* sexuality education. The majority, however, needs correct information about the true nature of sexuality education; otherwise, they are easily persuaded by the specious arguments of opponents. Both SIECUS and the Planned Parenthood Federation of America have developed "Action Kits" to assist individuals responsible for developing and maintaining community support for sexuality education programs (see Appendix C for contact information).

DEALING WITH YOUR OWN DISCOMFORT

Educator comfort with sexuality is a critical factor in the success of a sexuality education class or workshop (see Chapter 3). Comfort level affects the decision to teach the subject at all and which topics will be included.[17] Educator comfort fosters learner comfort, which in turn facilitates learning about sexuality.

In 1984, two researchers, Cheryl Graham and Margaret Smith,[18] asked thirty-two experienced sexuality educators to describe comfort with sexuality, based on their own observations with learners. From the responses, Graham and Smith developed a portrait of a "comfortable" sexuality educator (see box).

Evidence of Sexuality Comfort in Sexuality Educators

Sexuality educators who are comfortable with sexuality . . .	Example of Behavioral Expression
• Feel satisfaction with and pride in their own sexuality.	React confidently to matters involving biological or physical aspects of their sexual natures.
• Feel secure about their own sexual natures.	Respond openly and confidently when their sexual values are challenged.
• Communicate effectively about sexuality.	Use sexual vocabulary that is appropriate to the situation, in well-articulated thoughts.
• Express respect and tolerance for others' sexual values.	Challenge individuals who express enmity toward divergent sexualities.
• Are sensitive to and respectful of others' feelings and anxieties.	Support students who have difficulty using sexual vocabulary.
• Encourage others to explore sexual issues and their own sexual values.	Use values clarification exercises.
• Make opportunity for experiences that enhance their own sexuality comfort.	Confront sexual problems as they occur and mobilize resources to deal with them.
• Are concerned about how they influence others.	Seek evaluative feedback from students.
• Are confident in their teaching skills and knowledge about sexuality.	Appear poised in the classroom.
• Use methods that are effective in teaching sexuality.	Roleplay, sociodrama.
• Are discreet.	Use humor in appropriate situations.
• Acknowledge that sexuality is an important topic to people and is therefore a legitimate topic for intellectual inquiry.	Actively support school sexuality education programs.

(SOURCE: Cheryl A. Graham and Margaret M. Smith, "Operationalizing the Concept of Sexuality Comfort: Applications for Sexuality Educators," *Journal of School Health*, Volume 54, Number 10 [December 1984], 440. Reprinted with permission. American School Health Association, Kent, Ohio.)

Evonne's research using the Graham and Smith definition has delineated two kinds of comfort with sexuality:

- *General Sexuality Comfort* (GSC): having a positive view of sexuality in general, being tolerant of the sexual beliefs and life-styles of others (even if they are different from your own) and being supportive of sexuality education.
- *Personal Sexuality Comfort* (PSC): feeling satisfied with your own sexuality, moral standards, and behaviors and being open with peers about your sexuality and experiences.[19]

Interestingly, one's *general* comfort with sexuality does not necessarily overlap with one's *personal* comfort: a person can be generally comfortable with sexuality as a topic, or feel accepting about other individuals' choices or life-styles, but not feel at peace or resolved about his or her own sexuality. This finding contradicts assumptions by both professional and lay persons that effective sexuality educators are likely contented with their own sexuality and life-style.

Graham and Smith have outlined some specific actions educators can take to improve their own sexuality comfort (see box). We encourage you to seek out learning opportunities that enhance your teaching skills in sexuality education and increase your comfort level.

Sexuality Comfort as a Developmental Task

Experiences that improve sexuality comfort are those that . . .	Example
• Improve self-understanding.	Analysis of one's own sexual values; counseling.
• Desensitize.	Teaching experience; verbal satiation.
• Improve understanding/tolerance of divergent sexualities.	Discussion groups with peers; reading.
• Improve communication skills.	Practice group process; analyze communication competencies.
• Improve teaching competencies.	Learn new teaching strategies; improve (through practice) skill with "tried and true" strategies.
• Increase one's knowledge base about sexuality.	Reading; conferences; other educational experiences.
• Involve exposure to a role model of sexuality comfort.	Take college coursework or in-service training from an experienced sexuality educator.

(SOURCE: Cheryl A. Graham and Margaret M. Smith, "Operationalizing the Concept of Sexuality Comfort: Applications for Sexuality Educators," *Journal of School Health*, Volume 54, Number 10 [December 1984], 440. Reprinted with permission. American School Health Association, Kent, Ohio.)

What does semen taste like?

Why do some people rape other people?

How do people get to be fags?

Don't you agree that abortion is murder?

If you have ever fielded questions like these (see box also), then you know how disconcerting the job of teaching about sexuality and HIV can be. All of us receive questions that may throw us off balance or have us puzzling over the best response.

Actual Questions Posed to Sexuality Educators

- You know your private parts? Sometimes it gets stiff. (Male, age 9)
- How is a boy raped? (Male, age 6)
- When is it OK for an adult to touch me? (Female, age 7)
- But, my mom told me babies come from bellies! (Age 10)
- Why do men like to suck women's breasts? (Age 10)
- What if it (sexual abuse) feels good? (Female, age 13)
- How tough is that hymen thing? (Female, age 13)
- Is it true that when you have sex with a girl on cocaine you get a big knot in your penis? (Male, age 14)
- If you can get HIV from blood, why couldn't a mosquito give it to you?
- Shouldn't all people with AIDS be put on an island somewhere? (Female, age 15)
- Why does it feel so good when you ejaculate? (Male, age 16)
- I don't have any desire for sex. Is there something wrong with me? (Age 16)
- Have you ever had anal sex? Did you like it?
- Should I tell my partner I have herpes? (Age 16)
- My partner wants me to have oral sex and I don't want to. What should I do? (Female, age 30)
- Can you guarantee I won't get AIDS if I do first aid on a bleeding victim? (Adult)

(Source: Recollections of sexuality educators at the Northwest Institute for Community Health Educators, North Bend, Washington, August 1993.)

Learners want and need information about sexuality: they may have heard a rumor or a word and not understand; they may think they are the only ones who don't know something; they want reassurance about their own normalcy; and they are bewildered and confused by what they see in the popular media. They also may be curious about what you, the teacher, think, and are fascinated by the questions their peers ask. They may feel more comfortable asking their questions when they are assured of anonymity.

Questions posed in sexuality classes can be troublesome to educators for various reasons:

- You may not know enough about the topic and worry about giving misinformation or omitting essential information.
- You may be unfamiliar or uncomfortable with slang used or the *content* of the question (e.g., certain sexual behaviors).
- The student may be seeking information about your values and personal experiences that is inappropriate to share.
- The question may be intended to shock rather than be a sincere inquiry.
- The question may be of interest to the asker but developmentally or experientially inappropriate for the rest of the class.
- There may be a "question behind the question" that also needs to be addressed (see box for example).

Hearing the Question behind the Question

Evonne was observing a seventh-grade teacher giving a required unit on AIDS when a male student, known for being disruptive, raised his hand to ask the teacher a question.

"Hey, Mr. Roberts,* can you get AIDS from yourself?" The teacher dismissed the question, saying AIDS is a serious subject that deserves serious questions.

A few minutes later the boy posed his question again, albeit more tentatively. "Mr. Roberts, can a person get AIDS—uh—if he's *alone?*" This time the boy got a warning from the teacher that if he didn't behave, he would spend the rest of the period in the principal's office.

The boy looked discouraged, but raised his hand a third time anyway. This time he blurted out, "Can—can a person get AIDS *having sex with himself?!*" To my utter amazement, the teacher missed the question behind the question again, silencing the young man and banishing him to a corner of the room for the remainder of class.

The student apparently did not know the correct language with which to frame his question, but I'm certain he was worried he could get AIDS from masturbating.

*Not the teacher's real name.

Learner questions often seem straightforward, but in fact may have a variety of meanings.[20] Children's questions, in particular, are sometimes difficult to interpret because different children use the same words to communicate different meanings. Adults often attribute more significance to a question than is warranted. A humorous example of the latter is the father whose young son asked him to "explain to him about babies." Having anticipated this question for some time, the father offered a brief but fairly explicit explanation of the mechanics of conception—only to discover that all his son wanted to know was why "babies' heads flop over on their necks!"

Possible Motivations behind Children's Questions about AIDS

Information-seeking and general curiosity:
   What is AIDS? Why do people get AIDS?
Anxiety for one's own welfare:
   How do people get AIDS? Could I get AIDS?
Anxiety for the welfare of one's family:
   Will my mother get AIDS? Do all grown-ups know how to keep from getting AIDS?
Solution seeking (not unusual for children ages 7 or 8):
   Can we give someone with AIDS new blood to make them healthy again?
Exploring values, beliefs, and attitudes:
   Are people who get AIDS bad?
Seeking reactions from adults ("shock-value" questions):
   Don't queers deserve AIDS?

(SOURCE: Adapted from M. Quackenbush and S. Villarreal, *"Does AIDS Hurt?" Educating Young Children About AIDS* [Santa Cruz, Calif.: ETR Associates, 1988].)

Children's questions also vary depending on gender and developmental age. A 1987 study examined differences in questioning behavior among seventh, eighth, and tenth grade boys and girls and found that younger students had more questions about biology, intercourse, and clarification of slang terms, while older students were more interested in learning about birth control, health risks, and communication. Also, boys in general were more curious about slang and intercourse while girls were more interested in communication, relationships, and health risks.[21]

When students seek your personal opinion on a controversial, value-laden subject such as abortion, you may be tempted to share your view, especially if you feel strongly about the issue. However, avoid doing so. Revealing your own opinions with learners risks alienating those who do not agree with you or may unintentionally condemn someone's behavior. Students distanced from you in this way may be less likely to consider you a credible source of information.

In some circumstances, sharing your personal views may be appropriate, for example, with mature, responsible students outside of the session. However, if you are a public educator, your charge is to illuminate the range of values that exist in the community and to assist students in examining their own values, not to express your own philosophy unless it reflects a universal value. (See Chapter 9 for more guidelines for answering sexuality questions, especially those with a value component.)

When presented with a question that catches you off guard, try to maintain an external demeanor that does not expose your true feelings, for example, surprise, confusion, disapproval, or embarrassment. Try to react to challenging questions with the same straightforward, even tone you would use with the easier ones.

Also note the body language of the questioner. For example, the student in Mr. Roberts's class (see previous box) was red faced and squirming in his chair while asking what was assumed to be a frivolous question. Had Mr. Roberts been more observant, he might have ascertained that the boy's inquiry was sincere.

Answering student questions can be challenging when the group's knowledge varies widely—for example, a mostly sexually inexperienced group, with a few experienced individuals—and the latter students pose questions that should not be answered in front of the others. In this case, offer to talk with those individuals after class to address their questions more fully.

Soliciting written questions via a "question box" is a time-honored technique of sexuality educators for managing difficult questions (see Chapter 9). This process is less intimidating for learners who are disinclined to ask questions openly; it also gives the educator more time, if needed, to decide how to handle a question. A problematic question can be passed discreetly to the bottom of the stack while you gather your wits. If a student poses a deliberately disrespectful question, use this method to avoid responding at all.

Fielding difficult questions is one of the most challenging aspects of this work; however, practice leads to greater comfort and effectiveness. To improve your skills, practice answering questions (ones listed previously or others particularly troublesome for you) in front of a mirror or with a supportive friend, devising strategies that work best for you. Also review the guidelines provided in Chapter 9 and, for suggested responses to common difficult questions, see Marian Shapiro's "Answering Anonymous Questions in the Sexuality Education Class" in the summer 1995 issue of *Family Life Educator.*

RECOGNIZING LIMITS

Sexuality educators should know the limits of their capabilities and responsibilities and always work within them. Knowledge is one such limiting factor. Because learners typically have so many questions related to sexuality, do not comprehend the expansiveness of the topic, and rarely have the opportunity to talk with an "authority," they frequently pose questions that exceed the educator's expertise— a tendency one author has termed the "sexuality guru" effect. [22]

If you are a community health educator trained in HIV education or another specific subtopic within sexuality education, you may be less capable of answering general questions about sexuality than someone more broadly trained; on the other hand, a classroom teacher may not be able to answer questions about HIV in the same depth as an HIV education specialist, or about contraception as well as a family planning educator.

When presented with questions outside your expertise, admit your limitations, refer the learner elsewhere, offer to provide more information after further research, and/or, if feasible, procure a guest speaker who is knowledgeable on the topic.

Learners who are survivors of traumatic sexual experiences or who are currently experiencing crisis in a relationship occasionally may expect the educator to serve both as teacher and counselor. Likewise, they may treat the group like a therapy group. Such expectations are inappropriate for a setting with educational rather than therapeutic objectives. For instance, a student may approach you after a session to seek advice on a relationship problem, a suspected pregnancy, or concerns about his/her sexual orientation. Or, during a session, a student may become upset over a personal problem and request advice from the group. Or students may ask you directly if you would counsel them on sexual concerns. Each of these situations crosses the line between education and counseling.

Many sexuality and HIV educators join the profession out of a desire to help others; most, however, have not been trained as professional counselors. Furthermore, your job description may define your limits. Consequently, educators should not allow themselves to slip into a counseling role. Clarify your limits and role with such learners, make appropriate referrals, and suggest other resources when needed, while maintaining a supportive relationship; avoid fostering dependency on you as a "counselor."

Any sexuality educator may be asked to act beyond his/her expertise and proper role; community health educators are especially susceptible—in part because they are more likely to be viewed by students as sexuality "experts." Students may ask questions of a visiting health educator they would never raise with their regular classroom teacher. On the other hand, some students may be more likely to confide in their regular teachers by virtue of a long-term and trusting relationship with them.

Legal liability is another limiting factor for many sexuality educators. Most states have laws requiring educators to report any suspected case of sexual abuse, harassment, or assault. You also may be obligated by law to report if a student discloses that s/he is *planning* to assault or has already victimized someone. Even if the specific nature of a student's disclosure is not regulated by current law or policy, you can be required to violate the student's confidence if served with a court-ordered subpoena. These legal constraints on the educator supersede any agreement you made with learners about maintaining personal confidences shared in private or with the group. Discuss this exception to the ground rule about confidentiality during ground-rule setting, so that learners know what to expect.

Other limitations on the sexuality and HIV educator are inherent in differences existing between the educator and learners; some learners prefer that their teacher be the same as they are in gender, race, background, sexual orientation, religious beliefs, or political persuasion. For example, one black teenager advised sexuality education planners, "We don't want to hear sex education from white people."[23]

Matching educator and learner characteristics is desirable but rarely possible; educators most often work solo, with heterogeneous groups. Therefore, sexuality educators should work to enhance their respect for cultural differences and develop skills in relating well to *all* students by deliberately expanding their knowledge of different cultures, by inviting guest speakers who represent diverse personal and cultural perspectives, and by using materials that reflect many different perspectives.

A sexuality or HIV educator's own history may be a limitation or boon to effective teaching of certain topics. An educator who is a survivor of sexual abuse or assault, for example, *may* not be the best person to lead a class on this topic, if doing so provokes unmanageable emotional responses in him or her. On the other hand, if effectiveness is not adversely affected, s/he might be the most credible "witness" on this topic.

SEPARATING PERSONAL VALUES FROM PROFESSIONAL RESPONSIBILITIES

Sexuality education is never "value free," nor should it be. Sexuality and HIV prevention curricula have underlying values, many of which are "universal values" (see Chapter 2). Educators also have their own sets of values that guide their personal and professional lives. However, the educators' values should not interfere with effective teaching about sexuality.

Educator values affect a sexuality education program in a number of ways: the inclusion or exclusion of certain topics from sexuality teaching;[24] the extent to which certain topics are covered; selection of materials; how group issues are handled; and teacher interactions with learners, colleagues, and community members. For instance, educators uncomfortable with or negative toward homosexuality may have a difficult time providing correct and unbiased information about HIV; they may select materials that do not fairly address the perspective of gay, lesbian, or bisexual learners; or they may reveal their personal discomfort by their tone of voice, choice of words, inappropriate use of humor, or body language.

Sexuality educators should be especially careful not to impose their own values on learners. For example, one teacher told us about a colleague who uses the "values continuum" method, intended to reveal a range of student values on an issue, to promote his own views on abortion. This teacher reportedly solicits student comments, but then denigrates any that do not match his own views. Such abuses shut down learning and reduce the educator's credibility.

Expressing one's personal values outside of the classroom also can damage your program. No matter what the controversial topic, your beliefs are bound to conflict with those of some parents or community members; for example, aligning yourself with either "pro-life" or "pro-choice" views when advocating for a sexuality education program is likely to generate concern from one camp or another.

If parents or other community members ask you to reveal your position on certain issues, remind them that, although you certainly have your own views, your job is not to preach your own values to students but to teach an approved curriculum. Consequently, your personal values are not relevant to the discussion. Share instead the universal values addressed in the curriculum or program.

Obviously, you cannot divest yourself of values, nor should you strive to; however, you *can* monitor how your values affect your teaching. As a public servant, your responsibility is to promote universal values and foster tolerance for the philosophical pluralism in our society; a teacher who cannot or will not live up to this expectation should not be in the sexuality education classroom.

Dealing with Disclosure: Theirs and Yours

Handling personal disclosures—students' or your own—is sometimes a challenge in teaching about sexuality. Because sexuality education is personally meaningful and growth producing, learners and teachers alike may want to share personal information or experiences. Sexuality educators deliberately create a learning environment that is conducive to discussing sexual topics; however, we must walk a fine line between facilitating transformative learning experiences and providing therapy to learners (or ourselves). Having a class ground rule discouraging personal disclosures helps to define these boundaries.

Even when guidelines have been established, learners occasionally reveal personal information anyway, in front of the entire group, in small group activities, or in private communication with the teacher. For instance, a learner may disclose as a way of celebrating a decision (e.g., "coming out" as a bisexual), to facilitate healing from a traumatic experience (e.g., surviving a sexual assault), to challenge a perceived majority view in the group (e.g., being pro-life or pro-choice), or to seek group or teacher approval (e.g., for breaking off a relationship).

Once a disclosure is made, regardless of the motivation, the individual may feel embarrassed, vulnerable, or at risk of censure by the group or educator; others may feel uncomfortable as well. In any case, thank the individual for trusting the group with the information, return to the topic as soon as feasible (to discourage more sharing), and, if appropriate, offer to speak with the student after class. If it becomes necessary, remind students of the ground rule regarding disclosures.

As noted in a preceding section, some disclosures require follow-up, for example, regarding sexual abuse or harassment. Even if no policy exists, if you suspect that a student has been sexually victimized or is at risk of hurting someone or him/herself, consult with the school counselor or administrator about the appropriate course of action; be sure to document what action you take. Check with your local organization, school, state attorney general, or state office of education regarding laws and policies dictating the handling of such cases.

An Inadvertent Disclosure

I was visiting a class of fifth graders, answering their questions on sexual anatomy and physiology. One girl, taller and more physically mature than others in the class, was especially curious and energetic in her participation.

At first, she excitedly fired off one question after another, demonstrating knowledge beyond that of her peers. But as she began to comprehend some implications of what she was hearing that day, she appeared troubled.

Finally, she raised her hand one more time and asked, slowly and somberly, "Is it true . . . is it *true* that you can't get pregnant by having sex with your Dad?"

"No," I said. "It is *not* true."

She fell quiet, remaining so for the rest of the session. After class, I approached

the teacher to discuss the possibility the girl was being sexually abused by her father.
(Source: Evonne, 1994.)

If and when teacher disclosures are appropriate is the subject of ongoing, lively debate among sexuality educators. Some believe such personal sharing demonstrates that we, like learners, have had formative life experiences, which enhances our credibility; others feel it is inappropriate.

The AIDS educator who reveals that s/he is HIV-positive, for instance, indeed may increase the educative impact on the audience. Similarly, some gay or lesbian educators believe that "coming out" to learners provides much-needed positive role models for gay, lesbian, and bisexual learners. Many heterosexual educators talk openly about their relationships and children, yet do not consider this to be "disclosure"; to many lesbian or gay educators, who do not feel equally welcome to divulge such personal information, it is.

Clearly, some learners appreciate such revelations by the educator; others, however, may feel uncomfortable with the information. Also, you should weigh other potential risks: loss of credibility and goodwill with learners; decreased effectiveness; public gossip, censure, or stereotyping; misrepresentation outside of class or even attacks; and, finally, job restriction or loss.

Guidelines for Making Disclosures

Before sharing personal information or opinions with learners, consider the following:
- Is it *necessary* for me to make this disclosure?
- Is my disclosure appropriate in this particular group, for example, at the developmental level of learners?
- Will the disclosure enhance or detract from my effectiveness with this group? How will it effect my credibility, my interactions with certain students, and the general trust and comfort level in the group?
- Is my timing appropriate, that is, is it too early, inhibiting discussion, or too late, appearing to summarize?

In the following box, colleague Wayne Pawlowski relates how he answers the question, "Are you gay?" All sexuality educators can use this method to help learners assess their attitudes and feelings about sexual orientation. Students should be reminded how prejudice colors one's perceptions of a speaker and encouraged to separate the message from the messenger. The easiest course for a heterosexual teacher may be to say, "No, I'm not gay" (not risking being misperceived) but a teachable moment will be lost.

In the final analysis, personal disclosures regarding sexual issues, whether by a learner or the educator, always present a certain risk. Deciding how best to handle disclosures in the sexuality or HIV classroom will continue to be a dilemma for educators.

Classroom Teachers and Community Health Educators: Effective Collaboration

Classroom teachers of sexuality and HIV education frequently invite guest speakers to supplement the curricula or provide expertise they lack. Some schools, in fact, depend heavily on community health educators (e.g., from the local health department or Planned Parenthood) to provide the *only* sexuality education their students will receive that year.[25] These collaborations between classroom teachers and community health educators provide wonderful opportunities for enhancing sexuality education but also have some potential snags.

When the relationship works well, students benefit from having *two* teachers of sexuality and HIV education who complement and reinforce each other's messages. However, when the two miscommunicate or either party fails to meet expectations, the result can be a less effective program. Such failures also undermine the relationship between the school and the community organization, reducing the likelihood of future collaboration.

Community health educators have many "horror stories" about classroom visits that went awry because of teachers who did not provide proper support or even undermined their presentation (see first box). Likewise, some classroom teachers report having been disappointed or subjected to angry administrators or parents because of the inappropriateness or policy violations of a community educator's presentation (see second box). School requests occasionally offend community agency policies as well, as when schools request an HIV-positive speaker, but insist that the person be heterosexual.

"At the last minute, the teacher told me that another class would be joining us. I had brought handouts and planned activities for only half the number of students I ended up working with."

"The whole time I was presenting, the teacher was in the back of the room flipping noisily through a newspaper, obviously uninterested in what I had to say. I got the feeling I was substituting for the day."

"My sponsoring teacher left the room altogether while I was presenting. While he was gone, one student fainted and I was the only one in the room who did not know that her problem was drug related."

"While I was talking with the class, the classroom teacher kept interrupting and contradicting me."

"A group of students was disrupting the class and throwing things; the teacher did nothing to assist me, and eventually left the room!"

"I was invited to speak on a controversial issue, but was not told that parents would be attending and that I had been set up for a debate with people who oppose my agency's program."

"I was quite distressed when the community health educator did not address the topic we had agreed upon, making it difficult for me to follow up after her presentation."

"One visitor from a community organization handed out condoms and literature to students, in violation of our school's policy."

"One guest misrepresented his intention to present both sides of an issue, and then used his visit as an opportunity to 'preach' his own views to the students."

"I was very uncomfortable when, without consulting me, the guest speaker brought anatomically correct displays that I felt were inappropriate for the age level of my students."

The key to working effectively with another educator is the same as for maintaining any productive relationship—good communication. Each party needs to be clear regarding his/her expectations of the other and for the learning experience. The risk of miscommunication increases when students are responsible for inviting the guest (e.g., for a project). Guests should insist on direct contact with the teacher (and vice versa) to verify agreements made via the student.

In Chapter 6, we list specific questions to ask a host or guest to prevent problems.

Maintaining Personal Boundaries and Managing Transference

Freud described *transference* as an unconscious process in which a client "transfers" positive or negative feelings associated with previous relationships (e.g., with parents or other teachers) onto a helping professional. Transference can occur in any relationship in which the client's vulnerability is heightened by relinquishing some control over his or her own circumstances to an authority figure, for example, psychotherapist, doctor, dentist, social worker, judge, or educator. Such feelings may hinder or enhance the client-helper relationship.

A learner who has a difficult relationship with a parent, for example, may unwittingly project feelings of anger, distrust, or fear onto a teacher. Or, a learner may make unconscious associations between the teacher and a previous romantic partner, transferring unwarranted positive feelings or even sexual interest onto the educator.

Most teachers become the object for such unspoken feelings of conflict or attachment to some extent, but the phenomenon is often exaggerated in the sexuality education classroom. Because of the explicit nature of the topic and its personal significance, learners may feel especially vulnerable as they entrust their psychological safety to your care.

Transference also occurs in reverse—*countertransference*—that is, cases in which the educator unconsciously holds positive or negative feelings toward a learner based on experiences with others. In this case, you may have expectations of the learner based more on transference than on the objective experience of that learner; for example, if an irresponsible student reminds you of someone close to you who consistently fails to follow through on commitments, your anger at the student may be unfairly intensified. Or, in an extreme case, an educator may become romantically interested in a learner.

Obviously, transference in the classroom is an important issue; therefore, be aware that transference could be operating in your interactions with students, with either a negative or positive impact. Conscious, *responsible* use of transference can enhance your educative influence on some learners; irresponsible use could be perceived as improper fraternization, "flirting," or even lead to charges of sexual harassment.

Dealing with Stress, Grief, Stigma, and Personal Safety Issues

In sexuality education, positive stress ("eustress") comes from the joy of working with learners in a personally meaningful subject area, from the excitement of observing them learn and grow, from experiencing your own growth, from working with colleagues who stimulate you intellectually and personally, and from realizing the significant impact you have on others' lives (see box).

I became involved in sexuality education as a volunteer when, one day, I was riding the #48 bus and watching a number of teenage girls getting on and off the bus with their babies while headed to school. I stayed on the bus and came directly to Planned Parenthood to offer my services to my community.

(Jo Henderson, Planned Parenthood, Seattle–King County, Washington.)

When I think of all the people who have benefited from my work as a sexuality educator I have to say that I have benefited the most. There just isn't a more exciting field to be in. It's as old as humankind, yet only recently has it been accepted as a serious educational endeavor. I love the topic. I love the people. I love the issues. I can't believe I have all this fun on my job and am paid for it as well.

(Anne Terrell, Educator Director, Planned Parenthood of Tompkins County, New York.)

Negative stresses in sexuality and HIV education come from many sources: dealing with unsupportive colleagues, parents, or administrators; coping with organized opposition; trying to do a good job with inadequate time and materials; and hearing about the mistakes, tragedies, and ongoing struggles of learners. Many educators enter this profession in part because they have experienced sexual or relationship misfortunes themselves, or observed those of others, that are a consequence of sexual ignorance.[26] Sexuality and HIV educators are much more likely to hear the personal stories of learners and to grieve or celebrate with them.

HIV/AIDS educators, in particular, face several ongoing stressors as a daily part of their jobs: the depression and frustration that often accompany teaching about a devastating, likely fatal disease and, in many cases, the accumulated grief of actually losing friends, colleagues, and students.

Dealing with personal and professional stigma is a unique stressor associated with teaching about sexuality and HIV. Some people assume, for example, that anyone who undertakes sexuality education or research must have questionable, perhaps even voyeuristic motives; others suspect that sexuality educators are over-sexed, or endowed with extraordinary sexual prowess, or have a dysfunction for which they are trying to compensate.[27] A few accuse us of subverting "traditional" family values, or being antireligious, or promoting (perhaps even practicing) every behavior about which we teach. Many assume that AIDS educators are HIV-positive or gay; neither assumption should constitute a stigma, but it often does.

At the very least, colleagues and others may consider sexuality education not worthy of professional specialization. One of us, for example, was opposed for a college faculty position by a colleague who felt that her specialty area was not sufficiently "scholarly." Indeed, 32 percent of sexuality educators report that they have experienced occupationally related discrimination, including social ostracism, being the object of crude jokes, and loss of jobs or promotions.[28] Classroom teachers and community health educators who teach about sexuality or HIV as part of a broader subject (such as health education or social studies) are less likely to experience such negative responses; however, for those who specialize in sexuality or HIV education, stigmatization can be a subtle, persistent stressor.

The work of the sexuality educator also provokes intense reactions by some individuals, most positive (e.g., from learners) but some negative. In preceding sections, we described scenarios in which a sexuality or HIV educator could become the focus of irrational anger or obsession by others, for example, a community member adamantly opposed to sexuality education or a student who projects unresolved anger or sexual interest. Most people never go beyond civil disagreement or, in the case of a student, unspoken feelings; however, although it is *extremely rare,* an unstable person could become a threat to your privacy or your safety. We say this not to frighten you, nor to dissuade you from doing this important work; rather we believe that "forewarned is forearmed." Take precautions: avoid compromising situations, such as staying alone with individuals after class or community meetings; after evening sessions, ask someone you trust to escort you to your vehicle; keep your home address and phone number confidential, and install an answering machine to record calls; if you have reason to suspect someone is a threat to your safety, inform your employer and others of your concern, and discuss specific safety procedures in the event of trouble; and if you receive threats, report them and ask a colleague or administrator to serve as a "fair witness" to verify and help you document actions on both sides.

As a general rule, being aware of potential trouble, and taking precautions, will keep you safe and undisturbed as you go about your activities as a sexuality or HIV educator.

TRAINING NEEDS

Most preservice training programs for classroom teachers address neither the content nor the special methodology for teaching about sexuality and HIV.[29, 30] Preservice training programs for community health educators place greater emphasis on sexuality content, but often shortchange methodology. An ideal training program for sexuality educators provides both, preferably in separate courses.[31]

Many (if not most) sexuality educators are self-selected and self-taught as a matter of necessity.[32] Few schools or organizations provide adequate inservice training to their employees. Furthermore, because of the scarcity of appropriate materials for sexuality/HIV education, many educators have to develop their own, a task most are unprepared to handle.[33]

At the same time, information about human sexuality and AIDS is expanding and changing rapidly. New developments about HIV/AIDS, in particular, are almost a daily staple of the media, as changes occur in medical treatments, epidemiological trends, educational practices, and government policies. Likewise, textbooks on human sexuality are revised almost yearly in order to reflect the most current, accurate information.

Keeping up-to-date in this field, therefore, is often a struggle. More often than not, we must create our own "inservice" training programs, consisting of relevant formal education, independent study, "on-the-job" training, networking with colleagues, and professional conferences.

A plethora of professional organizations address specific sexuality topics including sexual abuse, sexual violence, HIV/AIDS, diversity, gender equity, teenage pregnancy, family planning, and education methods, to name just a few. Many hold national, regional, or local conferences, produce relevant journals or teaching materials, or provide training of use to the sexuality or HIV educator.

One professional organization for sexuality educators and trainers is *The American Association of Sex Educators, Counselors and Therapists (AASECT)*, which holds national and regional conferences each year, publishes a quarterly journal *(The Journal of Sex Education and Therapy)*, and offers a rigorous, expensive process for certifying sexuality educators. In our opinion, this organization does a better job addressing the concerns and needs of therapists and counselors than sexuality educators. Other national organizations of interest are the *Sexuality Information and Education Council of the U.S. (SIECUS)*, which serves sexuality educators primarily, and the *Society for the Scientific Study of Sex (SSSS)*, which focuses on sex research. (See Appendix C for a complete list of resource organizations that publish journals, newsletters, or sexuality materials, act as clearinghouses, and provide training.)

Depending on where you are, you may have a local or regional organization of sexuality educators that can meet your immediate needs for networking and information as well as if not better than a national organization. Good examples are the *Association for Sexuality Education and Training (ASSET)* in the Pacific Northwest region and the *Sex Education Coalition of the Metropolitan Washington (D.C.)* area. Many such organizations already exist, but if they are not yet in your area, you may want to help start one.

Professional journals are a valuable resource. The quarterly *Family Life Educator*, for instance, is a good source of teaching activities and abstracts of recent research. (See Appendix C for a list of organizations and their journals.)

From time to time, *SIECUS* or another organization sponsors a special training experience—the *Sexual Attitude Restructuring (SAR)* workshop—to assist sexuality educators in examining and reevaluating his or her own attitudes about sexuality. This several-day, intensive, often residential experience involves viewing a series of sexually explicit films and discussing reactions in ongoing, small groups facilitated by experienced sexuality educators. The *SAR* is a powerful way to increase one's sexuality comfort and change attitudes that may interfere with effective teaching about sexuality.

Other residential training experiences address skills for sexuality, family life, family planning, and HIV educators. The *Northwest Institute for Community Health Educators (NICHE)* is a week-long, residential, skill-based training in sexuality education principles and methods for both classroom and community-based educators. Similar institutes now operate all around the country, including

California (Western Region, or *WRICHE*), the Southwest (*SWICHE*), the Great Lakes region (*GLICHE*), and the North Atlantic region (*NATICHE*). Another residential training for sexuality educators is the *Annual Workshop on Sexuality* (Thornfield conference), held in upstate New York. Sponsoring organizations for these institutes are listed in Appendix C.

Dedicating time to professional development not only addresses gaps in knowledge and expertise, it also helps in revitalizing oneself. Spending quality time with other educators gives you an opportunity to reflect on current practices, gain fresh insights on old problems, and return to the work place with renewed energy and commitment.

Advocating for Sexuality Education

Many educators are content to focus their attention entirely on teaching and not concern themselves too much with school politics, outside forces, or administrators who may or may not support them. Sexuality and HIV educators do not have that luxury; we work in a field in which we must advocate actively and continually for programs, or perhaps lose them.

E. G. Guba has observed that successful educational programs move through three phases of development: (1) *institutional commitment,* in which school districts state their intent and enact policy; (2) *implementation,* in which schools put regulations into practice; and (3) *public reputation,* in which schools monitor and respond to community reactions to their program.[34] Community-based programs are subject to the same principles. Sexuality education programs are vulnerable at any point in the process.

Therefore, sexuality educators must be both vigilant and proactive: keep administrators informed so they can preempt or weather any controversy that might arise; keep communication open with parents and community members; garner support from colleagues and others; stop rumors cold; and work with local media to represent the program in a positive, or at least unbiased, light.

Because of the continuing controversy about the role of schools in sexuality education—mostly from organized, outspoken opposition—sexuality educators cannot be silent about the importance of this work to the health and well-being of learners. We all share a responsibility to educate the public about the true nature and value of comprehensive sexuality education.

PART TWO

SEXUALITY
EDUCATION METHODS

> A good meal, like a poem or a life, has a certain balance and diversity, a certain coherence and fit. As one learns to cope in the kitchen, one no longer duplicates whole meals but rather manipulates components and the way they are put together. The improvised meal will be different from the planned meal, and certainly riskier, but rich with the possibility of delicious surprise.
> —Mary Catherine Bateson, *Composing a Life*

The most effective sexuality educators don't just follow recipes; they know the basic ingredients for good teaching and then adapt or build their own recipes. Besides knowing sexuality content, the skilled sexuality educator knows and can adapt the basic methods. There are certainly plenty of "cookbooks" out there; some of these curricula, sets of strategies, and resource books are very prescriptive, even completely scripted, while others leave a great deal of room for teacher adaptation and utilization of skills. The effective teacher knows how to pull selectively from existing "recipes" and when to leave the recipe behind altogether. S/he knows how to respond to emerging needs of students, how to be flexible, and how to adapt the lesson plan to fit the setting, the group, and the time allotted.

Teaching about Sexuality is not a cookbook. Instead we analyze and describe sexuality education principles and processes with the hope that our readers will be better able to understand and utilize sexuality education strategies and curricula, and indeed develop their own.

Most sexuality education curricula and resource books are made up of a series of content-based lesson plans, strategies, "teaching tools," or activities, each with a purpose or set of objectives. We differentiate between these and *methods* as follows: methods are the basic building blocks of which individual lesson plans are made, for example, teaching procedures such as brainstorming, presentations, role play, reading, and videos. Activities, strategies, and lesson plans are constructed with basic methods, usually rooted in one or more key concepts or messages.

The *SIECUS Guidelines for Comprehensive Sexuality Education,* for instance, describe key concepts and important messages for sexuality education. But simply presenting those messages—telling them to our students—does not mean that learners will internalize them. For example, how can a sexuality educator teach the message "people always have the right to refuse any person's request for any type of sexual behavior"?[1] Teachers could say it, their students might believe it, repeat it back, even understand it on some level. But will they transfer *knowing* to actually using the *skills* to refuse? What teaching methods are most likely to help them *personalize* this message, *believe* it, understand its *importance, believe in their ability* to act on it, and then actually *act* on it when needed? How, when wanting to address a given topic, concept, question, or important message, can educators develop the best process for teaching to that purpose?

In this part of the book we hope to answer those questions by describing, analyzing, and giving examples of methods necessary for accomplishing the goals of effective sexuality and HIV education. We divide methods into learning-domain categories—cognitive, affective, and behavioral—to serve as a reminder to address each domain while teaching. Division by learning domain also facilitates analysis of the unique contributions of certain methods to the teaching of sexuality concepts and the special considerations for using them in this field. To emphasize our belief that no one method, for instance, a lecture, can alone be the means of effectively educating our young people, we begin Part II with considerations for planning and delivering integrated sexuality education lessons.

CHAPTER 6

Planning Sexuality Education Sessions

The challenges of designing effective lessons are different for a workshop leader or community educator who works with a particular group only once (like a host for a dinner), versus the ongoing classroom teacher who works with the same group over a long period (like cooking for a family). The workshop leader, like the host, seeks to provide an offering to the "guests" that will make a favorable impression and stand alone in its quality. The regular teacher, on the other hand, like the family cook, must consider not only the quality of a single day's offering but also how it will be integrated into the overall "diet" of the students. And when the teacher invites an outside speaker (perhaps a community health educator) into the classroom, they must work together to ensure that the guest's content and processes fit into the context of the class.

AFFECTIVE, BEHAVIORAL, AND COGNITIVE METHODS: BUILDING BLOCKS FOR PLANNING SEXUALITY EDUCATION

For the purpose of analysis, definitions, and descriptions, we divide teaching methods for sexuality education into three categories: affective, behavioral, and cognitive. Think of the learning domains as the ABCs of sexuality education:

A. *Affective:* Referring to feelings, attitudes, values—the heart and soul.
B. *Behavioral:* Referring to actions, involving the body (including verbal and nonverbal skills).
C. *Cognitive:* Referring to thinking, or the mind.

Apply the "ABCs" when planning lessons, using "A"ffective methods to help learners get in touch with feelings and values, "B"ehavioral methods to give skills and empower positive action, and "C"ognitive methods to give and gather information.

Affective methods help students focus on their own feelings, values, beliefs, and attitudes; often the goal is to motivate students. Affective methods include discussion, dyads, interviews, fish bowl, case studies, stories, and introspective methods (such as focus writing and guided imagery). We analyze introspective methods in a separate chapter, since they often are used as an introductory exercise.

Behavioral methods are intended to help students develop skills and practice cognitive learning. They include role play and other practice methods, problem solving, simulations, and "real-life" homework. Of course, components of these methods will have an impact in the affective and cognitive domains as well; sexuality educators' intent is not only to increase self-efficacy, but also to increase learners' expectation or belief that they can utilize needed skills.

Cognitive methods give information and help learners examine concepts, facts, and ideas. Cognitive methods include presentations, display of models and objects (e.g., contraceptives), videos, anonymous questions, task groups, reading, research, and so on. However, sometimes these methods have an impact on learners greater than increasing knowledge. For example, an effective presentation captures students' attention, helping them personalize information and perceive relevance for their lives. Occasionally, a very good video is more than a passive method, especially if followed with interactive activities. Also, when students handle displayed contraceptives, they begin to deal with feelings about using them.

Not only is the division among cognitive, affective, and behavioral categories of methods a bit fuzzy, the educator also cannot control the outcome. You might have a cognitive purpose for a lesson (e.g., that the students learn some information), use a cognitive process (e.g., a lecture), and probably have a cognitive impact or effect (they can repeat the information, have increased their knowledge). Or, you may have no impact at all; or, if your information disequilibrates a student, the effect for that person may be affective or even behavioral. You could have a behavioral goal in a lesson (learning skills for refusing sex), use a behavioral method (role play), but not change the behavior of those students who are already sexually active. The chosen methodology should fit the objective, which must be appropriate for the age, interests, needs, and abilities of the learners.

Nonetheless, the educational outcome of an "A" method is more likely to be affective (e.g., values clarification or increased tolerance); the outcome or impact of a "B" method is more likely to be behavioral (e.g., reduced risk taking, improved decision making, increased self-efficacy); and the effect of a "C" method is more likely to be cognitive (e.g., increased knowledge of facts or concepts).

ACTIVE VS. PASSIVE TEACHING

Throughout this text we have described ideal, effective sexuality education as being an experiential process that involves learners and facilitates dialogue and collaboration. In order to achieve this ideal, teachers must move away from traditional, authoritarian, teacher-directed learning systems to more learner-centered systems and replace passive learning methods with more innovative, *active* methods that involve the learner in his or her growth.

In the box we compare passive learning systems with active learning systems according to a number of key characteristics.

Learning Systems: Active vs. Passive

Characteristic	*Passive System*	*Active System*
Relationship of learner to educator	Dependent	Independent or interdependent
View of educator	Expert	Knowledgeable; directs process
View of learners	Ignorant, need to be controlled	Knowledgeable; their resources included, utilized
Whose ideas valued	Educator's only	Learner's and educator's
Emphasis on content or process	Primary emphasis on content	Emphasis on content and process
Lesson design	Rigid, strict format	Flexible format
Communication	One way: educator to learner	Fluid: educator to learner, learner to educator, learner to learner
Responsibility for learning	Learner's responsibility	Both educator and learner responsible for learning
Responsibility for design of content and process	Educator's responsibility	Both educator's and learner's responsibility
Evaluation responsibility	Educator's role	Educator's and learner's role
Evaluation focus	On learner	On learner, program, and educator
Whose needs and interests are reflected by design	Educator's	Learner's
Outcome	Little retention, skill acquisition, behavior change, or improved self-esteem	Good retention of content, skill acquisition, behavior change; learners feel affirmed

(SOURCE: Adapted from Michael Marlowe's "A Contrast of Active and Passive Learning Systems," unpublished [Seattle: Whitworth College/Leadership Institute of Seattle, 1981].)

In Chapters 8 through 13 we describe major sexuality education methods. Throughout these descriptions, if a method is typically passive, we describe ways that the method can be enhanced or made more active. For example, presentations, as described in Chapter 9, can be much more interactive than the traditional lecture if augmented with effective props or followed by a student-centered discussion. Other activities, such as the establishment of ground rules, can be very passive, with the educator listing rules and then soliciting participant endorsement of them; or it can be an active brainstorming activity. A physical intervention, such as changing the seating arrangements, can be active, involving all participants, or passive, done by the educator before learners enter the classroom. Videos are typically a passive method, but if they are used to "trigger" discussion, problem solving, or role play, they can have greater impact. Even teen theater can be passive for the audience, but if actors interact with learners and get them involved in role play, the method becomes more effective.

A Model for Planning: Designing Effective Sexuality Lessons and Workshops

Too many sexuality educators take an activity or exercise they enjoyed themselves and "do it to" the next group of learners without any thought as to how it fits into the curriculum or the lesson, how it meets learners' needs, or what political risks they are taking in the community. These educators fail to follow basic principles of effective sexuality education; in other words, they don't carry out a good planning process. The model we describe here is especially valuable for planning sexuality education sessions because it helps us put the theory of effective sexuality education into practice. It serves as a mental checklist for planning lessons and provides a framework for addressing each of the principles of effective sexuality education.

Our suggested planning model has six basic steps: conceptualizing the session, assessing learners, rethinking the lesson (or reconceptualizing), planning the environment, designing and sequencing activities, and planning for evaluation. Use these steps for planning various educational experiences, from individual lessons or workshops to an extended series or curriculum.

Step 1: Conceptualization

In the first step of the planning process, determine the most important concepts, facts, attitude components, and skills to cover about the topic you will be teaching. To accomplish this, ask yourself (1) what is worth knowing about the topic? and (2) what do my particular students most likely need to learn?

To answer these questions, draw upon your knowledge of sexuality content to brainstorm the most important concepts, facts, attitudes, and skills to address within topic areas, factoring in what you know about learners in general and your audience in particular. Use published curricula and guidelines for ideas and direction. The *Guidelines for Comprehensive Sexuality Education*,[1] for example, provide a complete set of topics and important messages for all developmental levels (kindergarten through twelfth grade) arranged in six conceptual areas: human development, relationships, personal skills, sexual behavior, sexual health, and society and culture.

Webbing is a useful planning method for generating content, concepts, values, or skills—whatever topics you want to address in workshops, lessons, units, or curricula. Beyond generating a simple list of possible subtopics within a larger topic, webbing helps reveal relationships among topics—shared concepts around which to organize an event. Use it also as a tool for assessing students' knowledge and interests (see Chapter 3).

An example of a *concept* web on the topic of gender is shown in the first box. In the second is a *content* planning web. There is no right or wrong way to construct a web; your webs on the same topic might have looked quite different from ours. Rather, webbing is simply a tool for stimulating and reflecting your own unique way of conceptualizing a topic.

Webbing is used to reveal many *possible* subtopics and conceptual approaches; it is unrealistic, however, to attempt to address all ideas generated in a web. Once you visually outline the possibilities, you can make a more informed decision about what is most important to include in your lesson or workshop, and the best beginning point with your particular learner group.

Regardless of the topic, choose a few key concepts, skills, or attitudes on which to focus your design. For example, when teaching about contraception, if you don't have a focus, you could spend hours teaching all the facts on every method without getting to what may be most important: how to ask a partner to use a condom, how to choose a method, or how to deal with one's nervousness about going to a clinic. Ask yourself the following questions:

- What are the few key concepts or skills to be addressed with these learners?
- Which concepts or skills are *central* and which are *corollary*?
- How do these key concepts and skills connect with concepts of previous lessons?
- What important factors do I know about my learners that will influence the concepts I choose and the lesson design?
- What attitudes or values do we need to explore?
- Where is the most important point to start?
- Again, what are the relevant skills that my students need?

Step 2: Assessing Learner Realities

The next step is to assess learners' needs and interests with respect to two broad criteria.

Knowledge, attitudes, and skills. What do the participants already understand, believe, and do related to this topic? You could simply ask them. But when assessing behaviors, use caution: do not ask learners to report sexual behaviors or personal sexual histories. By contrast, it would be appropriate to ask about skills or behaviors related to communication. Other subjective assessment methods

Conceptual Web on
Topic of Gender

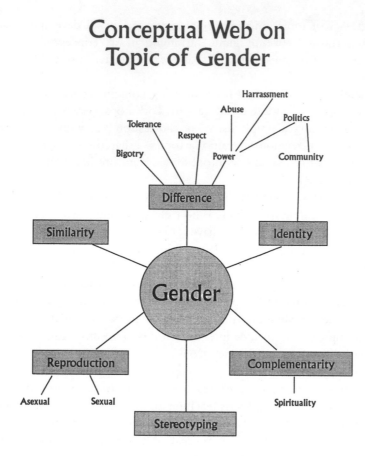

Content Web on Topic of Gender

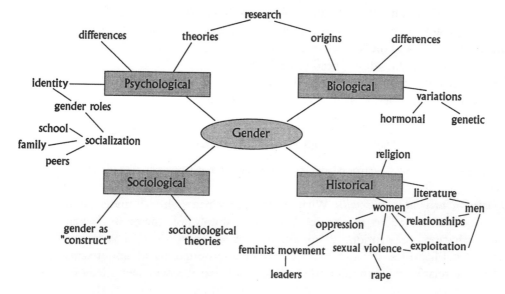

include brainstorming and observing and listening to individual students and groups. More objective assessments include anonymous questions, surveys, and polls (see Chapter 9), tests of knowledge, attitude and skills, evaluative games, and feedback forms (see Chapter 13).

Interests, needs, and special circumstances. What are the general and specific interests, needs, attitudes, personal histories, and special circumstances of these learners? Ask your students what they need to know and want to study. Observe what they talk about, read, watch, listen to, do to recreate, care about, hope for, and regret; talk with representatives or leaders of the group. Read about similar groups; watch television shows and commercials and read publications and literature aimed at that age or cultural group. Consult with teachers and other professionals who typically work with people like your learners. Observe or ask about the group's dynamics, that is, interpersonal conflicts, leadership roles, level of interaction, trust, and the like.

Besides ascertaining the specific needs, interests, and characteristics of a group, you can make certain assumptions about learners (as noted in Chapter 1): there will be survivors (or perpetrators) of sexual or other abuse, and group members who are gay or lesbian; there may be pregnant or parenting and sexually active members; there will probably be individuals who live in one-parent, adoptive, or foster families; some may have hidden disabilities. Assume differences, problems, conflicts, concerns, fears, sensitivities, and special circumstances, regardless of appearances, and use these assumptions to help shape your lessons and workshops.

Ideally, assessment of learner knowledge, interests, and group dynamics takes place before the lesson is actually planned. In the case of the regular classroom teacher, such assessment can be both ongoing and periodic prior to beginning new units. The community health educator or workshop leader, however, likely will not have the benefit of frequent contact with the student or participant group. In this case, s/he will have to rely on consultation with the regular teacher or group sponsor. In the box we suggest assessment questions to be asked of the teacher or group sponsor by the guest community health educator.

The Community Health Educator's View: Questions to Ask Your Host or Sponsor

If you are a community health educator who is invited to present to a class in a school or other setting, seek the following information before planning and presenting your session:

1. *About the student group.* What is their total number, age or grade level, level of maturity, previous lessons and current knowledge about the subject, and special needs (e.g., English literacy problems)? What are their expressed attitudes about your upcoming visit? What are their questions, feelings, and ideas about the topic? Have participants had experiences that will make them especially sensitive to your presentation?
2. *About the course.* What is the title and summary of the course for which you

are a guest? Is it an elective or required? What material have students already studied, and how will your presentation fit? What does the teacher or sponsor hope will happen?

3. *About prior planning and needs assessment.* What assessment has already been done? Will it be possible to do an on-site needs assessment, or could you do one prior to the day of the event?

4. *About organizational policy.* What are the policies and attitudes of the administration toward your topic or agency? Have mandatory approval or preview processes been conducted? Is there anything you should not say or discuss? What materials are appropriate or inappropriate?

5. *About logistics.* What is the time and length of the session? Will you have the necessary audiovisual equipment? Is there anything unusual about the classroom space? What interruptions can you expect? Will the teacher remain in the room with you?

6. *About group dynamics.* What teaching style are they accustomed to and how do they usually participate (talkative, reserved)? Do group members work well together? Are they accustomed to small group work? interactive methods? What roles do individuals take in the group? Are there individuals who dominate discussion?

7. *Miscellaneous.* Will there be any other guest speakers that day or following your presentation? Are you substituting for someone else? Will there be any parents or other guests in the classroom?

When prior assessment of learners is impossible, unreliable, or incomplete, conduct your own assessment within the first few minutes of contact with the group. Suggested methods for such "on-the-spot" assessments are described in Chapter 7.

Step 3: Rethinking the Lesson

Information gleaned in the assessment step may require you to revise your original plans. For example, you may discover that student understanding of a concept you considered key to the lesson is quite inadequate or, on the other hand, advanced beyond your expectations. Therefore, it may be necessary for you to start at a more basic or advanced level than you originally anticipated.

This step in the planning process requires adaptability on the part of the educator and curriculum. A prepackaged lesson from a published curriculum guide typically does not allow flexibility for making the adjustments necessary to address immediate or emerging learner concerns and interests. On the other hand, some curricula are very adaptable, even requiring the teacher to collect materials from current media and suggesting alternative activities. Such adaptations require skill and work, but go further toward meeting the needs of learners.

Step 4: Planning a Stimulating and Comfortable Learning Environment

This step requires the educator to consider the physical and psychological aspects of the environment, from both the facilitator's and the learners' perspectives.

To plan the psychological environment, address the following questions:

- What ground rules should I or the group establish that will facilitate the group's effective functioning?
- What existing group norms or issues might have an impact on the lesson?
- What general role (or combination of roles) do I want to play in this learning experience: expert? group facilitator? observer?
- What will enhance the learners' comfort and my own comfort?

To plan the physical environment, address the following questions:

- What room arrangement will be optimal for the kind of communications and activities planned for this class or workshop?
- What physical "props" (handouts, posters, etc.) will best support the lesson?
- What other environmental factors (e.g., light, sound, temperature, interruptions, distractions) might have an impact?
- What image should I as the facilitator project to the group? How should I dress?

Please see Chapter 3 for more discussion of the general principles of designing effective learning environments.

Step 5: Designing and Sequencing Activities

The effective sexuality education session is a balanced whole, the parts of which fit with each other and fit the learners' needs. To accomplish this, you must attend to how methods are formed into the whole activity, lesson, workshop, course, or curriculum. Carefully sequence a series of activities so that one activity provides a basis for the next, so that each activity builds on the previous one.

The most common sequencing order is *deductive,* that is, proceeding from the general and abstract to the specific and concrete. In a *deductive* lesson, learners proceed from concepts and information to analysis and specific inferences and applications:

1. The educator presents concepts and information and/or learners gather information. The teaching methods used here include presentation, videos, research, reading, question and answer, and so forth (see Chapter 9).
2. The learner works with the information (either alone or in groups), analyzing it, reflecting on concepts, ideas, and facts. The teaching methods used for reflection and analysis include introspection, discussion, worksheets, case studies, fish bowl, continuums, guided imagery, and so on (see Chapters 8–12).

3. The learner participates in experiences that illustrate the concepts. The teacher may provide educational experiences through interviews, panels, games, simulations, and so on (see Chapters 8 and 10–12).
4. The learner practices skills and experiments with the information through methods such as role play, simulation, skits, or "real-life" homework (see Chapter 11).
5. The learner applies information to his/her specific real needs or imagines such an application (perhaps with journal writing).

This format is similar in its deductive sequencing to the *Reducing the Risk* curriculum:[2] students are presented with information about abstinence, safer sex, and contraception; they are then asked to analyze, categorize, and explore that information; they examine various birth control and protective methods; they discuss social skills necessary for using protection or being abstinent; and they practice those social skills in role play and real-life homework opportunities.

To further illustrate deductive sequencing, let's analyze a specific activity. In Chapter 11 we have reprinted "You Would (Use a Condom) If You Loved Me" from *Teaching Safer Sex*,[3] which is sequenced as follows:

1. After an initial introduction of the topic (talking with a partner about using condoms), participants *gather information* from each other by brainstorming all the things people say as excuses for not using condoms; each excuse is listed at the top of a sheet of newsprint.
2. Learners then walk around the room to each of the posted excuses, think about them, and write a response to each excuse on each sheet. This requires them to *analyze* and *reflect* and *generate more information*.
3. Then volunteers read the posted responses aloud; they thus begin to *experience* feelings about using and hearing the language and to *practice* it.
4. Participants then view a video and discuss it, exploring their own feelings *(analyzing* and *reflecting)* as they project themselves into the vicarious *experience* of the scene in the video.
5. In the last step, pairs write and then read aloud a dialogue (at least the first two sentences) of a couple discussing using a condom, *practicing* and *experimenting* with the communication skills needed for safer sex.

We have taken this activity out of any context. In an effective curriculum it would have been preceded by other activities that prepared students for both the content and the processes. However, in and of itself, it follows an effective sequence starting with gathering information, analyzing and working with that information, reflecting on the feelings evoked by the information and the process, and finally practicing and experimenting with the information and related skills. In doing so, the activity uses a variety of cognitive, affective, and behavioral teaching methods and appeals to a variety of learning styles.

You can develop many variations of this sequence, given the specific needs of your group and your specific content. For example, you could spend considerable time giving, gathering, analyzing, and reflecting on information through a series of activities before beginning to practice and apply. Or you could reverse the process: begin with an individual or small group experience (e.g., a guided imagery that helps learners remember an actual experience from their past, or a simulation), introduce the key concepts verbally, help learners analyze the initial experience, and then present relevant information. This "reversal" of the deductive sequence, at least initially, is *inductive,* that is, proceeding from the specific and concrete (for the individual learner) to the general and abstract. Some have called this the "experiential learning cycle," because it starts with an "experience" (though some have started with a lecture and erroneously called that an "experience"). Whatever your sequence, it should proceed logically through a cohesive series of related steps.

Step 6: Planning for Evaluation

The last step of the planning process is to plan for evaluation on two levels: (1) assessing learner progress in attaining knowledge and skills; and (2) evaluating the success of the lesson or workshop in meeting the objectives of the educator.

Evaluation of learner progress provides feedback to the student and also further crystallizes concepts, facts, attitudes, and skills as they are reviewed and practiced during evaluation processes. Evaluation of the success of the lesson indicates what should take place in future lessons and allows student input into the progression of their sexuality education. (Please see Chapter 13 for a discussion of various methods for evaluating students and sexuality education sessions or programs.)

You probably will not follow the six steps of the planning model in a linear and rigid fashion. However, each step is important to the planning process, and when addressed consciously and separately, can significantly enhance teaching in sexuality education.

In the box we give an example summarizing the steps of the planning process for a workshop on gender.

A Workshop on Gender

Evonne was invited to present on gender (Step 1—initial conceptualization) to an ongoing class of psychology students that had been experiencing interpersonal conflict along gender lines. Both genders in the group were entrenched in their stereotypical views of the other gender, as well as in their firm belief that only their own gender experienced discrimination and pain as a result of being male or female.

In consideration of the rigid conceptions of gender and the hostile climate among this group of students (Step 2—assessing learners), a workshop was planned to facilitate a healing process between the two genders. Consequently, the concept of "similarity" was selected as the most appropriate entry point to gender (Step 3—rethinking and refining initial conceptualization), as opposed to exacerbating the students' current focus on "difference." An additional affective objective was to foster empathy for the other gender.

Evonne then designed a sequence of activities (Step 5). First she divided students into same-gender groups where they generated three lists: (1) what they liked about being their gender; (2) what they disliked; and (3) what they would give to the other gender if possible (either to get rid of it or to share it). This phase of the workshop allowed students to spend time talking about feelings and issues with their own gender (a rare opportunity, especially for men), and to vent some feelings out of the hearing of the other gender (Step 4—establishing a comfortable environment).

In the second phase of the workshop, the two groups shared their lists with the other gender, revealing three striking patterns: (1) marked similarities between the genders; (2) some qualitative differences in male/female responses (i.e., females tended to focus on physical attributes, males on psychological); and (3) a noted generosity of spirit between the two genders with respect to sharing qualities (especially among the males).

At the end of the series of activities, each gender expressed greater understanding of the other (Step 6—evaluation). Here are some sample comments: "I was really surprised that the men were eager to share their power and privilege with us." "Now I see that men have their own cross to bear as a result of strict gender role socialization." "I don't feel so defensive about being a male in this group anymore. I feel like I was heard for the first time."

The Ideal Lesson, Workshop, or Curriculum

The ideal sexuality lesson, series of lessons, curriculum, or workshop is composed of sequential learning activities that work together to accomplish the following goals:

- Introduce key concepts.
- Continually reassess learner needs, interests, attitudes, knowledge, and skills.
- Connect with participants' real lives.
- Introduce and/or reinforce positive social norms.
- Introduce or reinforce ground rules—guidelines for working and being together.
- Establish (or maintain) a comfortable environment while disequilibrating and motivating learners.
- Teach to all learning styles.
- Help participants expand their learning abilities.
- Present and gather information; correct misinformation and myths.
- Stimulate articulation and analysis of feelings, values, and attitudes while building respect and tolerance for others' different values.
- Help participants reflect, analyze, and draw conclusions.
- Help participants conceptualize, test theories, solve problems, and make or project practical application of new information.
- Help participants apply knowledge and skills.

CHAPTER 7

Facilitating Sexuality Education Sessions

> At the heart of the process of leadership is the communicative ability of the
> leader, and the core of this ability is the act of listening—not speaking.
> —Dominic A. LaRusso, "Listening: Missing Link in Leadership," 1970

Planning is one thing; *facilitating* effective sexuality education is quite another.
Having planned what seems to be an exciting sequence of activities and gathered all
the necessary materials and equipment—that will get you to the door. Knowing the
content, being comfortable with the language—that will help you get started. But
how do you guide interaction in ways that will enhance learning, enable positive
growth? How do you direct activities, make transitions? What do you do if unfore-
seen difficulties—negative reactions, lack of attention, interruptions—occur?

Effective teaching about sexuality is much more than giving information; "telling" learners what is right or wrong and lecturing to them about facts will accomplish few of the goals of an ideal lesson (see Chapter 6). Effective sexuality
education requires a dynamic relationship with learners. The skills needed for
nurturing that relationship, for enhancing individual learning about sexuality, have
to do with guiding and facilitating group processes. To do that, you need to listen.
You need to get beyond a focus on (and anxiety over) the sexuality content and
lesson plan to the relationship between you and individuals, between you and the
group.

In this chapter are suggestions for facilitating individual and group learning.
First we provide a brief background on group process. Then we present a somewhat chronological approach to delivery of sexuality education sessions—what to
do when you get there: making on-the-spot environmental adjustments, introducing self and lesson, continually assessing learners and group, establishing and
reinforcing ground rules, giving directions, facilitating activities in large and small
groups (including dyads and triads), making transitions between activities, intervening in problematic situations, staying flexible and adapting, and, last, making closure.

GROUP PROCESS

Educators should understand group process,[1] which has considerable impact on
individual learning. Since the impact of group dynamics seems to intensify when

the subject is sexuality, exploring strategies for facilitating group process is particularly important.

Groups are dynamic entities:

> A group is more than a sum of its parts, more than a collection of individual traits. A group is a social system distinct and different from the personalities of its members. While it is important to look at the individuals who energize group process and to understand how individuals learn, it is also important to see the group as a separate entity.[2]

Sexuality educators will recognize many common group characteristics, or dynamics, whether they work with ongoing groups and classes or do guest appearances and workshops with young children, teens, or adults.

Member contributions. Every member of a group brings individual experiences, expectations, and a personality, all of which influence the way the group deals with sexual issues. If an influential group member belittles others for asking questions, for being interested, or for expressing a particular opinion, the entire group may have difficulty with the process. If one member of the group is pregnant, this fact, if known, will influence how the group interacts about related topics.

Group history and shared experiences. The length of time a group has worked together and the ways they have been facilitated impact the process. Previous conflicts, prior lessons on related subjects, experience with interactive activities, and specific incidents (such as a gay student being publicly harassed) will have an influence on a sexuality lesson.

"Pluralistic ignorance." This term refers to a common occurrence in groups: individuals assume that all members agree with a particular opinion or idea—perhaps because it was voiced by a vocal, influential person—and do not speak up for fear of being a minority of one; or, one person assumes that all members agree with him/her, and acts on that false assumption, perhaps monopolizing conversation, or making unilateral decisions. Individuals in sexuality classes often hesitate to ask questions for fear of appearing "stupid." They think, "I'm the only one who doesn't know," or "I'm the only one who believes this way" and may be afraid to ask or afraid to share.

Audience effect. Learners are very aware of who is listening when they speak about sexual issues; what they say and how they interact varies depending upon who and how many people are listening.

Dynamics of numbers. Learners discuss sexuality very differently in a group of two or three than in a group of twenty.

Rank or prestige system. All members can identify the person(s) with power, whether quiet or very verbal, who have disproportionate influence (positive or negative) over group interactions.

Content dynamic. The content or topic being dealt with by the group is a major influence on group process. When the topic has to do with sexuality, the atmosphere usually intensifies, perhaps because individual interest is heightened and personal feelings are involved.

Furthermore, all groups go through *stages of growth.*[3] In early stages, members are concerned, consciously or unconsciously, with inclusion and are usually quite self-aware. Interaction is more constrained, less productive. A discussion about sexual content in such an immature group may be no more than a series of statements, questions, or responses directed toward the teacher, with little evidence of learners listening and responding to one another. A new group may not be ready to deal with certain sexuality content; likewise, a new or immature group may not be ready for certain activities that necessitate an atmosphere of group trust, such as role play. Consider the "maturity" of the group as you plan the content and processes of your lesson.

Gradually, the group becomes more productive as members begin to share experiences. They begin to take responsibility for group process (e.g., for including others), especially if the group is learner-centered rather than teacher-centered, and the process has been interactive rather than passive (see Chapter 6). Members begin to influence the atmosphere of the group, and participants become informal group leaders and facilitators.

As the group further matures, productivity is high. A group with a long history of interactive education methods and well-established ground rules is more likely to be able to discuss sensitive sexual issues and participate in demanding activities: learners feel more comfortable expressing feelings; individuals recognize trust and interdependence; individual differences are understood and utilized rather than seen as obstacles or objects of ridicule; and leadership is shared—group members pay less attention to established hierarchy and more to each other's ideas and abilities.

As you guide group process in sexuality education, consider how much control you should maintain, when and how often you should intervene and around what concerns, how much of yourself you should contribute and reveal, and how involved you should become with the group. As the group matures over time, reconsider these questions and change your involvement style and level to nurture leadership within the group.

Obviously, group process is very complex. There are many other factors that influence how a group interacts, including age, gender, gender mix, language, developmental level, and culture of group members; in other words, anything that affects individual learning and all characteristics of individual members affect group process.

ON-THE-SPOT ENVIRONMENTAL ADJUSTMENTS

You can improve a sexuality education setting in many ways, making it more conducive to learning and enhancing educator-learner and learner-learner relationships. Make the physical conditions that surround the experience of sexuality education as conducive to learning as possible:

- Change the seating configuration to increase the ability of participants to communicate as a group.
- Remove barriers, such as desks, tables, or podiums, between you and learners.
- Post attractive, relevant posters, charts, or pictures.

- Arrange visual equipment (flip charts, overhead projectors, VCR monitors) and display items so that all learners can see.
- Control room temperature, extraneous noise, and lighting.
- Plan ahead for known interruptions, and eliminate them as possible.

Make these changes yourself prior to the session; ask for volunteers to help you, involving at least a few of the participants; or involve the whole group during the session. When learners participate in the work of making physical changes, some individuals feel more included. Also, the noise and physical activity can break a heavy silence or heighten the group's energy during a lull.

If the environment is unsatisfactory for learning, make a "physical intervention" at the start or in the middle of a session: ask learners how they would be more comfortable ("Would you like to open some windows?" "How many would like to do the next two hours of this workshop outside?") or be more directive ("Let's move all the chairs into a circle"; "Everyone seems to be getting a little tired; let's take a two-minute stretch break"). Individuals may disagree on changes to be made; you will need to help the group balance personal needs with group needs. Facilitate by suggesting decision-making procedures, or deciding yourself.

Please see Chapter 3 for further discussion of productive, comfortable learning environments.

INTRODUCTIONS

Learners want to know who you are and whether they can trust you and feel comfortable discussing sexuality with you. You need to establish a sense of trust and comfort in the classroom (or other setting). How you appear, what you say, how you say it, how you make eye contact, and how you listen in the first few minutes will make a big difference in whether you capture attention and can hold it to build trust. (See Chapter 3 for more discussion on building credibility.)

As we mentioned in Chapter 3, part of the discomfort participants have during sexuality education sessions comes from not knowing what will happen. Learners want to see a framework for the session and be able to make a cohesive whole of it before, during, and after it happens. Give them this framework: post your goals or objectives, outlining key concepts for the lesson; post your agenda; do a needs assessment process that gathers their input on goals and agenda; and when you finish the session, reiterate all of this. In other words, discuss what you and they are going to do, do it, and then review with them what you've done together.

Not only do learners want to see that you have a sense of direction and a proposed framework, they also want to influence or have some sense of control over their own learning, especially in sexuality education.[4] As you introduce the goals, concepts, and agenda and reflect on the needs assessment data, consider whether your agenda meets those needs. If not, how can you be flexible, adjusting your agenda or planning for follow-up to meet those needs? Asking for input should not falsely raise expectations; negotiate changes, clearly state which needs or interests you can address and provide references or referrals for those you cannot.

Some education sessions can be planned with a built-in process for learner input on the agenda: (1) introduce the key concepts and goals for the session; (2) brainstorm learner needs and interests; prioritize those needs, and discuss or brainstorm ways of meeting them; (3) after learner input regarding their preferred methods of approaching key concepts (or skills), suggest two or three alternative activities that you can facilitate; and then, (4) allow learners to choose which alternative activities to carry out.

ONGOING ASSESSMENT

While you are talking, while they are talking, *listen*. In other words, pay attention to students, to their unique qualities, needs, problems, issues, learning styles. Watch the group and how individuals interact with you and with each other. Observe body language and other "silent" reactions to you and to the content. Pay attention to the effect of what you say and the effect of your directions for group activities. Continually reassess learner needs, interests, attitudes, knowledge, and skills, and listen so that you can connect with who they are there and then.

Besides keeping your eyes and ears open, there are more explicit ways of assessing learners: ask them—brainstorm ideas, needs, interests, current information. In Chapters 3 and 6 we discuss assessment prior to sexuality education sessions. In the box we give an example of an activity that utilizes a type of brainstorming to assess students for a lesson on STDs.

Graffiti Sheets

Objectives: (1) To allow the educator to gain insight into the knowledge of and attitudes about STDs within the group; (2) to allow the participants to express their attitudes about STDs.
Prerequisites: Literacy skills.
Age Group: 16+
Group Size: Ideally a maximum of 25.
Time needed: 30–45 minutes.
What You Need: Large sheets of paper, felt-tip pens; a sound knowledge of sexually transmitted diseases.
How You Do It
1. Take several large sheets of paper and, at the top of each one, write a different statement about STDs. Suggested statements:
   • You would know if you had an STD.
   • Only dirty people catch STDs.
   • You can't get an STD the first time you have intercourse.
   • You can catch STDs from toilet seats.
   • You can get an STD more than once.
   • You can't have more than one STD at a time.

- Condoms keep you from getting STDs.
- Kissing spreads STDs.
- There's a cure for STDs.
2. Display the pieces of paper around the room so that they can be written on.
3. Have the participants move around the room and write down their responses to the statements on the paper. Encourage free expression and creative graffiti, allowing the participants to write whatever they like.
4. When everyone has had an opportunity to write on every sheet, re-form the group.
5. Read the graffiti and discuss such things as fiction and fact, myths and misconceptions.

Variations
1. Have participants form small groups and give each group paper and pen. The educator reads statements and asks the group to write their reactions.
2. Form small groups and circulate the graffiti sheets for groups to write their comments.
3. Similar statements could be used referring to HIV/AIDS.

(SOURCE: Reprinted by permission from The Clarity Collective's *Taught Not Caught: Self Esteem in Education* [Australia: Spiral Press, 1983], 168.)

One of our colleagues uses the following stem sentences as headings for the graffiti sheets; they are more open-ended, leaving more room for student elaboration.[5] Note that these stem sentences form a logical sequence for a subsequent presentation, for example, discussing STD myths, causes, symptoms, prevention, and resources in turn:

- People who get STDs are . . .
- You can get an STD by . . .
- Some symptoms of STDs are . . .
- People sometimes don't know when they have an STD because . . .
- You can prevent STDs by . . .
- If I got an STD I could get help from . . .

ESTABLISHING AND REINFORCING GROUND RULES

The process of establishing ground rules for sexuality education sessions will enhance the educator-learner relationship and increase learner comfort and safety. (Please see Chapter 3 for a complete discussion of the purpose and need for ground rules. In this chapter we suggest methods for establishing ground rules and provide examples.)

Involving students in establishing ground rules acknowledges the importance of each person's input. The most common method for involving the group is to brainstorm ground rules. After introducing the goals, key concepts, and agenda for the session, ask learners, "What rules would you like to establish for how we are going to work together?" "What should we expect from everyone in this group?" "What guidelines shall we set for group and individual behavior that will make this session comfortable and meaningful for everyone?" Resulting ground rules should cover issues of confidentiality, right to pass, tolerance and acceptance of others, and so forth (see Chapter 3).

Post all contributions to the brainstorm. Ask learners to clarify and elaborate: if someone suggests "confidentiality," ask that person (and others) to describe what that means in terms of concrete behavior. Categorize rules and clarify your expectations for each one as necessary; add any important provisions the group neglects to include. In a short session, when group generation of ground rules may not be feasible, post suggested ground rules, seeking agreement from the group in carrying them out.

In a series of lessons or a longer workshop, you may want to use a small group process to brainstorm initial lists for ground rules. Groups could develop skits to illustrate ways people commonly (if unintentionally) violate the ground rules and then enact the skits for the whole group and discuss the issues illustrated. Or small groups can clarify and add concrete behavior descriptions to a whole-group ground rule list.

New Methods for Puberty Education[6] provides an effective method for developing ground rules for a series of lessons or a complete puberty education curriculum. Students read a series of cases describing problematic situations in family life classes, such as one student being derogatory of another's curiosity, or students asking questions of others that are too personal. Students then respond to discussion questions (e.g., "Why do you think Sally became angry?" "What are some reasons why people make insulting comments to others?" and "What makes people curious about other people's personal experiences?"); they then relate the situations to the goals for their class and together formulate ground rules for class interactions. See Chapter 3 for a similar case study used to generate ground rules.

To illustrate the kinds of interaction guidelines typically generated by different age groups, we provide (in the boxes) three sample sets of ground rules for use with young children, with older children and adolescents, and with adults.

Ground Rules for Teaching Sexuality Education to Young Children

1. There are no dumb or silly questions.
2. No one has all the answers.
3. If we can't answer a question, we'll look it up.
4. Try to use correct words.
5. No put-downs are allowed; everyone has different ideas and questions.
6. Listen to each other.

Ground Rules Suggested by Teachers for Sexuality Education in Schools

1. Everyone has the right to "pass" on activities or on answering questions they do not wish to answer. The teacher also may choose not to answer a question in front of the entire class.
2. All points of view are worthy of being discussed. No preaching; no put-downs of others' values.
3. No question is "dumb." Questions only indicate a desire for knowledge; they do not tell you anything else about the person asking the question.
4. When possible, correct terminology should be used. When you do not know the correct term, use the term you know. Teacher or other students can supply the correct term.
5. No asking of personal questions to the teacher or to the class.
6. No talking about class members' comments outside the classroom.
7. Teacher will respect the confidentiality ground rule as well, except where s/he is required by law to disclose information, for example, sexual abuse. (Some teachers also include in this ground rule that they will not be able to maintain confidentiality if what is shared is illegal or dangerous to the students.)
8. Speak for yourself. Use "I messages" to state opinions or feelings.
9. If you or people you know have a complaint about the class, come directly to the teacher to discuss it.
10. Discuss the issues raised in class with your parents and give an accurate accounting of what the class is about. Do not sensationalize.
11. It is all right for the teacher to blush, feel embarrassed, or not know all the answers.

(SOURCE: *Beyond Reproduction: Tips and Techniques for Teaching Sensitive Family Life Education Issues* [Santa Cruz, Calif.: ETR/Network Publications, 1983].)

Sample Ground Rules for Sexuality Education and Training with Adults

We hereby agree that we will do the following:
1. Practice effective communication in this group by listening when an individual speaks and by trying to involve all group members in discussions.
2. All accept responsibility for how well this group works.
3. For the most part, operate in the "here and now" as opposed to dwelling on past personal experiences.
4. Show respect for diverse opinions, values, life-styles, personal backgrounds, and sexual orientations that will be represented in this group or among our invited guests, whether or not we agree with or embrace those views or perspectives ourselves.
5. Respect the right of individuals to "pass" on some questions and activities if they so choose.

6. Exhibit common courtesies to others (such as arriving on time) and respect building rules (such as refraining from smoking in the building).
7. Challenge each other to think in new ways and to grow personally and intellectually while operating within the previous general guidelines.

(SOURCE: Adapted from Barbara Fuhrmann's "Education of the Self" class at the Open High School, Richmond, Va.)

GIVING DIRECTIONS FOR GROUP ACTIVITIES

Most educators experience difficulty getting learners to understand what they want them to do; or, as learners, they have themselves been confused and frustrated by badly worded directions. Confusing directions may reflect poorly conceived or designed learning processes, a lack of preparation, or poor articulation.

Confusion also may indicate anxiety or excitement on the part of learners regarding the sexuality content of the lesson; such content-centered anxiety may be compounded by group process issues or by being asked to participate in interactive learning methods. A lot is going on inside learners that affects their ability to pay attention!

Some learners are experienced with a wide variety of interactive group processes, for example, some know how to move easily (physically and psychologically) into small groups, with little resistance or anxiety. Other learners, experienced with a more traditional passive learning process, may be uncomfortable, resistant, and confused when instructed to work in small groups. An adequate assessment of your learners (see Chapter 6) prior to the session should give you clues about their group process sophistication and learning styles. As you give directions, continue to observe group and individual responses and adjust accordingly.

As you design a learning activity or plan a lesson, think through the entire process, imagining what you will say, not only in content, but also how you will direct learners verbally and with body language. Prepare the simplest phrases to direct people; think of how you can rephrase instructions in case you are not understood the first time, but don't complicate the process with too much repetition. Visualize how people will move, how the process will look physically. Plan ahead how you will divide the whole group into subgroups (see our suggestions that follow) and practice the verbal instructions you will use to achieve this.

Many published learning activities and curricula include specific content suggestions; some also include suggestions for process instructions. Practice and alter these statements, making sure they fit your style and manner of communicating. Be sure that you can paraphrase them if learners are confused.

FACILITATING LARGE GROUP DISCUSSIONS

The unique dynamics of the particular group become apparent during a discussion. There will be differences in participation, participation shifts, and norms for the treatment of silent members. Leadership (or influence) by members and subgroups will emerge. Other group norms, such as subgrouping, exclusion and inclusion of members, decision-making procedures, and acceptance of feelings can be observed.

An effective discussion seems to improve these dynamics. The group seems to be "healthier" in its functioning and more productive following what members perceive to be a "great discussion." Effective discussions are usually *learner centered,* rather than teacher centered (see Chapter 6).

We make the following suggestions for facilitating interaction among learners in discussions:

- Arrange seating so that learners can see and interact with one another; chairs aimed at the front of the room will aim the interaction in that direction. If you are a guest speaker leading a discussion and chairs are in rows, consider asking group members to rearrange chairs with you.
- Pose open-ended questions or topics; do not limit your questions to subjects for which only you have the answer, and resist always having to have the last word.
- Draw out a number of perspectives. Wait for participants to bring up your ideas; get involved in the content of the discussion only when you can interact without suppressing learner involvement.
- Use a flip chart or board to record main points; the resulting list becomes the group "memory" and shows progress.
- Facilitate participant leadership by modeling and then asking learners to take on "group functions": paraphrasing, summarizing, asking for or giving information or opinions, mediating conflict, encouraging others' participation, expressing group feeling.
- Move away from center stage. Sit in the group or move to the back, and tell them what you are doing and why.
- When a learner is speaking, try looking elsewhere than just at that person; encourage him or her, verbally and with your body language, to speak to the group, not to you.
- Don't reply to all learner input; wait for group members to reply. If necessary, ask, "Any reaction to that comment?"
- When appropriate, redirect questions asked directly of you, saying, "What do the rest of you think?"
- If someone rambles, ask that person or another group member to summarize or paraphrase the main point of that person's comments.
- Act as gatekeeper, watching the body language of quiet participants; when someone seems to want to speak, invite him or her to do so.
- Refer to ground rules when necessary, especially with regard to respecting others' values and beliefs.
- Never disparage someone for an opinion, and don't allow group members to do so, whether by humor, condescension, sarcasm, or cross-examination.
- Please see Chapter 10 for specific interactive discussion methods and activities.

FACILITATING SMALL GROUPS

In Chapter 9 we describe the use of task groups (any subgroup of the whole that convenes to do a task) in sexuality education and offer examples of task group activities. Here we describe ways of facilitating or guiding all types of small group activities.

The purpose of a small group activity may be as simple as to discuss reactions or share memories but usually includes some assigned task that will be reported on to the whole group. When well facilitated, task groups become "cooperative learning groups," where the focus is not only on the content, but also on the interactive process. The effective use of such groups is doubly important in comprehensive sexuality education, since one of its broad goals is to increase communication and relationship skills.

Small group work allows more opportunities for learners to share information, feelings, and attitudes than does large group discussion; small groups also are important for the practice of skills. Individuals who are usually silent in large groups may feel more comfortable about speaking or even take active leadership roles in small groups. Most people find it more difficult to remain silent and totally nonparticipative in a small group.

Individuals may carry out (or be assigned) specific roles or functions, including leading, facilitating, initiating activity, gathering opinions or information, recording, reporting, gatekeeping (helping all give input), standard setting, mediating, decision making, summarizing, harmonizing, evaluating, relieving tension, diagnosing, testing for consensus, or expressing group feeling.

Individual commitment to the group can depend on many factors, including previous knowledge of each other, prior shared experiences (e.g., group-building activities), level of trust, and any current issues, concerns, and special circumstances that each member brings to the group. Commitment to the group and individual investment in the task can have a tremendous positive impact on group productivity.

Small group activities, as a means of more intensely involving all members, will usually help build a feeling of cohesiveness and productivity in the large group as well as within the small group. However, power struggles or unmet inclusion needs can adversely affect group productivity. Time limits, competition among groups, or pressure to perform can also affect productivity, positively or negatively. Task groups utilize the collective knowledge, experience, and skills of group members, yet productivity may be greater than that collection would suggest because of the synergistic effect of group dynamics.

You may assign tasks to groups and take an inactive role, observing and clarifying directions as needed; or you may work more actively with the groups, consulting, offering resources and suggestions, clarifying, stimulating, mediating, answering questions, and arbitrating. Do not use task groups as a method if you believe that only you have the correct answers, since the product of the group is "owned" by the group.

Use small groups for many of the same kinds of activities you would use with large groups:

- To brainstorm a list and then rank order or prioritize the list.
- To write definitions, mission or goal statements.
- To carry out a defined problem-solving process.
- To role play with set scripts, write their own scripts, or produce a skit.
- To discuss case studies and role play the characters described therein.
- To do research and write reports.
- To study or analyze information or discuss a question or topic, with or without reporting back to the whole group.
- To make recommendations or decisions for which they have been empowered by the whole group.
- To design teaching activities.
- To evaluate or analyze information on a worksheet.
- To interview one another.
- To participate in simulations or games.
- To do forced choice, continuum, and quadrant activities.

We offer the following suggestions for directing small groups in sexuality education and training sessions:

1. Introduce the topic and the goals of the activity.
2. Describe the entire process, clearly defining and posting the task(s), describing expected quantity and quality of the outcome, time constraints, reporting process, and member roles.
3. Divide the whole group into subgroups:
   - For a random division, have participants count off by the number of groups you will form (i.e., if you will have five groups, count off by fives; all "ones" work together, all "twos" together, etc.); this separates people who sit together and seems by all to be an unbiased method of division.
   - Allow participants to choose their own groups: state the number of groups there will be and the number you want in each group. Many participants will be distressed by this method of division, not knowing where to go, feeling anxious about not being chosen, especially when the topic or content is sexuality. You may need to be directive, dividing groups that are too large or combining ones that are too small.
   - Preselect and assign groups, posting names of individuals in each group, or using color-coded name tags or other symbols given to participants as they arrived.
   - Have participants form groups where they are sitting.
4. Start the process, acting as timekeeper, observer, and consultant as appropriate.
5. Reconvene the whole group. Don't expect instantaneous compliance; you will have to ask for attention at least three times.

6. Manage the reporting process by timing task group reports, asking only one person to speak from each group, or asking the whole group to question, evaluate, or otherwise react to each report. Reporting can take several forms:

- Each group reports a summary of their process and presents their entire product (e.g., a list, a definition, a description).
- Each group presents a skit depicting (verbally or nonverbally) the feelings, values or opinions of the group.
- The first group gives a complete report; following groups add whatever they had that was significantly different ("report plus add-ons").
- Poll each group with a prepared list of questions.
- Ask each group to report only their most important item ("cream-off-the-top" reporting).
- Invite "minority reports" or clarification from members who are not the groups' official spokespersons.

FACILITATING DYADS AND TRIADS

The dynamics of dyads and triads (groups of two and three) are significantly different from larger groups. They can be used as task groups, but are small enough to facilitate sharing of feelings and opinions. They are much different from task groups when the focus is on the persons involved rather than on the task: members share an experience rather than create a product. These small groups can be used for getting acquainted, self-disclosure, values clarification, skills practice, and many other purposes in sexuality education and training. Participation in dyads and triads help individuals feel included and can reduce performance anxiety.

The facilitator cannot completely control the individual's experience during a dyad or triad, or recapture it afterward. Ask learners to summarize, generalize, draw conclusions, or make conceptual connections, but do not expect them to report their experiences—what was said or felt during the dyad—except in summary (e.g., "After hearing the speaker talk about his HIV status, some of the feelings we discussed in our group were . . .").

The close sharing of dyads and triads may feel risky for some individuals; the content of what is discussed should be carefully designed for the developmental level of the group, with serious consideration of the characteristics of each individual involved. Ask yourself if everyone in the group will be comfortable sharing ideas or opinions about sexual issues with one other person, and on what level. Also consider the whole group's dynamics around inclusion, control, and sharing of feelings.

You may wish to consider participating in one of the dyads or triads you are facilitating, but only if you can work with the group as a peer (for example, if you are conducting a professional workshop). Also, consider whether you are able to keep time while you participate in short dyad/triad activities. Circulate among groups to monitor process, but do not interrupt or eavesdrop; respect the confidentiality and intimate nature of the groups. Be less controlling of the process for mature groups; allow them to work with fewer interruptions and directions than you must give groups less experienced in small group interaction.

We suggest the following steps for facilitating dyads and triads:

1. Introduce and discuss the goals of the activity.
2. Post and discuss the topic(s). Describe the process, including the time format and how (or if) you will interrupt to give further directions.
3. Give directions for preliminary introspection, allowing participants to gather their thoughts and "rehearse" before focusing on their discussion partners.
4. Discuss sharing and listening roles: participants should understand how to focus on one person at a time and how to do active listening. Or, try "uninterrupted listening," where one person talks about him or herself for a prescribed period of time and the listener does not interrupt, even with nonverbal nods or grunts. Uninterrupted listening is an excellent communication skill for use in ongoing relationships; it allows the speaker to take an idea or feeling wherever s/he wishes, without the direction that even the most subtle communication from the listener can impose.
5. Form groups: allow participants to choose partners, count off for random groupings, or assign dyads/triads. The more risky the topic, the more we recommend allowing people to choose their own partners. On the other hand, for some people the choosing of partners is the most distressing part of the process; they would rather the facilitator be directive, asking them to choose someone they don't know, or someone with whom they haven't been in a group before, or to turn to their neighbors. You may want to describe the dyad/triad process early in your program (before it takes place), suggesting that participants begin to think about potential small group partners or asking for input on the process.
6. Suggest that participants move their chairs to a private space and face each other; help them facilitate communication by removing desks, tables, and other barriers.
7. Direct participants to decide who goes first, second, or third.
8. Direct the groups to begin; announce time as appropriate. Allow time for all to share, or call time as each individual should be finishing.
9. In a triad, the interaction sometimes can be between two people, with the third person acting as observer. The observer role can be particularly important in a skill practice exercise (see Chapter 11). Describe the responsibilities of the observer and clarify how this role will rotate through the triad before you begin.
10. Debrief a dyad/triad experience with discussion or other methods. Ask how participants felt about their interaction or for generalizations about what they learned.

Please see Chapter 10 for further discussion of the use of dyads and triads in sexuality education, and for examples of dyad/triad activities.

TRANSITIONS

Transitions should make explicit the connection between methods and activities in your sexuality lessons and workshops. Learners do not automatically perceive the connection, not having spent time thinking about the entire design. Helping them see the logic, flow, and connectedness of various parts not only shows your respect for them but also subtly increases their comfort and feeling of involvement with the process and their respect for you as an educator. Learners want to know where they are going, what they are doing, and why, especially in sexuality education.

Announce transitions with simple statements that summarize or mention the just completed segment and then state how it will be debriefed or followed. If an activity will not be debriefed, that should be stated as well. Here are some partial sample statements for acknowledging transitions:

> "If you remember just one thing from this activity, I hope it is . . ."
> "Now let's use this information to . . ."
> "Let's set this aside; we'll come back to it . . ."
> "We just looked at *why* people might want to prevent an STD; now let's talk about *how*."
> "I would like to leave this to you to reflect on at your leisure; let me suggest that you . . ."
> "In order to practice this, let's . . ."
> "Let's reflect on what we just experienced . . ."
> "How did you feel about . . ."
> "What were the key elements . . . Let's brainstorm . . ."
> "What were the most powerful, effective behaviors in that role play?"

PROCESS INTERVENTIONS AND FLEXIBILITY

Interventions are actions educators or trainers use to control, influence, direct, or guide process or content. Interventions can be more or less educator driven, that is, more or less controlling: the educator can make a decision internally and enforce it; s/he can ask for input and then make a change or give a direction; or s/he can become less controlling or directive, giving feedback on what s/he is observing or making open-ended suggestions and allowing learners to direct some of their own process.

A *content intervention* focuses on the content (or topic) under consideration: for example, during a brainstorm, the educator may contribute his or her own ideas to the brainstorm list, share an opinion, or describe a personal experience. However, the teacher should try not to preempt a learner who was getting ready to say the same thing, taking ownership of the content away from the learner, reducing group productivity, and decreasing potential learning. Since the educator has a great deal of power, being too active, too vocal, and too controlling can diminish learner involvement. Sometimes the best intervention is waiting, being patient, or enduring silence until learners make contributions themselves. Furthermore, pay attention to cultural norms for this and other group processes; the need to fill quiet time with words is a distinctly Anglo-American trait and can stifle learners.

Process interventions focus on the progress of the group, the course of action, how the group is formed, how subgroups are formed and work together, how content is discussed or otherwise handled. Therefore, *giving instructions* for a group activity is a process intervention. How those instructions are given, that is, whether they are imposed or suggested, general, or very specific and controlling, depends on the control needs of the educator and the educator's perception of the needs of the group. For example, during a dyad sharing exercise, the educator may state the total time allowed for the activity at the beginning, allow dyads to proceed uninterrupted, and then ask participants if they are finished, allowing more time at the end as necessary. Or, for a more controlled dyad process, the educator calls time when the first person in the dyad should finish and the second person should begin, and calls time at the end.

Level of control also may depend upon time factors, resources within the group, or the educator's tolerance for ambiguity. Learners want direction and typically look to the educator for leadership, yet they grow more when they have legitimate influence on group process, when they practice leadership skills. Look for a balance between autocracy and anarchy.

Changing the agenda is another type of process intervention. If you perceive that learners are not responsive to the topic, or seem uninvolved with the activity, or are anxious about the process, propose an agenda change or ask for group suggestions. Likewise, if time is running out and the agenda cannot be completed, make an internal decision about what to leave out and how to conclude, and then announce that decision; or ask for group input—what are their priorities for the time remaining?

Asking for feelings is an effective way of guiding the process. Asking how learners feel about group process and content gives legitimacy to feelings, helps release tension, and leads to increased participant involvement, all of which enhances learning about sexuality. For example, after a fishbowl exercise on gender (see Chapter 10), ask observers how they felt about not being able to say anything to inner circle members during their discussion. Or, following an "uninterrupted listening" dyad exercise, ask learners how they felt while talking without immediate feedback.

Diagnosing is another way of intervening during uncomfortable group process. If you perceive something problematic about the group atmosphere, such as an underlying current of tension, sudden tiredness, or inattentiveness, state your perception and ask for input: for example, after showing an emotional video about HIV, "You've all gotten very quiet; that was pretty intense—how should we proceed?" or "Would you like a quick stand-up break?"

Giving direct feedback to individuals or the group also guides the process: comment on an individual's behavior or skill; compliment the group or subgroup about their progress or productivity; thank a participant for a question. Positive feedback thoughtfully given is, of course, more beneficial for the learner-educator relationship and learner productivity than negative feedback.

Performing group functions means helping people get acquainted, involving individuals, suggesting a decision-making process, making group decisions, asking for input, and so on. In an educational setting, especially early in the life of the group, the educator is usually the one who performs such group task and maintenance functions. One such function, controlling a person who monopolizes discussion, is particularly difficult for participants to handle by themselves. Most are appreciative when the teacher intervenes by thanking the person for his or her input, redirecting the conversation, and emphasizing giving everyone a chance to share. As the group matures, turn these "task and maintenance" functions over to group members, fostering improvement of group communication skills.

Finally, facilitate learning by *protecting individual learners:* divert or stop severe negative feedback from others; interrupt actions that put one learner or small group on the spot, making them anxious; help individuals keep their own identity in the face of pressure to conform; and, as noted in Chapter 5, prevent learners from "overexposing" themselves by sharing too much.

Use the preceding general process interventions to facilitate interaction when things are going well and to prevent or deal with problems as they occur. Here we illustrate their use in specific problem situations:[7]

One problem that sometimes occurs in sexuality education sessions is nonresponsiveness. The reasons may lie in incidents that occurred before you arrived: a community educator colleague discovered that the classroom teacher had told the class that if any students opened their mouths when the guest speaker was there he would flunk them! Or students may be unresponsive if your materials or activities are developmentally inappropriate for them; other reasons are peer pressure, embarrassment, disinterest, or lack of trust. Ask learners what is going on; do an anonymous feedback questionnaire; talk with other teachers or parents. Remember, learners are more likely to participate when the session is relevant to their lives. Remember also that your assessment of nonresponsiveness may reflect a cultural difference; they may be highly responsive by their own measurement—you just don't see it!

If students are disruptive or if subgrouping develops, you may need to draw limits on what behavior you will or will not accept, reiterating groundrules as you do so. You could even open the issue to group discussion, though it may be more effective or appropriate to talk to the disruptive person(s) privately.

Deal with hyperactivity, silliness, and giggling in some of the same ways: describe the problem as you see it; reiterate ground rules; discuss the source of the problem; gradually use definitions and activities to help learners develop comfort with the topic (see Chapter 3); or talk privately with the individuals involved. A strategy that works especially well to reduce tension in younger groups is a "one-minute giggle" session.

Even the most experienced educators have had that sinking feeling of losing a group's attention, or suddenly realizing that the planned agenda, for whatever reason, is inappropriate. Making immediate changes is most often avoided because of anxiety, a lack of trust in the group to guide its own work, or a feeling of inability (warranted or not) to produce anything different without more preparation. Deliberately plan alternative activities in case you must shift the agenda. However, external factors, such as the demands of a school administration or insufficient time, sometimes preclude making changes on the spot.

CONCLUSIONS AND CLOSURE

For the end of a sexuality education session, we recommend a brief concluding process:

1. *Summarize the session.* Include a summary or reiteration of key concepts, skills, and information (make summary statements yourself, or solicit statements from learners—see "Learner Declarations," Chapter 13).
2. *Assess learner understanding.* A final assessment or evaluation of learner understanding and retention of key concepts, skills, and information may be appropriate (see Chapter 13).
3. *Solicit learner feedback.* You may want learner feedback about the content, the process, and/or your competence (see Chapter 13). Don't project or impose your assessment on the group by saying such things as, "Now, wasn't that fun?" Instead, ask for their assessment first and give your feelings only as part of the feedback discussion.
4. *Give resources and referrals.* Further suggestions of resources (e.g., referrals to meet expressed or assumed learner needs) enhance and augment participant learning (see Chapter 9).
5. *Follow-Up.* Describe your plans and ask learners for suggestions for follow-up; reiterate any promises made to get additional information you couldn't provide during the session.
6. *Thank participants* for their attention and involvement during the session or unit.

As you close, remember that because your topic was sexuality, a highly charged subject for most people, the session may have brought up unpleasant memories and personal issues (e.g., incest or an unwanted pregnancy) for some participants. They may feel uncomfortable, embarrassed, or excited, and their learning and disequilibration may continue long after the session. As you close, you may wish to acknowledge that feelings may linger and give an opportunity for learners to express those feelings. After the session, remain in the area, available for individual questions, comments, expression of feeling, or requests for assistance.

CHAPTER 8

Introspective Methods: Helping Learners
See Relevance

One of the most important tasks of the sexuality educator is to help learners connect vital concepts or messages to prior experiences, interests, feelings, beliefs, and needs—to personalize. To do that, educators ask learners to think and reflect or, more specifically, to *introspect:* to look inward, examining or observing one's own mental and emotional processes.

The main purposes of introspective methods for sexuality education are to focus learners on the topic, to help them find significance in the material, to "warm up" the group, to begin to gather information, and to do mental rehearsal for subsequent sharing.

With introspective methods, learners are asked to remember, visualize, reflect, or imagine in response to questions, topics, questionnaires, stem sentences, pictures, or descriptions. Learners' responses can be internal (thought only) or can involve writing, diagramming, or drawing. Though content is often processed in dyads, small groups or large group discussion, introspection is solo in nature; the sexuality educator encourages the learner to control his or her own experience and should not expect to recapture the content of the experience for the whole group.

Ideally, the use of introspective methods gets all learners involved. If a teacher asks, "Who can name an STD?" only selected individuals will respond. However, if the question is reframed to "Everyone think for a moment of three facts you know about STDs, and be prepared to share with your neighbor," most if not all learners begin to focus on the topic.

Introspection helps individuals learn about themselves and prepare for subsequent activities. All learners have a chance to participate, have privacy and confidentiality, and can work at their own levels of risk and thought. Therefore, as long as learners know what use will be made of the products of their introspection, these methods are especially useful for reducing anxiety about the sexuality content of the session.

On the other hand, introspective methods may be stressful and risky for individuals who can't write, draw, or form mental images. Others find it distressing to be asked to think about their own responses to sexual issues or topics.

Any sexuality topic, issue, or concept can be used for introspection. The educator cannot predict exact content, since the topics used will provoke many memories and perspectives in learners. Care should be taken in the phrasing of a question or topic to make it appropriate for the goals, key concepts, and time constraints of the lesson; the developmental level of the group; the political climate of the community; the interests, needs, and culture of the learners; and the subsequent sharing process, if any. Ensure safety and comfort by including a variety of levels of questions and various ways of recording and processing the introspection. For example, when asking a group of adults to remember their adolescence, give them a list of questions to which they respond; then, during dyad sharing, individuals can discuss only those questions that they are comfortable sharing.

STEPS FOR FACILITATING INTROSPECTIVE ACTIVITIES

We suggest the following steps for facilitating activities involving focus writing, questionnaires, stem sentences, drawing, responding to pictures, guided imagery, or journals:

1. Introduce the goals of the activity, connecting it to previous activities and concepts.
2. Clearly state what will be done with whatever learners write or draw during introspection; give a general description of follow-up activities. This is especially important for most sexuality topics. If an element of surprise is needed for follow-up activities, at least assure learners of what *won't* be done with their writing or drawing (i.e., they won't have to show it to anyone).
3. Describe the complete process: post questions or topics, hand out materials, tell how the activity will be timed, and reiterate ground rules as appropriate.
4. Suggest alternative variations to the activity; that is, focus writing will not be shown to anyone, so it need not be coherent; learners can write random notes on scratch paper, make a list, or actually write sentences and paragraphs. Or, in the same set of instructions, give learners the option to just think about the questions.
5. Begin the process, quietly clarifying the task for confused individuals, observing and keeping track of the time.

FOCUS WRITING

Learners may be asked to write, or "focus write," in response to questions, statements, case histories, or topics. Educators often use this method at the beginning of an activity, to help learners gather their thoughts for subsequent discussion or other processes.

For example, pose the following questions at the beginning of a lesson on the concept "gender roles":

- What qualities are considered masculine?
- What qualities are considered feminine?
- Of the qualities from both your lists, which do you want to have?

Follow this focus writing activity with dyad sharing, perhaps in same-gender pairs, and then a fishbowl (see Chapter 10) or large group discussion.

For a "stream of consciousness" variation on focus writing, the facilitator instructs participants that they will have an allocated period of time to write whatever comes up: "You have three minutes; don't stop writing; just put your pen to the paper and keep writing until I say stop."

QUESTIONNAIRES

Asking learners to complete questionnaires is a more formalized type of writing introspection. The questionnaire takes the form of a handout and learners complete it for their own introspection and perhaps for subsequent discussion. Care should be taken with sensitive sexuality topics to protect learner anonymity.

One example of a questionnaire is "Thrill Seekers," in *Entering Adulthood: Coping with Sexual Pressures*.[1] Learners are asked to think about how much of a risk they would take with such behaviors as walking alone at night, staying out past their curfew, smoking cigarettes, and so on. This activity is part of a larger lesson on risky sexual behaviors and could be used as an anonymous survey (see Chapter 9), that is, to gather data for use by the group.

See the box for an example of a questionnaire that gives students the opportunity to personalize abstinence and pregnancy protection information they have previously received.

How Will You Avoid Pregnancy?

Directions. This worksheet is for your own use and information. It is not for class discussion and will not be turned in to the teacher.

1. Which method(s) for preventing pregnancy would you like to know more about?
2. How will you find that out?
3. Which method seems most convenient?
4. Which method has the fewest side effects that worry you?
5. Which methods are effective enough for you?
6. Which method do you think your boyfriend or girlfriend will be most interested in using?
7. Which method would your parent(s) be most likely to approve?
8. Share your conclusions from this self-exam by circling the numbers that show which methods seem best for you. (*Note:* Each of the following methods is rated on a scale of 1 to 3, with 1 the "best choice," 2 an "OK choice," and 3

the "worst choice": abstinence, condoms, foam, condom + foam or sponge, sponge, pill.)

(SOURCE: Richard P. Barth, MSW, Ph.D., *Reducing the Risk: Building Skills to Prevent Pregnancy, STD & HIV* (Santa Cruz, Calif.: ETR Associates, 1993), Worksheet 8.3, page 127. Reprinted with permission; for information about this and other related materials, call 800-321-4407.)

STEM SENTENCES

Another introspective writing method asks learners to complete stem sentences. For example, when asked to respond to "A person who gives someone an STD is . . ." learners might respond, aloud or on paper, with a variety of opinions and feelings about such a person. You can develop any number of stem sentences for a given concept or topic and use them to get a group warmed up and focused, as a way of stimulating discussion, as a dyad or triad activity, or as a solo thinking activity.

Here are some sample stem sentences on a variety of topics:

1. *Relationships*
   - I feel best about myself when I am with . . .
   - The person who makes me think the most is . . .
   - I think it would be really risky for me to spend much time with . . .
   - I most admire people who . . .
   - The person who gives me the best advice is . . .
   - The characteristics I look for in a best friend are . . .
   - I can trust people who . . .
   - I am hurt or frustrated by friends who . . .

2. *Gender differences*
   - I am most hurt when a person of the opposite gender . . .
   - Women trust men who . . .
   - Men trust women who . . .
   - The ways boys and girls are alike are . . .
   - Gender role stereotypes are harmful when . . .

3. *Contraception*
   - The best method of contraception for teens is . . .
   - The best method of contraception for me right now is . . .
   - Under no circumstances would I ever use . . .
   - People who have sex and don't use protection are . . .

4. *Body image*
   - The aspect I like most about my body is . . .
   - I am really pleased with my physical ability to . . .
   - What I would like to change about my body is . . .

5. *Love*
   - Loving someone means . . .
   - I would most appreciate someone showing love for me by . . .
   - The qualities I would look for in someone I could love are . . .

DRAWING

Drawing pictures, symbols, and diagrams can substitute for writing and may be particularly useful for younger or less literate learners, and to appeal to a variety of learning styles. Drawing ability, for the purposes of sexuality or family life education, is unimportant, for which some learners will need reassurance. The intent is to provide a medium for expressing ideas and feelings. For example, children may be asked to draw the ideal family, or a picture of "a best friend." Or, in an activity used more to increase comfort or assess knowledge (rather than introspection), groups may be asked to diagram male and female reproductive systems.

One example of a drawing activity is "Girls and Boys" in *When I'm Grown: Life Planning Education for Grades 3 & 4*,[2] the purpose of which is to identify children's attitudes about gender roles and stereotypes. Following a whip exercise (see Chapter 10, where this activity is reprinted), the teacher asks the children to make drawings showing what they think is the *best* thing about being a girl or a boy. Students then complete a series of stem sentences about stereotypes (e.g., "girls can't . . . ," "boys are so . . .") and discuss the harmfulness of stereotypes.

RESPONDING TO PICTURES

Many sexuality educators use pictures to analyze messages from the popular media. Since much of the media, particularly advertising, is subtly or even blatantly sexual, such activities could be used to enhance critical thinking skills.

For example, during the lesson called "Media Messages" in *New Methods for Puberty Education*,[3] students bring in magazines with a variety of advertisements showing male and female models. They then analyze the differences among the models in the pictures; afterward they discuss their own reactions to the pictures, the standards of beauty portrayed there, and how the pictures made them feel about their own bodies. You could ask older students more specifically to judge whether some aspect of an advertisement gives a negative or a positive message about women, gender roles, relationships, or other aspects of sexuality.

In another activity in *New Methods for Puberty Education*,[4] groups of students make collages of pictures of individuals representing a range of body types, styles, and ages. Students then complete a "Picture Survey" that asks a variety of questions (e.g., "Which person seems the most self-confident?") and discuss the factors that influence their opinions.

GUIDED IMAGERY

Guided imagery recruits and uses all the senses, synthesizing images in the mind of the learner. The images are often visual or kinesthetic (involving body movement), but sometimes are also aural (i.e., the learner remembers or imagines a sound or spoken words), or involve smell and taste memories.

Sexuality educators sometimes use guided imagery to help learners clarify values and feelings or to imagine themselves successfully using a skill. Use it also for teaching about decision making, or for relaxation.

The story "A Friend Discloses" (see box) is used in lessons on HIV/AIDS to teach tolerance and empathy. The facilitator should control the environment for distractions and interruptions, make sure that all learners are comfortable and attentive, and then say the story, with pauses for learners to follow their own thoughts.

A Friend Discloses

Close your eyes; or, if that makes you uncomfortable, look down. Get comfortable; relax. Take a deep breath and let it out.

Imagine that you have a very good friend. You really like this person; he or she is very nice, very considerate. This friend has all the characteristics you admire and like in people. You have lots of fun together. You do lots of things together.

Imagine some of the times you have together. You talk a lot with this friend; you share things, talk about things you have never shared with anyone before. You trust this person.

One day you are just hanging out—walking around one of your favorite places. Notice where you are. Notice what is going on around you, who is there, what noises you hear, what smells you smell. You are talking about things, and suddenly your friend says, "I have something to tell you. I have AIDS."

You had no idea; you are very surprised. How do you feel, hearing what your friend has told you? What do you say? What is the first thing you do? How does your friend feel about your reaction?

Think about your feelings for a few minutes. When you are ready, come back to the present and open your eyes.

The facilitator should follow this story with a process for helping learners articulate their feelings, perhaps doing some introspective writing, then sharing in dyads or triads. Or proceed with a whole group discussion.

Another example of a guided imagery exercise is in "Where Does Violence Come From," a lesson in the high school curriculum, *Life Planning Education: A Youth Development Program*.[5] Students brainstorm factors that cause violence among teens. The educator then focuses on anger as a cause of violence and asks participants to close their eyes and recall recent incidents during which they became angry. Then they discuss the feelings, including physical sensations, associated with those events.

When sexuality educators use guided imagery, they usually use a combination of two types: *remembering* and *imagining*. While *remembering,* the learner thinks about his or her past; for example, teens or adults may be asked to think back to a specific incident that gave them their first information about puberty changes.

When we ask learners to *imagine,* we help them develop awareness of specific feelings regarding a hypothetical or potential situation; for example, learners may be asked to imagine themselves in a situation they presumably have never experienced and to examine the feelings evoked. While imagining a potential problem situation, the learner can turn insight into a rehearsal of action by clarifying feelings, looking at options, choosing an option, affirming the choice, creating a concrete plan, and doing rehearsal in his or her mind.

The successful facilitator of a guided imagery must be accepting, compassionate, permissive, attentive, patient, relaxed, and trusted by the learner. The facilitator must not evaluate or interpret the experience for the learner.

The use of guided imagery in public school education may be objectionable to some. With this method, after all, teachers deliberately ask students to use imagination. However, guided imagery and imagination are considered acceptable within many contexts: with athletes, to visualize an action to improve performance; in television and movies, which use intense visual and aural bombardment to stimulate imagination; in the health field for behavior change (e.g., smoking cessation) and pain control; and even in some religious settings as a form of prayer. Furthermore, teens have active imaginations; their current fantasies may include images and scripts that motivate sexual risk taking and serve as obstacles to well thought out behavior. Skillful use of guided imagery enhances learning in a variety of settings and, in our opinion, is appropriate for public school classrooms.[6]

JOURNALS

The purpose of journal writing is to encourage students to reflect on the content and processes of their sexuality education program and to help them express personal reactions, values, attitudes, beliefs, and feelings. A useful method for longer workshops, courses or seminars, journal writing may include reactions, feelings, note taking, response to specific questions, action plans, and so on.

Advocates for Youth's *Life Planning Education: A Youth Development Program* includes a journal process throughout. The program suggests a variety of ways for using journals:[7]

- Build in 5–10 minutes at the end of sessions for teens to record their reflections on what happened.
- Assign 10–15 minutes at certain times during sessions when journal writing is most useful.
- Structure journal writing so teens respond to specific questions, or leave it unstructured so they can write about their experiences in any way they choose.
- Journals can be shared with the teacher, the whole group, or kept confidential.

Another colleague, in her human sexuality course, uses journal writing as a series of self-awareness exercises for students. For example, students may be asked to describe how they feel about their own sexuality; or, in a section on gender development and gender role socialization, they answer the questions, "What is your earliest memory of being treated differently because you are a boy/girl?" "In your home, what is expected of girls/boys?" "In elementary school, what did boys/girls get to do that you didn't get to do?" "Who are the three people of your own gender you most admire?"[8] Students may discuss their responses in dyads.

The *Human Sexuality: Values and Choices* curriculum[9] provides a "Student Thought Book" for a variation on journal writing. This "journal" is actually a series of questionnaires, inventories, stories, and other guided writing activities students can use throughout the curriculum.

CHAPTER 9

Giving and Gathering Information and Examining Concepts, Facts, and Ideas

In this chapter we examine methods for teaching in the cognitive domain, that is, ways of giving and gathering information, facts, and ideas, and ways of encouraging examination and learning of concepts.

Sexuality educators must have effective means of presenting and gathering information for a variety of reasons:

- To help learners review what they already know.
- To give learners information they need for understanding their own susceptibility.
- To give learners information they need for effective decision making and other life skills.
- To correct misinformation, myths, and misunderstandings.
- To assure them of the efficacy of protective methods (e.g., condoms, effective communication skills, etc.).
- To ensure a common group vocabulary for the lesson.
- To address learner questions, concerns, and anxieties.
- To disequilibrate learners.
- To encourage sharing of learner-held information.

Some cognitive methods, particularly lecture, are ineffective. Unfortunately, lecture and presentation are the predominant teaching methods in this culture and often seem to reassure school administrators, teachers, and parents that learning is taking place. Many seem to think that if we just tell our students the right message, loud enough, often enough, and with enough scary stories, then they won't have sex.

However, learners need practical, relevant information that will be related to affective and behavioral growth. New information is very important if it builds on learners' existing concepts of the world and if it can become operative (see Chapter 4). To meet learner needs, educators must offer information about sexuality in a variety of forms, using a variety of teaching methods.

Since learners have considerable misinformation about sexuality and related topics (e.g., contraception), it is important that educators find ways of assessing learner knowledge for several reasons: to provide a baseline needs and interest assessment, to enable the educator to correct misinformation, and to aid in the assimilation and accommodation of new information. Therefore, several of the methods presented here focus on gathering learner-held information; also, please refer to Chapter 13 for a discussion of student evaluation.

PRESENTATIONS

We begin this section on cognitive methods with a discussion of presentations, the mainstay method for imparting information. We suggest that you follow the following steps as you prepare and make sexuality presentations:

1. *Be well prepared, clear, concise, accurate, relevant, and honest.* Do your research well, and don't exaggerate facts in an attempt to manipulate behavior. Again, focus your content on learner needs and interests, giving information that has significance and relevance.

2. *Assess and adapt the physical environment.* If possible and necessary, rearrange seating to facilitate the attention of all learners.

3. *Assess the needs of individuals and the group,* both to give yourself needed information and to help students focus on the topic and get involved; in the box are two examples of brief assessments.

Assessment Example 1. In a lesson on contraception, begin by asking all learners to do the assignment you have posted, for example, "During the next two minutes, write down all the birth control methods you can think of and be prepared to share." While students are writing, you might take care of attendance or other necessary paperwork. Or, if you are a guest speaker, you have valuable time to observe group and individual behavior and to gather your thoughts. Follow this activity by asking learners to volunteer their information, by calling on a few to share what they have written, or by asking learners to form small groups and discuss their responses with other learners. This activity has an advantage over simply asking the group to review methods of birth control, in that it demands the involvement of all individuals.

Assessment Example 2. In a lesson on relationships, begin by asking the group to brainstorm all the different kinds of relationships they can name; post these as they list them. (See other ideas for on-the-spot needs assessment in Chapter 7.)

4. *Focus on the learners.* Many educators, especially those who are nervous about speaking in front of groups, are tempted to focus on content. By knowing your material well, you can focus more of your attention on individuals and the group.

Assess learner needs and interests before, during and after your presentation; remain attentive to learner responses (verbal and body language) as you talk.

5. *Capture their interest.* Not all of us can be charismatic, but we can make an attempt to connect with our learners, to touch them in some way. Try telling a story, one that is culturally appropriate and with which learners will identify. Give a startling statement ("Within ten years, fifteen of you will have had at least one STD, and two of you will be sterile"). Use a quotation from music, poetry, philosophy, or literature and build on it. Role play someone who is famous to your students, or act out a mini-drama. Use humor; tease the learners—gently, and only if they respond in kind!

6. *Build your presentation around a few key concepts* and stick to them. As you introduce your presentation, post your objective(s) and describe the key concepts to be examined in this session. Describe the logical relationship between this lesson and previous lessons; describe the relationship between your information and learner knowledge or misinformation. For the community educator who is a guest speaker, this necessitates both the ability to think and act spontaneously and prior discussion with the host classroom teacher.

7. *Remember that what you say is not necessarily what they perceive or comprehend.* Learner understanding of information may be inaccurate, depending upon the nature of the material and individual receptivity. Learners may selectively ignore, misread, mishear, or forget information that does not fit their current understanding or perception of the world. Check understanding periodically by asking open-ended questions and listening to learners during other active and interactive activities.

8. *Focus on the positive.* Much of the misinformation learners have focuses on the negative. For instance, many people believe that contraceptive pills are dangerous, when in fact they are safer than many over-the-counter medications and are protective for certain types of cancer. Such negative information doesn't reduce risk taking; it makes people scared risk takers! Positive information, focusing on pros rather than cons, is more effective than negative information.[1]

9. *Consider aloud the broad range of values and beliefs* on any issue (particularly controversial topics) and acknowledge them. Show respect for diverse family and religious perspectives and teach a respect for diversity and pluralism (see Chapters 2 and 5). Your opinions, and the opinions and beliefs of your sources, should be declared as such. Be clear about the connections you make between facts and theory or opinion.

10. *Anticipate special circumstances and conditions of individuals.* For example, as you give information about problem pregnancies, be aware that there may be a pregnant girl or teen father in the classroom. As you teach about relationships and intimacy, assume that there are gay, lesbian, or bisexual participants and use language that is inclusive. Also, take into consideration that some learners may have disabilities that make presentations a difficult method for them.

11. *Use clear language, and anticipate language differences.* Define your terms, post key definitions, and ask for participant definitions. While you use what you think is common terminology, consider that learners may use idioms and euphemisms from their families and subcultures. For example, some young children may not know the words "penis" or "vagina," having only heard "wee-wee"

and "bottom." Ask learners to share their words in ways that do not embarrass them: "Let's brainstorm all the words *people* use for 'penis' " (not "all the words *you* use"). Have learners say (or shout!) new words aloud. Consider learners for whom English is a second language.

12. *Remember that many sexuality topics can heighten learner feelings about prior personal experiences.* For example, as you present a lesson about sexual abuse, incest, inappropriate touch, date rape, or other sexual exploitation, know that some of your learners will have had these experiences. Be prepared to deal with the consequences of discussing these topics (e.g., disclosure by a student that s/he is currently experiencing incest, and subsequent reporting requirements). Be sensitive to the feelings that such information can raise, feelings that can make learners inattentive or feelings that will enhance learning by disequilibrating them. Please see Chapter 5 for a review of this issue.

13. *Pay attention to learning style differences.* Many students learn better kinesthetically; combine hands-on experiences with your presentations (see Chapter 12). Many need visual cues; use plastic models, show samples, post key words, give handouts, use flip charts, overhead transparencies, or posters. Encourage learners to take notes.

14. *Show enthusiasm for your topic and for the group* in a way that is consistent with your comfort and style. Try getting out from behind the podium, tables, desk, overhead projector, slide projector; walk among learners, back and forth in front of them. Convey your message with energy in your posture, movement, and expression. Vary the rate, pitch, and volume of your voice. React honestly to the group; show your feelings and that you are human too! Use humor appropriately.

15. *Follow your presentation with activities* that help the learner process, review, and remember the information, with methods that help learners analyze the material (e.g., worksheets, following later in this chapter) and articulate their feelings and values (affective learning methods—see Chapter 10), and with methods that help learners apply the information (behavioral learning methods—see Chapter 11).

The person who speaks is the person who learns; when the sexuality educator does all the talking, learners have less opportunity to analyze, discuss, ask questions, get ideas and input from other learners, and otherwise process the information. Presentations are less passive if you involve learners by a number of means, including making eye contact, showing enthusiasm, using appropriate humor, making process observations, asking process questions, asking informational and open-ended questions, and utilizing other methods that are visual and kinesthetic. We suggest that you focus on developing a relationship with your learners; your presentations can become a conversation, a basic part of that relationship.

Several of the best sexuality education curricula include suggested scripts for presentations; here are some examples.

1. *F.L.A.S.H.* All the *Family Life and Sexual Health* curricula provide background notes for teachers that can be adapted for presentations. For example, in *9/10 F.L.A.S.H.,*[2] Lesson Plan 13 on "The Developing Baby" includes six transparencies of physiology diagrams, extensive background notes for use with each transparency, and a transparency that reviews important vocabulary for understanding the physiology of pregnancy.

2. The curriculum *Postponing Sexual Involvement*[3] is built around a series of scripted presentations. Some of the presentations are given as the audio portion of a video; or, with the sound turned off, the script can be spoken by trained older teens.

3. The *Reducing the Risk*[4] curriculum includes, in each class lesson, step-by-step presentation suggestions for introducing, delivering, and processing all the activities.

PROPS: MEDIA AND EQUIPMENT FOR ENHANCING PRESENTATIONS

Visual and "hands-on" props, including models, displays, slides, charts, posters, flip charts, and overhead transparencies, augment presentations and activities.

Many excellent models of sexual and reproductive anatomy are available to sexuality educators and are useful if only because many people learn visually. Others need visual input to enhance aural understanding. We offer the following suggestions for their use:

1. Be cautious; some people are offended by seeing realistic models of human genitalia.
2. Make sure models are accurate, complete, and easily explained and understood. Check learner interpretation; what may look like a uterus and fallopian tubes to you could represent a plastic ear to others. Many children find it difficult to perceive, for example, that the plastic model they see represents an *internal* organ.
3. Allow learners to handle and explore models; remember, some individuals learn best through kinesthetic or tactile means.
4. Do not waste limited budgets on expensive models; use or make less expensive ones. Even better, have learners make models (see Chapter 12 for examples of kinesthetic and tactile methods, including ideas for making models).
5. Use models that reflect diversity. For example, if you use models of human anatomy, make sure some have dark skin, others light.

Sexuality educators often can borrow models from local family planning clinics and Planned Parenthoods; or call them for information about commercial sources. The following activity (see box) uses a model—an apple—as an abstract, three-dimensional representation of the earth.

Earth: The Apple of Our Eye

Procedure. Ask students to consider the earth an apple (hold up an apple). Slice the apple into quarters. Set aside three of the quarters. What do these represent? (They represent the oceans of the world.)

What fraction do you have left? (1/4). Slice this land into half. Set aside one of the portions. This set-aside portion represents the land area that is inhospitable to people: the polar areas, deserts, swamps, very high or rocky mountains.

What fraction do you have left? (1/8). The piece that is left is land area where people live but not necessarily where they grow the foods needed for life.

Slice the 1/8 piece into four sections. Set aside three of these. What fraction do you have left? (1/32.) The 3/32 set aside represents the areas too rocky, too wet, too cold, too steep, or with too poor soil to actually produce food. They also contain the cities, suburban sprawl, highways, shopping centers, schools, parks, factories, parking lots, and other places where people live but do not necessarily grow food.

Carefully peel the 1/32 slice of the earth. This tiny bit of peeling represents the surface, the very thin skin of the earth's crust upon which mankind depends. It is less than five feet deep and is a quite fixed amount of food-producing land. Protecting our land resources is very important. Advanced agricultural technology has enabled the world to feed many of its people. But, with a fixed land resource base and an ever-increasing number of people to feed from that fixed base, each person's portion becomes smaller and smaller. It is essential to protect the environmental quality of our air, water, and land.

(SOURCE: Reprinted by permission from Zero Population Growth, Inc., as printed in *For Earth's Sake: Lessons in Population and Environment*, copyright 1989.)

The classic display items for sexuality education programs are samples of contraceptives for lessons on birth control, and condoms and other barriers for STD/HIV risk reduction lessons. We suggest the following guidelines for the display of contraceptive and safer sex materials:

- Some school districts or programs do not allow any display of contraceptives or barriers; others do not allow them to be handled by students. Ascertain policies before your presentation.
- Allowing learners to handle display items can be an excellent learning experience, especially for those who are tactile in learning style.
- An effective way to teach condom use is to have learners practice putting them on models of erect penises (or other representative objects). This practice takes the lesson beyond cognitive learning into the behavioral domain.

Our recommendations for use of graphs, charts, slides, and other visual aids are similar to those for all other sexuality education materials:

- Make sure that all visual aids are accurate, complete, and free from bias. For example, anatomy and physiology charts often exclude the clitoris, reflecting a reproductive bias and ignoring sexual response for females.
- Use only those materials that are approved by your program.
- Understand your materials thoroughly, and be prepared for learner questions and misunderstanding.
- See Appendix A for other guidelines for reviewing materials.

Here are some ideas for the use of slides and posters.

1. Showing slides and photos of STD infected genitals is a classic scare tactic in sexuality education. The risk is that students will say, "This grosses me out. It's

obviously not me—so why should I listen?" However, a colleague uses slides and skillful humor to jar students out of their complacency, at the same time getting them to personalize their own susceptibility. Rather than approaching the slide presentation as a serious warning, she says, "None of you have teflon-coated genitals. Your genitals are part of your body—they can get colds just like the rest of you. You get a runny nose? You can get a runny vagina!" She assures students that they don't have to look at the slides and also intersperses photos of healthy and infected genitals with pictures of landscapes, using the interim to give information she wants them to hear without being distracted. Her main goal is to get adolescents to pay attention to their genitals as they would any part of their body: to take care of them, look at them, understand their important functions.

2. The curriculum *Human Sexuality: Values and Choices*[5] is built on seven values essential for maintaining positive human relationships: equality, self-control, promise keeping, responsibility, respect, honesty, and social justice. A poster listing these values is available from that book's publisher for use in the classroom.

Skilled educators make effective use of chalk or dry erase boards, flip charts and easels, or overhead projectors to enhance their presentations and discussions. We offer the following ideas for sexuality educators:

1. Label or color overhead transparencies of reproductive anatomy (with a washable overhead pen), part by part, as you go through your presentation.
2. Many curricula offer excellent overhead transparency masters, among them *F.L.A.S.H., When I'm Grown,* and *Taught Not Caught.* The latter has anatomical drawings that appear three-dimensional. Watch for gender inequities in anatomical drawings; some include the glans and penis on the male, but not the clitoris on the female; others include the anus on the female but not the male.

VIDEOS

Videos too often are used as a substitute for good sexuality education. However, if they are used selectively, skillfully, and appropriately, videos can complement a sound program or curriculum.

We suggest the following steps for using sexuality education videos:

1. Preview *all* sexuality education videos. If you are a classroom teacher and your guest speaker is bringing a video, be sure to preview it. If your school district or program has restrictions on use of preapproved materials, follow those restrictions.
2. Choose a video that is less than half of your allotted time (or select a cut from a longer video) to allow time for processing issues, concerns, questions, values, and key concepts.
3. Start your session with an activity that involves learners and helps them focus on the topic: an introspective focusing exercise, a brainstorm, or a small group discussion of concerns related to the content of the video.
4. Introduce the video by discussing or presenting the following: its title; its intended purpose, and your purpose for using it; key concepts or facts to look

for; how it relates to previous learnings; suggestions on how to view it; issues in the video the group will explore later; unique or interesting facts about the video; what activities will follow the video.

5. Be sensitive to learners' comfort levels and warn them about video sequences they may find distressing, such as childbirth scenes. Discuss these feelings before and after showing the video.

6. Show the video, or a segment of it.

7. Be sure to allow time to debrief the video. Don't end a program with a video, since much of its benefit lies in adequate processing. Learners will have varying experiences of the video, and may have misconceptions about information received, depending on how its content relates to previously held concepts. Lead a discussion, starting with specific questions about video content and proceeding to more general, open-ended questions about values, policies, cultural context, or action needed. Address questions and concerns raised by learners. Relate the video to previous learnings. Follow the video with other appropriate learning methods that help learners examine and retain information and concepts, analyze and reflect on values, feelings, and attitudes, and practice skills or new behaviors.

Use videos in creative ways that engage learners actively; here are some ideas:

1. Show one vignette, stop the video, discuss the behaviors shown, and role play or practice skills. For example, *Human Sexuality: Values and Choices*[6] provides a video to be used at various points in the curriculum; some segments are vignettes that students view, discuss, and then role play, taking on the roles and practicing the refusal skills shown in the video.

2. Stop the video before a crucial point; discuss or role play possible conclusions.

3. Play a segment of the video with no sound, discussing the meaning of video characters' body language as it is happening; for example, after viewing a vignette of one person trying to get another to have sex, discuss whether or not the person who was resisting used body language consistent with his or her intent.

4. Show a short vignette; stop the video, give an assignment of what to watch for ("What are Sally's options in this problem situation with her parents?"), and immediately show it a second time.

5. Show just the crisis point; ask learners, "What do you think brought the characters to this point?"

6. Show segments of informational videos at different times in your program, allowing time after each segment to process and augment information.

By themselves, videos are a passive educational method, and as such are received by many learners as entertainment, a time to "vegetate" or think about other concerns. Television is omnipresent in our culture, and many viewers have become desensitized, because of daily bombardment, to whatever is seen there; passive viewing of many programs no longer reaches many of our learners.

However, good videos skillfully incorporated in a series of activities can expose individuals vicariously to a wider range of values, cultures, behaviors, dilemmas, and choices than might be available in the group. This wider range of vicarious experiences may present options that are appealing to learners, disequilibrating, or even offensive, causing rejection.

Furthermore, videos allow safe introspective time. They may be appropriate for introducing subjects that groups have difficulty discussing, such as HIV/AIDS. Videos provide a common vocabulary, a common experience for group interaction following viewing. In a mature group, videos can provide an excellent focus for discussion, disagreement, and debate with less risk of personalizing conflicts; the focus can be kept on the video rather than on group members.

Videos also can lend authority and credence to your message. They can fill holes in an agenda and give you a break from being "on stage," but can't substitute for your skills as a discussion leader and activity facilitator. Don't depend on videos as a substitute for more active sexuality education methods; most learners benefit much more from direct interaction with the educator and with each other.

When deciding to use a video, consider the content of your sexuality or HIV lesson:

- Does the video "fit" the context within which it is viewed?
- Are you using it at the right time in the program?
- Does it provide information or viewpoints that build on earlier learning?
- Does it present information or viewpoints in an appealing way that will capture viewers' attention?
- Is it too long or short? Can you show only the segments needed?
- Does it augment your program? Or does it duplicate content covered in other ways?

Evaluate the content of the video itself. Is it appropriate, accurate, efficient, inclusive, appealing, and effective? Does it address sexuality and HIV issues and promote universal values? SIECUS, the Sex Information and Education Council of the U.S., publishes *HIV/AIDS Audiovisual Resources,*[7] an excellent guide to selecting, evaluating, and using videos. Also, see other guidelines and tools for evaluating sexuality education materials in Appendix A.

ANONYMOUS QUESTIONS

Addressing learner questions is basic to the educator's role. Providing opportunities for anonymous questions is uniquely important in sexuality education because of our culture's discomfort with the subject. Use of this method elicits questions and clarifies misunderstandings that otherwise might not be addressed directly in the class.

To facilitate the anonymous question process, distribute 3 x 5 cards to all learners and ask them to write their questions on the cards. To protect anonymity, all cards (or other paper) should look alike, and all learners should write a question (or, if they can't think of one, a comment). Classroom teachers may find that anonymity and confidentiality are difficult to protect in a question box kept in the classroom; we recommend the repository be kept accessible to students (so they can add questions at any time) but in a place where it would be difficult for students to break into and look for familiar handwriting, such as on the teacher's desk. Or, have question cards completed all at once and collect them immediately. Questions may be collected on one day and answered at the next session or lesson. The educator then has the opportunity to study questions and rehearse responses.

The *F.L.A.S.H.* curricula utilize a set of manila envelopes pinned to a bulletin board and labeled with the topics to be covered in that particular series of lessons. For example, in *9/10 F.L.A.S.H.*,[8] the envelopes are labeled as follows: (1) touch, abstinence, and general questions; (2) reproductive system; (3) puberty and adolescence; (4) sexual exploitation (including rape); (5) pregnancy; (6) planning to parent; (7) unplanned pregnancy; (8) contraception; (9) sexually transmitted diseases, including AIDS; and (10) sexual health care. The process for eliciting questions is given in the box.

Anonymous Questions

You will have prepared, in advance, ten large manila envelopes (and optionally, a bulletin board), labeled [with unit topics]. In fact, you may want a separate set of manila envelopes for each period of the day.

Show the class these envelopes and give each student several small pieces of scrap paper. Ask them to write at least one question and drop it in the appropriate envelope. Explain that they should not write their names on the slip, unless they prefer to talk with you privately about their question. Have them write only one question per slip (to facilitate your sorting the questions into logical order, later), but give them as many slips as they need.

If people are unsure about which envelope is appropriate for a particular question, they can use their judgment and you can rearrange them later. (Or, if they express concern that others see which envelope they choose, they can drop them in a folder you can sort out later.)

Explain that, as each lesson arrives, you will answer the questions from the appropriate envelope, so it's OK to add questions as they think of them, in the days to come. Allow about 5 minutes for the writing of questions. You may want to assist the class by jotting some sample question roots on the blackboard: "Is it true that . . ."; "How do you know if . . ."; "What causes . . ."; "What do they mean by . . ."; "Should you worry if . . ."; "What should you do if . . . ."

(SOURCE: Elizabeth Reis, MS, *9/10 F.L.A.S.H.* [Seattle: Seattle–King County Department of Public Health, 1989], 5; reprinted with permission from Family Planning/STD Program, Seattle–King County Department of Public Health.)

Our suggestions for responding to questions apply to anonymous questions as well as those that are asked openly:

1. Try to respond to or acknowledge all questions.
2. Paraphrase the question to change slang, correct terminology, or check your understanding. Ask learners to help you understand confusing questions: "Do you think this question means . . . ?" If you decide it could mean more than one thing, address all possibilities.
3. Affirm the asker and legitimize the question: "I am very glad you asked that"; "Many people ask this question"; "This is an important question." Do not laugh at or belittle a question; it may be funny to you but serious to the questioner. React positively; a negative response (e.g., "You are too young to be asking this") can diminish further communication.
4. Answer the factual part of the question, if there is one.
5. Turn the question back to the group, asking for group input to stimulate discussion. The purpose of anonymous questions is not just to give and clarify information; the process can also help students begin to use the words, be capable of talking about sexuality.
6. Describe the range of beliefs and values on the topic, asking for learner input.
7. To check for understanding, ask learners to paraphrase your answer.
8. Always preserve confidences and anonymity; if a question seems to give enough details to enable others to know who is asking, rephrase it and leave out details. Invite students to put their names on the question cards if they want to talk with you privately, but assure them that if they do so, you will keep their confidences (see Chapter 5 regarding legal limits to confidentiality).
9. Pay attention to your language: be inclusive; don't assume that all your students will someday have children, will get married, know who their grandparents are, are heterosexual, are sexually active, or aren't sexually active; don't use sexist, racist, or heterosexist language, or communicate disdain for certain age groups, classes, cultures, disabilities, and so on.
10. Be aware of possible underlying issues; often, there is history to a question. For example, if a sixteen-year-old girl asks about fertile cycles, she may have been having intercourse during what she thought was her infertile period and might be worried she is pregnant. Likewise, frequent questions about condoms may be based on the school district's recent decision not to distribute condoms in the school health clinic. But try not to jump to conclusions or make assumptions about a person's behavior or history based on his or her question. Please see Chapter 5 for a review of some of the special challenges sexuality educators confront when answering student questions.
11. Monitor your nonverbal behaviors while responding to questions; you could be communicating powerful judgments and assumptions.
12. Decide on the nature of the question and respond accordingly:

   • *Requests for information.* Be honest; all requests for information should be answered by giving the information. If you don't know the answer, say so; say that you will find out or refer the questioner to someone who can answer. Consider the age and developmental level of questioners; different age groups require different levels of information and answers at various levels of sophistication. Pre- and early adolescents need simpler, more concrete answers. Don't give too much unnecessary information.

- *Questions about your beliefs, values, or behavior.* "Do you think teens should have sex?" "How old were you when you first had sex?" "Doesn't teaching about sex turn you on?" Remind learners of ground rules about everyone's right to privacy and discussion of personal behavior; redirect discussion to the issue behind the question. The intent of such questions may be to obtain your permission or approval for a particular behavior; your response should reflect some universal values and a broad range of opinions and beliefs. Never discuss your own sexual behavior.
- *Questions that reflect concerns about normalcy.* "When do most boys start shaving?" Validate the question ("Lots of people are curious about that") and provide necessary physiological, developmental, legal, and medical information.
- *Questions intended to shock the educator or the group.* Remind learners of ground rules. Reserve the right to change language used for shock value to "correct" language, making sure your vocabulary is understood by all.
- *Values questions.* Consider the values components to all questions, and give all viewpoints; for example, all responses to questions about masturbation (like any controversial topic), even though fact-seeking on the surface, should address the broad range of values on masturbation. Do not impose your own personal values, but do express positive regard for universal values (see Chapter 2). Encourage children to discuss values with their families. In the box is a suggested protocol for answering values questions.

Values Question Protocol

1. Affirm the student for asking: "Good question"; "That's an important issue"; "I'm glad you asked"; "A lot of people wonder that."
2. Identify it as a belief question (distinguishing it from factual questions): "That's a value question. We can't look up the answer, because every person, family, and religion has a different answer."
3. Answer the factual part, if there is one. "Before we look at beliefs, let's examine a few facts. Most people masturbate as babies. After that, some continue on and off for the rest of their lives and others decide to stop. Another fact you need to know is that masturbating doesn't hurt a person's body. People used to think it would make you go blind, or give you warts, for example. It doesn't do those things."
4. Help the class describe the range of beliefs . . . not theirs, but society's. "Different people believe different things about masturbation. What do you think some people believe?" Here, the teacher has two jobs: (1) to ensure that as complete a range of beliefs as possible is described, and (2) to ensure that

each belief position is expressed in as fair and even-handed a way as possible, preferably in the way the person who holds it would describe it if s/he were there.

5. State your own belief, if it is asked for and if it is relatively universal. Thus, on the topic of masturbation (or abortion or homosexual behavior, etc.) it would not be appropriate for a teacher to express his or her own belief. Whereas, if the question had been, "What do you think about people teasing a classmate who they think is gay?" the teacher could very legitimately say, at this point in the protocol, "You asked my opinion; I think that's wrong," because all persons, regardless of gender identity, role, or orientation, are unique (entitled not to be stereotyped), valuable, and deserving of equal and considerate treatment.

6. Refer to family, clergy, and other trusted adults. "Since people have such different beliefs about masturbation, I would encourage all of you to find out what your families believe. Talk about it with people you trust, especially adults. For example, if you belong to a church, synagogue, mosque, or temple, find out what they teach."

(SOURCE: Elizabeth Reis, MS, *11/12 F.L.A.S.H.* [Seattle: Seattle–King County Department of Public Health, 1992], vi–vii; reprinted with permission from Family Planning/STD Program, Seattle–King County Department of Public Health.)

USING BOOKS

Though there are many excellent curricula, we know of very few good, comprehensive sexuality education textbooks for use in grades K–12.[9] Indeed, the sexuality education components of many health education texts have been censored recently,[10] even to the extent of removing diagrams showing techniques for breast and testicular self-exam, which were considered too sexually explicit.

However, many other good books, covering a broad range of topics, are available for teens and younger children. Many of the best sexuality education curricula include extensive lists of these books, for example, *New Methods for Puberty Education, Teaching Safer Sex, Positive Images: A New Approach to Contraceptive Education, Streetwise to Sex-Wise: Sexuality Education for High Risk Youth,* and all the *Life Planning Education* and *When I'm Grown* curricula. SIECUS provides a number of annotated bibliographies, and ETR Associates publishes and distributes a number of books and pamphlets (see Appendix C for addresses); other bibliographies are listed in the Selected Bibliography. The *F.L.A.S.H.* curricula list sources of books. Also, your local Planned Parenthood or health department may have a resource library and/or book store.

We suggest that sexuality educators use a variety of resource books (including short stories and novels), brochures, pamphlets, and handouts. Review the many materials available and collect a library of resources and lists of references for your learners.

An activity in *New Methods for Puberty Education* offers a rationale for students to own their own family life education book; we reprint the lesson here (see box), the lesson's assignment sheet later in this chapter, and, in Chapter 13, the form students use for evaluating their books.

Owning a Family Life Education Book

Objectives
1. The students will be able to evaluate their usage of a family life education book that they personally own.
2. The students will be able to analyze others' responses to their owning a family life education book.
3. The students will become aware of parents' support for them to acquire accurate information about sexuality.

Grades: 7–9.

Time: Thirty-minute introduction and 30-minute follow-up session.

Materials: A family life education book for each student (see Rationale), "Assignment Sheet," "Book Evaluation Form."

Rationale: Books and written materials are an integral part of the educational process. It is hard to imagine history, language arts, or mathematics being taught without the use of books. The time has come to get beyond the barriers that prevent schools from using books in their family life education courses.

This is a proposal for schools and parent organizations to present a gift of a family life education book to every student who participates in the school program. Parent organizations often have a budget for educational materials or the capabilities for raising funds for special projects, such as sales or raffles. We recommend that these funds be used to purchase the books for the students.

In these times of economic difficulties, it is convenient to use finances as an excuse for not utilizing books on sexuality. The real barriers, however, involve fear of negative community response and concern over how the students will use the books. This proposal offers a different perspective, emphasizing the positive values for obtaining information from reliable written sources. By involving parents in the gift-giving process, it bridges the gap that often exists between school and parents and provides students with the message that family life education is an area of study that is valued in the community.

Procedure
1. Tell the class that today's discussion will focus on what it's like to own a family life education book.
2. Discuss with the class some possible things that happen to family life education books. Write the following list on the board or have students brainstorm their own list:

Possible Things That Happen to Family Life Education Books:

- Pictures or slang words are sometimes written in the book.
- The book is read from cover to cover.
- Only certain parts of the book are read.
- The book gets lost or stolen.
- The owner hides it in his or her room.
- The owner discusses it with friends.
- The owner discusses it with parents.
- The owner lends the book.
- The book is thrown away.

Discussion Questions

> What things does the owner have control over?
>
> What are some of the reasons why family life books sometimes get defaced?
>
> Why do people sometimes feel embarrassed to own a family life education book?
>
> How do you think others would react if they saw you carrying a book about sexuality?
>
> What are some reasons why people read only certain parts of books?
>
> How might a person take care of a book that he or she owns?

3. Tell the students that they are going to receive books that are a gift from parents in the community. The books are theirs to keep and care for. Explain how the book was selected and why parents wanted them to have their own books. Distribute the books and have students write their names in them.

4. Distribute the "Assignment Sheet." Have the students select one of the alternatives for a final project.

(SOURCE: Carolyn Cooperman and Chuck Rhoades, *New Methods for Puberty Education* [Hackensack, N.J.: Planned Parenthood of Greater Northern New Jersey, Inc., 1992], 41–43; reprinted by permission from Planned Parenthood of Greater Northern New Jersey.)

OFFERING RESOURCES

If you are a classroom teacher, a community educator, or a professional trainer, you should know your community and where to refer people for additional resources, help, materials, information, or professional services. Often the most valuable piece of information learners glean from a presentation is where to go for help or answers to their questions. They may not remember any of your key concepts or facts, but they might remember the organizations mentioned as resources. Prepare handouts listing any of the following: local, state, and national AIDS hotlines; AIDS prevention, education, and support organizations; local, state, and national STD hotlines; county health department; school, college, and public libraries; STD and family planning clinics; Planned Parenthood; teen-parent support organizations; gay, lesbian, and bisexual youth support organizations; local chapter of PFLAG (Parents, Friends and Families of Lesbians and Gays); rape relief and sexual assault centers; state child abuse and neglect hotlines; domestic violence hotlines and women's shelters; community health center; migrant health center; crisis phone line; sex information line; private physicians, mental health therapists, nurse practitioners. Many city and county governments publish resource guides; you may wish to make your lists more narrowly focused, to correlate with the topics of your lessons.

ASSIGNMENTS: READING, RESEARCH, AND LEARNER PRESENTATIONS

Reading, research, and presentations can be done individually or in small groups. The educator should consider, when assigning reports, whether the information to be reported is necessary for the large group. Also, since learner reports often give misinformation, the educator must be prepared to correct inaccuracies and help learners distinguish opinions from facts in their reports.

A research and presentation assignment could follow these steps:

1. Assign for presentation only those topics necessary for the large group's learning. Several students could research and report on each of the contraceptive methods (condoms, vaginal spermicides, pills, abstinence, cervical cap, female condom, etc.); then other students could report on each of the common STDs in a later unit. Or, groups of students could research and report on *categories* of contraceptives (barrier methods, hormonal methods, etc.).
2. Whenever possible, allow learners to select topics in which they are interested.
3. Suggest that students include interactive methods in their presentations. Ask students to study and prepare not only the content of their presentation, but also the process, the teaching methods.
4. Look at student presentation outlines to assure completeness, correctness, and relative freedom from bias. Suggest students be ready to answer questions.
5. Give time limits; suggest that students practice and time their presentations.

New Methods for Puberty Education provides an assignment sheet (see the box) as part of the activity "Owning a Family Life Education Book" (reprinted earlier in this chapter).

Assignment Sheet II:4:A

Select one of the following and complete it by _____ .
A. Read and discuss a chapter of your choice with a parent. Write a brief report about this experience.
B. Carry the book with you, to and from home and around school, for one day. Write about how you felt doing this. Describe other people's reactions, if any.

C. Find a section of the book that you have strong feelings about. Write a report about why you think this section is important.
D. Make a collage about something you learned from reading the book.
E. Think about a topic area that you are interested in that is not included in the book. Write a statement about why you think this topic should have been covered.

(SOURCE: Carolyn Cooperman and Chuck Rhoades, *New Methods for Puberty Education* [Hackensack, N.J.: Planned Parenthood of Greater Northern New Jersey, Inc., 1992]; reprinted by permission from Planned Parenthood of Greater Northern New Jersey.)

Local organizations such as Planned Parenthoods often have information packets on contraception, STDs, sexual abuse, date rape, and many other topics that can be of help to students doing research. Many Planned Parenthood clinics or education departments have an extensive sexuality education library and experienced educators who are prepared to help students in research and presentations. Other organizations and youth serving agencies have extensive materials on a variety of topics. For example, American Friends Service Committee chapters have resources on sexual orientation issues; rape relief organizations and women's shelters have information on sexual abuse and exploitation; most health departments have a wide variety of brochures and other materials on family planning, STD, pregnancy, and other topics as well as experienced health educators who can be consulted.

WORKSHEETS

Educators often use "worksheets" to reinforce retention of figurative knowledge; we call them "tests" (see Chapter 13). Worksheets, by our definition, should provide opportunity and structure for students to analyze information, that is, to examine, question, evaluate, categorize, extrapolate, generalize, synthesize, compare, and contrast. Many curricula make excellent use of worksheets, among them *New Methods for Puberty Education* and *F.L.A.S.H.*

We offer an example of an activity (see the box) that utilizes two worksheets, one that provides information and the other that asks learners (in groups) to analyze that information and categorize it in an expanded format; there is also opportunity for learners to express their own opinions and to draw conclusions.

Sexuality Through the Life Span: Sex Is More than Intercourse

Objectives
1. Students will explore how sexuality develops and changes throughout the life span, from birth to death.
2. Students will learn that sexuality encompasses much more than sexual intercourse and includes all our attitudes, values, and behaviors related to being male or female.

3. Students will understand that outercourse (intimacy without intercourse) is a possible option for sex without risk of pregnancy.

Rationale: In today's society, "sex" usually refers to intercourse. As young people internalize this message from their environment, they may feel pressured to experience intercourse as an affirmation of their sexuality. This lesson is structured to heighten awareness of sexuality as an intrinsic part of every person's life, including their gender identity, gender role behavior, interpersonal relationships, and family life. By examining ways humans express their sexuality throughout the lifespan, students can broaden their understanding of their own sexual experience.

Materials: Worksheets "Sexuality through the Lifespan" and "Sex Is More than Intercourse"

Procedure
1. Note that humans are sexual beings from before birth until death. Discussion questions:
   a. What questions do young children ask about sex?
   b. What play activities do young children create to find out about their sexuality?
   c. Can you give any examples of sexual curiosity from your own childhood experience?
2. Divide the students into small groups and distribute both worksheets: "Sexuality through the Life Span" and "Sex Is More than Intercourse." The groups should work to reach consensus in completing the assignment.
3. Review the worksheets with the entire class. Discussion questions:
   a. What stage are you in? How does sexuality in the stage you are in compare with sexuality in other stages of the life span?
   b. How is sexuality in childhood similar to sexuality in old age? How is it different?
   c. (Explain that the word "outercourse" is used to describe intimate sexual relations without intercourse.) Describe some possible forms of outercourse. What are some of the reasons people choose to have outercourse rather than intercourse?
   d. What could parents do in raising children that would help them develop positive attitudes about their own sexuality?

Worksheet: Sexuality through the Life Span

Early Childhood (birth–3 years)
• Learns about love and trust through touching and holding
• Sucking (need for oral satisfaction)
• Boys: erection of penis
• Girls: vaginal lubrication
• Gender identity develops (child knows "I am a boy" or "I am a girl")

- Exploration of own body (hands, feet, genitals, etc.)
- Toilet training
- Possibility of orgasm
- Curiosity about differences between boys' and girls' bodies
- Curiosity about parents' bodies

Late Childhood (4–8 years)
- Childhood sexual play (i.e., "doctor")
- Sex role learning: how to behave like boy or girl
- Learns sex words: "bathroom vocabulary"
- Asks questions about pregnancy and birth
- Begins to distinguish acceptable and nonacceptable behavior
- Possibility of masturbation
- Becomes modest about own body
- Media influences understanding of male/female family roles

Early Adolescence (9–11 years)
- Puberty begins (growth of genitals, breast development, etc.)
- Possibility of masturbation
- Closeness of same-sex friends
- Possibility of body exploration with others

Adolescence (12–18 years)
- Pubertal changes continue
- Menstruation or sperm production
- Greater interest in sexuality
- Pleasure from kissing and petting
- Greater awareness of being attracted to people of same sex, opposite sex, or both
- Possibility of sexual intercourse
- Possibility of pregnancy or impregnating
- Possibility of birth control decisions
- Strong needs for independence

Young Adulthood (19–30 years)
- Possibility of sexual relationships (intercourse or outercourse)
- Possibility of mate selection (homosexual or heterosexual)
- Decision making about marriage, family life, and careers
- Possibility of masturbation
- Possibility of pregnancy, childbirth, and parenting
- Possibility of birth control decisions
- Possibility of ending relationship

Adult (31–45)
- Possibility of mate selection (homosexual or heterosexual)

- Maintaining relationships (sexual and nonsexual)
- Possibility of masturbation
- Possibility of parenting responsibilities (sex education of own children)
- Decision making about birth control
- Possibility of ending relationship

Adult (46–64)

- Menopause
- Possibility of grandparenting
- Possibility of sexual relationships (intercourse or outercourse)
- Possibility of mate selection
- Possibility of masturbation
- Possibility of birth control decisions
- Possible divorce or death of a loved one

Adult (65 + years)

- Body still responds sexually, but more slowly
- Possibility of grandparenting
- Need for physical affection
- Possible sexual relationships
- Possible masturbation
- Possible mate selection
- Possible death of a loved one

WORKSHEET: Sex Is More Than Intercourse

Directions: Human beings are sexual from birth to death. Sexuality, however, changes throughout the life span as a person grows and develops. Place a check on the column that indicates the time in the life span that each of the following needs or behaviors might occur.

Human Sexuality is . . .	Early Childhood Birth-3 yrs	Late Childhood 4-8 yrs	Early Adolescence 9-11 yrs	Adolescence 12-18 yrs	Adult 19-30 yrs	Adult 31-45 yrs	Adult 46-64 yrs	Adult 65+ yrs
1. Love								
2. Touch and affection								
3. Sense of being male or female								
4. Curiosity about body difference								
5. Need for friends								
6. Males: erection								
7. Females: lubrication of vagina								

Human Sexuality is . . .	Early Childhood Birth-3 yrs	Late Childhood 4-8 yrs	Early Adolescence 9-11 yrs	Adolescence 12-18 yrs	Adult 19-30 yrs	Adult 31-45 yrs	Adult 46-64 yrs	Adult 65+ yrs
8. Possibility of orgasm								
9. Possibility of masturbation								
10. Menstruation								
11. Sperm production								
12. Awareness of attraction to members of same sex, opposite sex, or both								
13. Possibility of intercourse								
14. Possibility of outercourse (kissing, petting, etc.)								
15. Possibility of pregnancy or impregnating								
16. Possibility of birth control decisions								
17. Possibility of becoming a parent (parenting)								
18. Divorce or death of a spouse								
19. Possibility of ending a relationship								
20. Need for independence								

1. Which stage in the left span seems most exciting?
2. Write the letter "P" next to the items that are pleasurable.
3. Write the letter "C" next to the items that involve choice and decision-making.

(SOURCE: Peggy Brick and Carolyn Cooperman, *Positive Images: A New Approach to Contraceptive Education* [Hackensack, N.J.: Planned Parenthood of Bergen County, Inc., 1987], 17-19; reprinted by permission from Planned Parenthood of Greater Northern New Jersey.)

POLLS AND SURVEYS

Although the two words are often used interchangeably, polls count votes (i.e., the number of people who agree with a certain statement) and surveys typically gather narrative information. Anonymous polls and surveys provide information to stimulate thinking, that is, for class discussion. When using surveys and polls to gather information, the sexuality educator must take care not to solicit information from K–12 students about their own behaviors; also, be cautious about asking learners to give their *own* values or beliefs. In our first example (see box), note that students are asked about the values and opinions of *their friends*.

Sexual Exploitation Poll

Directions: Here is a list of statements. For each one, ask yourself whether you think most of your friends (not your acquaintances, but your friends) would agree or disagree.

Most of my friends would say . . .
1. It is OK for a guy to hold a girl down and force her to have intercourse if he spent a lot of money on her.
2. It is OK for him to hold her down and force her to have intercourse if he's so turned on he can't stop.
3. It is OK for him to hold her down and force her to have intercourse if she's had sex with other guys before.
4. It is OK for him to hold her down and force her to have intercourse if she's high or drunk.
5. It is OK for him to hold her down and force her to have intercourse if she lets him touch her above the waist.
6. It is OK for him to hold her down and force her to have intercourse if she agrees to have sex with him and then changes her mind.
7. It is OK for him to hold her down and force her to have intercourse if she had led him on.
8. It is OK for him to hold her down and force her to have intercourse if she gets him sexually excited ("turns him on").

(Source: Elizabeth Reis, MS, *9/10 F.L.A.S.H.* [Seattle: Seattle–King County Department of Public Health, 1989], 181; reprinted with permission from Family Planning/STD Program, Seattle–King County Department of Public Health.)

Here are two ideas for the use of surveys.

1. In "Parent Survey," an activity in *Postponing Sexual Involvement: An Educational Series for Parents of Preteens,*[11] parents can compare their own predictions of teen responses with actual teen responses to questions about why teens become sexually involved, why they postpone sexual involvement, and what they think are some unexpected results of early sexual involvement.

2. One of our colleagues has taught an eight-week college course on human sexual behavior for many years. She describes gathering anonymous data from students through surveys. For example, in a "First Knowledge of Sex" survey,[12] she asks, "Who first told you about sex?" "How old were you?" "What did they say?" "How did you feel?" "How adequate and complete was the information you

received?" The data is summarized, reported to the class, and then extensively discussed.

TASK GROUPS

In Chapter 7 we discussed the processes of forming and facilitating small groups, which may be used for many purposes in sexuality education. Here we focus on task groups, defined as any subgroup of the whole that convenes to do a task. The purpose of a task group may be as simple as to discuss reactions or share information, but usually includes an assigned task that will be reported to the whole group. Educators now call such task groups "cooperative learning groups," recognizing that the goal of this method is not only to accomplish a task, but also to improve skills in interpersonal relationships.

The educator may assign tasks to groups and take an inactive role, observing and clarifying directions as needed; or s/he may work more actively with the groups, consulting, offering resources and suggestions, clarifying, stimulating, answering questions, and arbitrating.

Next, process the data produced in task groups with the whole group. You can manage the reporting process by timing reports, asking only one person from each group to speak for his or her group, or asking the whole group to question, evaluate, or otherwise react to each task group's report. Various types of reporting are described in Chapter 7 in the section "Facilitating Small Groups."

A colleague describes a task group activity she does in her eight-week human sexual behavior course:[13] students meet in two gender-segregated groups to list the standards they would include in a "Code of Sexual Behavior"; they then work in smaller integrated groups to try to come to consensus on the behavior code; then the entire class works to resolve any remaining differences.

In the next example (see box), groups are asked to come to consensus on qualifications for the "job of parent," analyzing information given in a worksheet in relation to their own values and opinions; the worksheet used in this activity is not reprinted, but is described in detail following the box.

Planning to Parent: Am I Qualified?

Student Learning Objectives: To be able to . . .
1. Describe at least three qualifications he or she believes are important for the job of "parent."
2. Recognize that people have differing beliefs about which qualifications are important.

Introduction: "If you were choosing a hairdresser or barber, you wouldn't just go to the first one in the phone book. You would have some criteria, things you'd look for in choosing the best person for the job. Give me some examples of things you'd look for . . .

"If you were hiring someone to clean your house, you wouldn't just offer the job to the first one you ran across in the phone book. You would have some criteria, things you'd look for in choosing the best person for the job. Give me some examples of things you'd look for . . .

"There is one job that almost anybody who wants to is allowed to do. Nobody checks people's qualifications. It happens to be one of the most important jobs in the world. No, it's not president of the United States. It is 'parent.' Today we'll examine the qualifications for the job. We'll look at who should be 'hired' as parents."

Hand out the worksheet entitled "Possible Qualifications for the Job of 'Parent.'" Have volunteers read it aloud, but make sure everyone knows not to fill it out yet.

Divide the class into groups of four or five. Explain to them: "Each group is the Board of Directors of a different adoption agency." Give each group one set of small group instructions. Give each group a large sheet of paper and a marking pen.

Small Group Instructions: "Your agency will have 25 infants to place in adoptive families this year. About 1,000 families will apply to adopt these infants, so only a few will actually get to adopt. Your staff will be interviewing all 1,000 families, deciding which families to approve and which are "best" for the babies whose futures you hold in your hands. Only the families your staff approves will be listed for birth parents to choose from." Remember to show respect for differences of opinion. What are the minimum qualifications you want your staff to look for? Talk it over with the rest of your "staff." Then do the following:

1. On the large paper, with marking pen, list the qualifications that anyone in your group thinks should be required of every adoptive family.
2. Now, each of you, put a star to whichever items you think ought to be required. So, some items may only get one star, if one of you wants to require them. Other items will get two stars, and so forth. Talk about it. Try to convince one another. Only items that get at least three stars will be required of every family that wants to adopt a baby from your agency.
3. Each of you, on your own paper, put three stars next to those same items (the ones that got three or more votes by your fellow Board members).

(SOURCE: Elizabeth Reis, MS, *9/10 F.L.A.S.H.* [Seattle: Seattle–King County Department of Public Health, 1989], 332, 335, 339–340; reprinted with permission from Family Planning/STD Program, Seattle–King County Department of Public Health.)

Consider the diversity of your particular students and the broad range of your community's values as you develop the worksheet you use with this activity. The *9/10 F.L.A.S.H.* worksheet includes the following categories of criteria; you and your students may want to add others:

1. Culture, race, religion, beliefs: statements about discipline, setting limits, work ethic, culture, race, ethnicity and religious beliefs (for example, "shares my religious and moral beliefs").

2. History of serious problems: police record, mental illness, alcohol and drug problems, etc. (for example, "has no police record").
3. Finances: ranges of income (for example, "has a steady income of at least $30,000 per year and owns a car").
4. Relationships and support systems: family, extended family and friends (for example, "married for at least three years").
5. Mental and physical health: disabilities, illness, emotional problems, intelligence, fitness (for example, "if physically disabled, has considered how child would be cared for").
6. Personal, professional, and educational situation, responsibilities, and plans: interests, community relationships, time, education level, etc. (for example, "is active in the community").
7. Parenting skills and interests: expressed likes for each age group (infants, toddlers, young children, teens) and statements about home and family interests (for example, "would encourage a child's questions").
8. Age, personality, maturity: other character traits (for example, "has a lot of patience and flexibility").

FIELD TRIPS

We distinguish "field trips" from "real-life homework" as follows: the purpose of "field trips" (e.g., to family planning clinics and other organizations) is to gather information; the purpose of "real-life homework" (which often includes field trips) is gaining and practicing skills (see Chapter 11). Depending on the needs of the learner at the time of the field trip, the line between the two definitions may be only arbitrary.

In the *9/10 F.L.A.S.H.*[14] curriculum, students receive an "Individual Field Trip" assignment at the beginning of the thirty-lesson unit. Students give oral reports on their trips throughout the unit, and must turn in a written report accompanied by a brochure, agency card, or other evidence of the visit. Students also must answer several study questions for the site and topic area chosen. Here are the suggested topics and sites, with sample study questions:

1. Child sexual abuse: a rape crisis center or sexual assault center ("Who sexually abuses children? Why?").
2. Date and statutory rape: a rape crisis center or sex information line ("What is 'date rape'? How does the law in our state define 'statutory rape'?").
3. Other sexual assault: a rape crisis center, the police department or a legal aid organization ("How does the law in our state define 'incest'?").
4. Prenatal health and drugs: the March of Dimes, a prenatal program, or an obstetrician ("Can this drug harm the sperm or egg before conception?").
5. Other birth defects: the March of Dimes, the Red Cross, a prenatal program, or an obstetrician ("What is this birth defect and how does it affect a baby?").
6. Birth and infant health: childbirth education association, La Leche League, a parenting program, or a childbirth class ("How can this agency help a pregnant woman or couple?").

7. Prescription birth control: a family planning clinic, such as a health department or Planned Parenthood, or a community clinic ("Who comes to this clinic for birth control? Is there a charge?").
8. Nonprescription birth control: a pharmacy, a family planning clinic, or another outlet for nonprescription contraceptives ("Are the contraceptives openly displayed, or kept behind a counter?").
9. Religion and birth control: a clergy or other religious leader ("What does this faith teach about birth control?").
10. Sexually transmitted diseases—tests and treatment: an STD or AIDS clinic ("Does a teen need a parent's permission to come to this clinic?").

COMPUTERIZED LEARNING PROGRAMS

Computerized learning programs[15] offer some benefits in teaching about sexuality: many learners are quite computer literate and seem to get very involved in good programs; programs can be taken home and used by family groups, enhancing family communication on sexuality topics; and learners can work at their own pace, with privacy and safety on sensitive content, and taking a path determined by their own needs and interests. For example, some computerized learning programs on HIV offer a risk assessment questionnaire and allow the user to choose a variety of sections based on his or her level of risk and "need to know."

However, we urge caution: review all programs thoroughly for accuracy, completeness and freedom from bias as you would videos and other materials. Some programs are incomplete or emphasize certain aspects of a topic to the exclusion of others; for example, we reviewed an HIV program that emphasizes shared needle transmission of HIV to the exclusion of sexual transmission, and another program that ignores heterosexual transmission. Such programs can be augmented more easily than others containing pervasive, subtle bias, inconsistencies, and inaccuracies. Use only those programs that are approved by your school district or other governing body, or refer learners to appropriate programs available at local libraries and other agencies. Use computerized programs to *augment* other sexuality education methods. And, finally, be prepared to help learners with questions about how to run the program and questions and issues raised by the sexuality content.

CHAPTER 10

Helping Learners Reflect on Attitudes, Feelings, Values, and Beliefs

A teacher who can arouse a feeling for one single good action . . . accomplishes more than one who fills our memory with rows on rows of natural objects, classified with name and form.

—Johann Wolfgang von Goethe

In this chapter we address teaching in the affective domain: how to help learners understand their feelings and values; how to encourage individual and group analysis of attitudes, feelings and values; and how to affect or change unhealthy attitudes.

In order to affect behavior, an important goal of effective sexuality education, educators must be able to deal with individual, community, and cultural values and feelings. Many people, particularly adolescents, do not always make rational decisions, that is, decisions based on knowledge of facts and consideration of long- and short-term consequences. Rather, decisions about personal sexual behavior are often based on *feelings:* a desire for immediate gratification; low self-esteem and low self-efficacy; overwhelming love or attraction; ambivalence about options; a need to prove oneself; or a sense of invulnerability. Learners often fail to perceive information as relevant to their lives. They often do not see themselves as susceptible to negative consequences of their behaviors; indeed, they may reject the oppressive nature of messages about sexuality that focus only on negative outcomes. Sometimes they believe themselves incapable of acting or controlling a situation. Sexuality educators must utilize effective methods for addressing these and other feelings, attitudes, values, and beliefs.

Many states restrict teachers from asking K–12 students about their beliefs, values, and practices. Sexuality educators, in particular, face criticism for conducting student discussions on beliefs and values. However, educators can frame the questions to make the discussion of values more general: "Do you think your community agrees with this idea?" "What are the reasons that some people . . . ?" You also can use introspective methods (see Chapter 8), with which students consider their own beliefs without making them public. Know your state laws and be cautious. This caution does not apply so strictly to those working with adults and children outside the public school system, but even educators with these groups should consult with sponsoring organizations and be aware of the political climate of the total community.

As we noted in a previous chapter, the line between cognitive, affective, and behavioral learning methods is not always clear. In Chapter 9 we discussed many cognitive methods that also are used for teaching in the affective domain: videos can be used as "trigger" material to initiate discussion of values and behaviors; computer learning programs often have values components; effective presentations may contain consideration of values, feelings, attitudes, and behavior, and speakers can raise issues that touch learner emotions and beliefs; and anonymous questions usually contain value and feeling elements. Furthermore, an "affective learner" may need an affective method to learn in the cognitive or behavioral domains. We describe these methods in this chapter as primarily affective in intent, but remind you to integrate a variety of methods into your teaching about sexuality.

DISCUSSION

Teacher-centered discussion—when students direct all questions and conversation toward the teacher—is primarily a cognitive teaching method, used to assist clarification and retention of information. However, in sexuality education, discussion often elicits feelings and opinions and is a valuable teaching tool in the affective domain as well. *Group-centered* sexuality education discussions are more effective, with learners interacting with each other as well as with the teacher.

Guide a group discussion using the following steps.

1. *Review data.* The first step in discussion after learners share a common experience—for example, hearing Magic Johnson announce his HIV status, brainstorming on a topic, participating in a simulation or role play, seeing a video, or hearing a guest speaker—should be an opportunity to reflect on the experience, review information, share feelings or reactions (feelings are data too!), declare opinions, add group member information, define terms, and share perspectives. Each person's memory and experience of "what happened" will be different; therefore, a "review of data" from the experience of watching a video includes review of the actual content of the video (about which there will be disagreement) and review of individuals' feelings and reactions.

2. *Process the data.* The next step is to step back from all the data and to analyze it: look for recurring themes; look for commonalities, differences or categories; ask general questions about key concepts; listen for trends and key terms; ask for meaning.

3. *Generalize.* In this step, ask, "So what?"; ask what principles can be generalized to "real life," to other similar situations; ask what individuals have learned from the experience. Some learners may jump to generalizing at the beginning of a discussion, which may be productive or may lead to disagreement or conflict if data have not been clarified first.

4. *Apply the data.* Last, learners should consider how the experience applies to their own lives, both as members of the group and individually. The group could brainstorm actions they can take as a group. Individuals could think about and discuss actions they will take on their own. Or follow the discussion with behavioral methods such as problem solving and role play.

The following techniques make discussions more specific and concrete and increase learner involvement:

- Encourage learners to use "I" statements rather than ascribing a personal belief to the whole group.
- Listen for generalizations and vague statements, and ask for more specifics and examples.
- Help learners discriminate between inferences, values, opinions, and facts; correct factual errors, or encourage group members to do so.
- Encourage diversity of opinion.

The following activities also augment and enhance discussions:

- Brainstorm and post a list of adjectives that describe learners' feelings at specific points in the discussion: "How did you feel when the girl in the video said she was pregnant?"
- Post key discussion questions or issues to give learners a visual reminder. For example, "In what way do kids your age conform with each other?" "What would you do about a relationship with a romantic partner who is unwilling to communicate?" "Why do teens and parents/adults often have conflict?" "How would adults you know answer this question?" "What aspects of sexuality are uncomfortable to discuss? With whom?"
- Ask all participants to rate items listed in a previous brainstorm or on a handout; tally and average the ratings; discuss.
- Do a "whip" (see section following), for example, ask "What do you see in this picture?" and quickly go around the circle asking people to give unrehearsed one- or two-word responses.
- Turn the discussion process over to the group, and step away to observe: "I'd like you to spend the next 20 minutes discussing the question I've put on the board; at the end of that time I'd like you to give me a list of five reasons . . ." There are two types of group-centered discussion: one that focuses on a task or a product (as this example illustrates), and one in which the primary goal is sharing opinions, ideas, and feelings.[1]
- Ask subgroups to discuss (see "Task Groups," Chapter 9) a topic and to bring their conclusions to the large group for processing, analysis, and generalizations.
- Hand out quick questionnaires (see Chapter 8) that focus learner ideas; discuss responses.
- Post a series of stem sentences (see Chapter 8) and ask learners to complete them aloud, for example, "Teen pregnancy is . . ." or "The most important thing to know about HIV is . . ."
- Ask everyone to write an "I learned" statement, or ask volunteers to share a sampling of "I learned" statements aloud (see Chapter 13).

Most of the best sexuality education curricula and resource guides include questions or points for discussion with each lesson or activity. For example, in a lesson on media messages about women and men, *Postponing Sexual Involvement* suggests the discussion questions in the box.

- How do the "looks" and behaviors of women in the media—TV, movies, ads—compare with those of the women you know, like your mother, teachers, or women in your neighborhood?
- How do the roles or characters played by women on TV compare with the kinds of jobs and life-styles of the women you know?
- Who is your favorite female character on TV? Why? How does that character handle her sexual behavior? Do you think if the people in real life did that, it would work out the same way?
- Name some females in music, TV, or movies who are influencing teens today—their dress, manner of speaking, way of wearing their hair, career choices (give example).
- What other things besides the media influence how we feel about ourselves?

- How do the "looks" and behaviors of men in the media—TV, movies, ads—compare with those of the men you know, like your father, teachers, or men in your neighborhood?
- How do the roles or characters played by men on TV compare with the kinds of jobs and life-styles of the men you know?
- Who is your favorite male character on TV? Why? How does that character handle his sexual behavior? Do you think if the people you know in real life did that, it would work out the same way?
- Name some males in music, TV, or movies who are influencing teens today—their dress, manner of speaking, way of wearing their hair, career choices (give example).
- What are some of the everyday responsibilities men have in life that usually are not shown by the media?

(SOURCE: Marion Howard, Ph.D., and Marie E. Mitchell, R.N., *Postponing Sexual Involvement: An Educational Series for Young Teens* [Atlanta: Emory/Grady Teen Services Program, 1990], 27–28.)

WHIP

A whip is an exercise in listening; its most valuable effect is that the group hears a pattern of responses, or hears an overall feeling in the group, or more easily hears contrasting feelings and opinions. To facilitate a whip, the educator poses a question, usually one addressing an opinion or feeling, and asks each learner to respond quickly in turn, either one after another around the circle or when pointed to at random (allow individuals to pass if they choose). Before starting the whip, the teacher should ask the group to attend to each person's response, listening for commonalities or contrasts.

In the boxed example, stem sentences first are used in an introspective exercise (see Chapter 8); then a whip activity allows the whole group to hear everyone's completion of each sentence in turn. Note that the statements in this illustration are phrased negatively; the effect of hearing all the negative attributes of boys and girls may be rather distressing. Try rephrasing them in positive language (e.g., "Girls like boys who . . ."), or do the negative version first, then the positive. Also, whips can become tedious if they go on too long; you may want to select only a few of these stem sentences to process in a whip and address others in a discussion.

Girls and Boys

Purpose: To identify children's attitudes about gender roles and gender-role stereotypes.

Materials: Handouts, "The Best Thing about Being a Girl" and "The Best Thing about Being a Boy"; crayons.

Time: 30 minutes (Session One); 30 minutes (Session Two).

Procedure: Session One

1. Begin the activity by explaining that today's discussion focuses on what the group thinks about girls and boys. Ask them to complete the following sentences:

    Girls don't like boys who . . .
    Girls don't like girls who . . .
    Boys don't like girls who . . .
    Boys don't like boys who . . .
    A girl is weird if she . . .
    A boy isn't cool if he . . .

2. Using a "whip" format, ask the children to give their responses quickly as you move around the circle. After each statement, discuss the similarities and differences in the responses. Point out any stereotypes that come up.

Procedure: Session Two

1. Distribute the appropriate handouts (following) and crayons. Explain the handouts. Ask the children to complete the sentences. Then they should make a drawing to show what they think is the best thing about being a girl or a boy.

2. After about 10 to 15 minutes, have volunteers share their drawings. Review the sentence completions. Encourage children to ignore those messages that say "Girls can't" or "Boys can't." Stress the fact that girls and boys can do whatever they want as long as they prepare themselves.

3. Close the activity by using the Discussion Points (following).

Discussion points

1. What is a stereotype? (The belief that all members of a group—all girls or all boys—should think and act alike.)

2. Why is it harmful to accept stereotypes about girls and boys?

Handout for girls
1. The *best* thing about being a girl is: (space for drawing)
2. I *hate* it when people say:
   Girls are so . . .
   Girls shouldn't . . .
   Girls should . . .
   Girls can't . . .
   Girls never . . .

Handout for boys
1. The *best* thing about being a boy is: (space for drawing)
2. I *hate* it when people say
   Boys are so . . .
   Boys shouldn't . . .
   Boys should . . .
   Boys can't . . .
   Boys never . . .

(SOURCE: Advocates for Youth [formerly the Center for Population Options], *When I'm Grown: Life Planning Education for Grades 3 & 4* [Washington, D.C.: Advocates for Youth, 1992], 25. Reprinted with permission. Call 202-347-5700 for more information.)

DYADS AND TRIADS

Dyads and triads (or "pairs" and "groups of three") can be used for sharing feelings, ideas, values, attitudes, experiences, or beliefs in a sexuality education session, whether in the classroom or a workshop setting. This sharing process can be preceded by a variety of preparatory activities: an introspective activity (see Chapter 8), where learners prepare their thoughts for sharing; or a panel presentation, fishbowl, discussion, role play, simulation, game, or video, for which the dyad experience becomes a way of processing reactions. Also use dyads or triads for "get acquainted" exercises or as "study groups" for the review of information. Follow a dyad or triad activity with a variety of methods, depending on the sequencing of your lesson or workshop (see Chapter 6) and the need for drawing conclusions or generalizations from the dyad experience.

In Chapter 7 we thoroughly described the process for facilitating these special small groups. Here we give a few examples of dyad/triad discussion questions with the assumption that nearly any sexuality topic may be adapted to use in small groups:

1. What are the advantages and disadvantages of being your gender? As an adolescent? As an adult?
2. What one question would you like to ask an adult who is part of your family or is important to you?
3. What plans and dreams do you have about family in your future?

4. Who most easily influences your behavior?
5. List at least two reasons why teens should not have sexual intercourse.
6. Describe your first memory of realizing the differences between males and females.
7. What do you think people mean when they say, "I love you"?
8. Describe the skills and attributes required for the job of parent.
9. How and from whom did you get your earliest information about sexuality?
10. If you could turn the clock back and correct one serious mistake you have made in your life, what would that be?

A variation of dyads called "revolving circles" or "wagon wheels" is used in the activity "When Race Is the Issue."[2] Students arrange their chairs in two circles, one inside the other. The inner circle chairs face outward; outer circle chairs (the same number as the inner circle) face in, paired with inner circle chairs. After each partner has addressed the topic, the outer circle rotates one seat to the left (moving bodies, not chairs) so that each person has a new partner. Topics in this particular activity focus on racial and ethnic issues (differences, stereotyping, discrimination, etc.) and begin with easy, "get acquainted" topics. Topics then become increasingly challenging, such as, "Share with your partner how you feel when you hear someone speaking a language other than your own," and "Share with your partner at least one thing you can do to challenge racism."

INTERVIEWS

In an interview, one person asks a series of prepared questions; the respondent answers from his or her own perspective. Interviews can take place in the classroom, and the person interviewed can be the teacher, a volunteer learner, a guest speaker, or, in a role play interview, someone who has assumed a role or character. You also can ask learners to interview family members, other students, or significant adults outside the classroom.

Set ground rules prior to beginning the interview. Questions should come from a real intent to explore issues and understand differing perspectives. Asking about feelings, opinions, and values is appropriate; however, do not allow questions that ask the respondent to reveal actual or intended sexual behavior or experiences. Care should be taken not to allow an attack on the respondent's values and beliefs. Questions can be probing, but must not be accusatory, based on assumptions, or intended to hurt or denigrate the interviewee. We deplore the "talk-show host" technique of assembling opposing groups as an audience and then attacking the interviewee: "Why do you promote the killing of babies?" Intervene if ground rules are broken or discomfort is too great.

You can prepare the questions, which become a script for the interview; or individuals or groups of learners can write the questions; or they can be brainstormed by the whole group. In a classroom interview (e.g., of a guest speaker), prewritten questions often become moot given particular responses, and interviewers should be prepared to proceed to other questions. Educators and learners also can ad-lib questions if they are careful not to break ground rules.

Several variations on the following sample interview (see box) have been used with middle school and high school students for many years.

Interview for the Job of Parent

The purpose of this interview is to explore the concept of "parenting" and to clarify values regarding parenting. It can be carried out in triads, with an applicant, an interviewer, and an observer/recorder. Here are some suggested questions:

1. **What previous related experience have you had?**
2. **What related training and/or education have you had?**
3. **Describe the references you have from previous employers in related jobs.**
4. **Why do you want this job?**
5. **How will this job change your life?**
6. **What is your basic philosophy of parenting?**
7. **How do you work with other people in teams?**
8. **How do you feel about working with children?**
9. **What are the occupational hazards? How would you cope with them?**

The preceding role-play interview elicits the expression of real and in-role feelings. It is one of the few in which we would allow "why" questions (#4), which are based on an assumption and may sound accusatory, but in this case are based correctly on the role-play assumption that the interviewee wants the job. This interview can be altered and used as a take-home assignment for learners to interview their own parents or parents of a friend; change the questions to past tense, add other questions, and consider eliminating questions 4 and 5.

Here are some more ideas for interviews.

1. In "Talk to Your Parents" in the *Reducing the Risk* curriculum,[3] students interview their parents about adolescent sex and protection. In Part A, students explore their own ideas and indicate what they think their parents believe about the same topics. Then, in Part B, they interview their parents using a questionnaire, talking and listening, not just giving the sheet to their parents to fill out. The content of interviews is kept confidential; students turn in only a parent-signed form verifying the interview took place. Since not all learners have parents, and some have parents who for many reasons cannot be interviewed, we suggest that this activity be altered to include "other trusted adult" or "adult mentor" as possible interviewees.

2. In an activity in *New Methods for Puberty Education* called "Professionals as Resources,"[4] students use a worksheet to discuss how they think a professional (such as a nurse or doctor) might feel about answering questions about puberty; then they practice interviewing a professional in the classroom; finally, they con-

duct actual interviews in the community. This lesson takes learning out of the classroom and into the community, enabling students to acquire skills for asking questions of professionals and analyzing the information received.

3. In "Adult Households" from *When I'm Grown: Life Planning Education for Grades 5 & 6,*[5] the purpose is to increase children's awareness of the variety of adult relationships and household compositions, such as living with a person of the same or other gender in a romantic relationship. The culminating activity in this lesson is for students to predict, using a worksheet, how their family members feel about various adult household situations; they then ask their family members and discuss their opinions.

FISHBOWL

In a fishbowl activity, observers surround an interactive group. For example, women in the inner circle can express their feelings about being female while the men around them listen; then the two groups switch, and the women listen to the men. The audience effect seems to heighten awareness and expression of feelings and values by both the inner group and, in their turn, the outer group. Because of the observation role taken by the outer group, feedback on the inner group's process and content, *how* they interacted as well as *what* they said becomes valuable information for discussion after the fishbowl. The most effective topics for fishbowls are those that air opposing views or differing perspectives.

Follow these steps when facilitating a fishbowl:

1. Introduce and post the topic; discuss the purpose and the process.
2. Divide into two groups; division depends somewhat on the topic. The whole group may be divided in half, or smaller groups can represent perspectives. Generally, the inner group should be no more than eight to ten people.
3. Reintroduce the topic, reminding learners that the inner circle is discussing while the outer circle observes. Observers must be silent.
4. Suggest that outer circle members write down observations regarding process and content to increase their attention and facilitate follow-up discussion.
5. Enter the inner circle to start and facilitate the discussion as appropriate. Or you may "huddle" with inner circle members for a few minutes prior to the activity to discuss their process. Allow the discussion to proceed for 15 to 20 minutes, depending on the group. Timing is important; stop the fishbowl while interest is still high.
6. Discuss the first fishbowl. At this point you can ask questions related to group process (see Chapter 7), but restrict discussion on the content until after the second group has its turn: "What did observers note about how the inner circle interacted?" "How did observers feel about enforced silence?" "How did inner circle members feel about being observed?"
7. Switch groups and proceed with the second fishbowl discussion.
8. Debrief the experience with a whole group discussion, dyad or triad sharing, introspective writing, or other activities.

The following fishbowl activity (see box) has two purposes: (1) to help students identify and debunk myths and stereotypes about their own gender, and (2) to examine how gender role extremes and stereotypes damage people of both genders.

Gender Roles

Use a "fishbowl" exercise to address role extremes and stereotypes. Here's how.

Put a circle of four chairs, facing one another, in the center of the room. Whichever gender is to be first, invite four volunteers of that gender to sit on the chairs in the "fishbowl." They will have a 5- or 10-minute conversation, in response to a question or questions you will pose.

At first, observers may only listen. However, after everyone in the fishbowl has had at least one opportunity to speak, you, as the facilitator, may decide to stop the conversation long enough to invite others of the same gender to tap a fishbowl participant on the shoulder and take his or her place. Whenever the conversation seems to need a boost, you may pose another question. You may also, at some point, add a fifth chair and invite people of the other gender to take that chair in order to ask a question of the four people in the fishbowl.

Ask the guys' fishbowl, for example: What myths and stereotypes about men make you most angry or frustrated? What do you think are the facts—what accurate information should replace those myths and stereotypes? Do you think some young men grow up believing those fallacies? Why? Men have higher rates of homicide, successful suicide, and heart disease than women. Do you think that is partly a function of gender role extremes? Why or why not? How else do guys get limited or hurt or even killed by gender role extremes or stereotypes? What do you wish women understood about men?

Ask the girls' fishbowl, for example: What myths and stereotypes about women make you most angry or frustrated? What do you think are the facts—what accurate information should replace those myths and stereotypes? Do you think some young women grow up believing those fallacies? Why? Women have higher rates of anorexia and bulimia than men, both of which can be fatal. Do you think that is partly a function of gender role extremes? Why or why not? How else do girls get limited or hurt or even killed by gender role extremes or stereotypes? What do you wish men understood about women?

(SOURCE: Elizabeth Reis, MS, 11/12 F.L.A.S.H. [Seattle: Seattle–King County Department of Public Health], 37. Reprinted with permission from Family Planning/STD Program, Seattle–King County Department of Public Health.)

You may use the fishbowl method spontaneously in a group discussion when you observe strong differences in viewpoint on a topic. One perspective is thoroughly discussed in the inner group; then individuals representing a differing perspective go to the middle. Utilize the whole group discussion that follows to summarize differences and commonalities.

Some facilitators use an "empty chair" technique: an empty chair is placed in the inner circle, and members of the outer group can drop in to make comments or ask questions (as in the previous boxed example). We sometimes find this technique to be confusing, interruptive, and unproductive, especially when outer group members use it to ventilate feelings. Another technique that allows outer group members to ask clarifying questions or suggest another tangent is to ask them to pass written questions to the facilitator, who screens them and passes them on to an inner group member for possible consideration.

Continuum, Forced Choice, and Quadrant Methods

These three methods are used primarily to increase awareness of the range of opinion on an issue; the learner has opportunity to examine his or her own values in relationship to others. These methods also energize the group and provide a means of getting people out of their chairs and moving.

A *continuum* is a method used to elicit public or private statements of values or opinions; the learner makes this statement by placing him or herself on a line between two extremes. Public statements are made by standing on an imaginary line on the floor; private statements are made by marking on a line continuum worksheet. The line represents an issue with two opposing viewpoints and the gradations between (see Figure 1).

In a continuum, an issue and its two polar positions can be suggested by the facilitator or by the group. A continuum used as a public statement of a value can be risky; begin a series with less risky topics. Do not use these methods unless you want to elicit and can facilitate adequate discussion on a broad range of opinions and values.

Here are some sample continuum statements on a variety of topics:

- People should avoid sexual activity before marriage.
- Information on birth control techniques should be made freely available to all people.
- Avoiding pregnancy is primarily the woman's responsibility.
- Women tend to be more emotional and less able to think clearly in an emergency than men.
- Most women who are raped have probably done something to entice or arouse the rapist.

Figure 1: Continuum

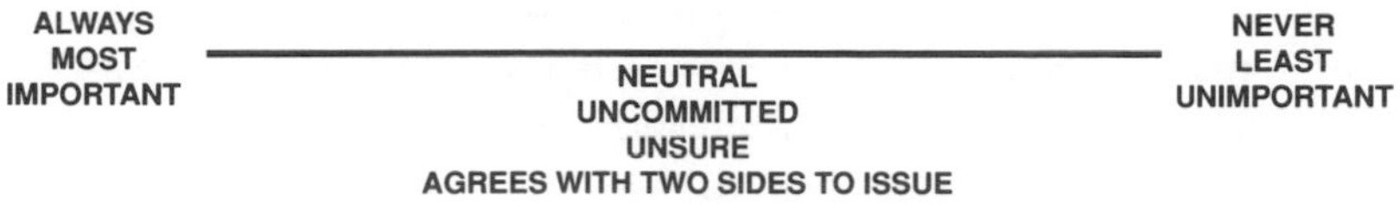

```
ALWAYS                                                              NEVER
MOST                                                                LEAST
IMPORTANT                      NEUTRAL                              UNIMPORTANT
                             UNCOMMITTED
                                UNSURE
                     AGREES WITH TWO SIDES TO ISSUE
```

Describe two extremes to each statement, for example, "Avoiding pregnancy is the woman's responsibility," and "Avoiding pregnancy is the man's responsibility"; participants place themselves on the continuum and then discuss why they placed themselves where they did. Follow these steps for a public continuum:

1. Remind learners of ground rules; a continuum can polarize individuals and lead to judging or criticizing others; adherence to ground rules must be enforced, particularly in respecting differing views.
2. Introduce the topic for each continuum and describe the two poles of opinion. Describe an imaginary line on the floor and indicate which end is for which pole of opinion. Curve the imaginary line to a semicircle so each person is visible to all and to facilitate discussion.
3. Ask group members to stand on the continuum in the spots that represent their opinions about the issue (closer to or farther from each end).
4. Invite (do not require) brief public statements of reason for placement on the line, reflecting how they interpreted the statement, what unstated circumstances they considered, and their basic values. Encourage participants to move during the discussion, reaffirming the right to change one's mind.
5. Ask for statements from both poles and from the middle area. Support people with unpopular or minority views. Ask learners to role play opinions not represented by the group, or play "devil's advocate" yourself. Model communication skills that enhance understanding and acceptance, including paraphrasing and active listening.
6. Go on to the next continuum. Participants usually get tired of standing through the process after discussing five or six issues.

You may wish to precede a continuum exercise with a discussion on values and tolerance for others' opinions. You can protect student confidentiality by asking participants to put their views on paper and hand them in; shuffle the written continuums, redistribute them, and then ask participants to put themselves on the public continuum to express the views written on the papers they hold. Many individuals will find expressing someone else's viewpoint very difficult and will find a way to disavow that perspective; however, this can be a valuable lesson in understanding different opinions.

If the exercise is to be done privately on paper, hand out continuum worksheets. In a large group, all participants can complete worksheets at their desks while eight or ten volunteers "put their bodies on the line" in front of the group; discuss each continuum item, with seated participants questioning standing volunteers.

Here are some sample continuum activities.

1. In *Postponing Sexual Involvement*,[6] the lesson "Setting Limits on Physical Affection" uses a continuum to describe six levels of affection, from "give friendly looks and smiles" to "have sex." Students are asked to move to the place on the continuum that describes the level at which they think 13–15-year-old teens should stop when expressing physical affection; then they move to the level where they believe parents would want them to stop.

2. During the activity "Mixed Messages," in *Teaching Safer Sex,*[7] students examine the messages about their sexuality that they are receiving from various individuals, groups, and institutions. Using a worksheet, they write the major messages from a number of sources, create a written continuum on each expressing their degree of agreement, and then participate in a public continuum expressing degree of helpfulness of each message.

3. *Teaching Safer Sex* also uses the continuum method in a cognitive, analytical manner. In the activity "Continuum of Probabilities,"[8] students describe behaviors that reduce their chances of acquiring an STD to as close as possible to 0% and compare them with behaviors that give closer to 100% probability of getting an STD. This activity effectively emphasizes abstinence and monogamy without preaching or communicating a sex-negative attitude.

Forced-choice activities are a variation of the continuum method. With a forced choice issue there is no gradation of opinion; participants choose between only two viewpoints. Forced-choice activities demonstrate that many people see choices as forced, often with no good options. However, this method often causes unresolvable polarization and stereotyping, and should be used with caution.

To facilitate a public forced-choice exercise, label one side of the room "agree" and the other side "disagree." Read each statement to the group and ask learners to move to the side of the room that represents their position for each statement, emphasizing that there are no right or wrong answers. Discuss: "Which choices were hard to make? Why?" "How did it feel to be required to choose?" "On what basis was the choice made?" "How did individuals interpret the statement differently?"

Here are some examples of forced-choice statements regarding contraception, parenting, adoption, and abortion:[9]

- Lack of information is the primary cause of failure to contracept.
- Teens do not make good parents.
- Any reason for an abortion is an acceptable reason.
- A birth parent should not be able to change her/his mind once a child is placed for adoption.
- A parenting teen should forget about finishing high school for now if it means she/he won't have enough time to be a good parent.

A *quadrant* exercise adds a second dimension and consists of two continua at right angles, graphically forming four quadrants on paper or in the four corners of the room. See the box for an example of a quadrant activity.

Personal Styles

A simple "personal style quadrant" can be used in a session on relationships. This exercise asks participants to place themselves on two consecutive continua that are drawn crossing each other at right angles (see Figure 2). The horizontal continuum asks participants to decide whether they are more "Feelers" or "Thinkers," depending on how they initially respond to relationship situations—with rational thoughts or with feelings. The vertical continuum asks whether they respond by primarily waiting and listening or by talking—"Listener" or "Talker." Each participant's style is described by one of the four quadrants. For example, if someone's first continuum style is "Feeler" and second continuum style is "talker," this person's overall style is "Feeler-talker," arbitrarily called "Supporter." Other people will fall in the "Analyzer," "Controller," and "Promoter" quadrants. Some people will describe themselves close to the middle on both continua; these individuals may have elements of all four styles. The facilitator should emphasize that these labels are quite arbitrary; they are only used as an exercise, a way of looking at ourselves. Furthermore, no one style should be seen as more important or valuable than another.

Discussion about the meaning of individual placement in the quadrants can take place in small groups seated in the correlated four corners of the room. Groups can then present the positive aspects of their quadrant's style to the whole group. Emphasis should be placed on listening to other styles and understanding differences. Participants could also discuss possible misunderstandings between two different styles and ways of communicating that could bridge the differences.

(SOURCE: Adapted from "Behavioral Characteristics Matrix" [Portland, Oregon: Northwest Regional Educational Laboratory, 1978].)

Figure 2: Quadrant

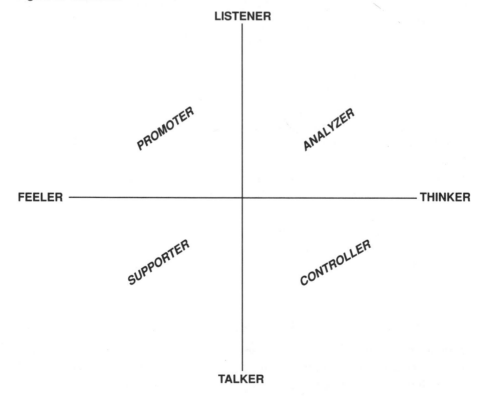

> "Remember only this one thing," said Badger. "The stories people tell have a way of taking care of them. If stories come to you, care for them. And learn to give them away where they are needed. Sometimes a person needs a story more than food to stay alive. That is why we put these stories in each other's memory. This is how people care for themselves. One day you will be good story tellers. Never forget these obligations."
>
> —Barry Lopez, *Crow and Weasel*

Storytelling is a strong tradition, particularly in some segments of our diverse culture. Stories can form the basis of effective sexuality education lessons and are particularly important in younger grades where language arts form the basis of many learning processes. During a story, listeners and readers often undergo a shift of consciousness, letting the story live in their imaginations.

Educators can write and use stories to teach key messages. For example, in family life education, use a series of stories about different families—adoptive family, single parent, gay/lesbian parent, extended family, and so on—to teach tolerance and understanding of the diversity of family configurations. In puberty education, use stories to stimulate discussions about students' concerns, for example, a story about a girl buying tampons, or a boy experiencing his first nocturnal emission. For young teens, abstinence-based stories about potential problem situations in which couples need to negotiate their behavior may help learners personalize and explore communication skills. In HIV education, a story about a girl who contracts HIV from her boyfriend at age 16 and dies at 28 (a true incident in our experience) may help learners recognize their own risks, if any.

To differentiate between the use of stories and case studies, we note that commonly listed synonyms for "story" are "tale," "narrative," "romance," "fable," "allegory," or "parable"; in contrast, a "case" is an "incident," "situation," "event," "example," "circumstance," or "illustration." Case studies in sexuality education use a hypothetical or actual description of a situation that is analyzed by the whole or subgroup and utilized in a series of activities. Ask learners to describe the facts of the case, report their feelings or opinions, brainstorm a list of the key issues, discuss the feelings of the characters in the case, apply problem solving to the main issues, or role play the relationships.

In the example of a case study activity (see box), the goal is to enable high school or college students to critically analyze and discuss ethical issues society faces with respect to the HIV epidemic.

Challenging Attitudes toward HIV/AIDS

Audience: High school and college students.
Goal: To enable and encourage students to critically analyze and discuss ethical issues society faces with respect to the HIV epidemic.

Planning and materials: The facilitator/teacher should have an accurate and up-to-date knowledge of HIV/AIDS to facilitate this exercise. (Additional readings are listed at the end of the article.)

Make a copy of the case studies for each student. As an alternative, an overhead transparency of the case studies can be used and students can copy their assigned case study.

Time required: Approximately 70 minutes or one 50-minute class period if given as a homework assignment in a previous class.

Directions: Divide students into five groups of five to eight. Divide groups so males and females are represented in each and friends do not form a group. Give each group one of the case studies. Have each group choose a chairperson and a separate recorder. The responsibility of the chair is to solicit opinions from each member of the group and to make sure that no one monopolizes the discussion. The recorders should take abbreviated notes of the group's discussion and decisions. (As an alternative, students could be divided into groups and given this activity as an assignment. Presentations could then be made in class on an assigned date.)

Instructions for the facilitator/teacher: Instruct each group that the goal is not for everyone to agree with how the case study is resolved. Thus, there may be a dissenting report that the recorder will also provide. Give groups 15 minutes to discuss their case study and 10 minutes each to discuss what decision(s) they reached.

Encourage questions and challenges from other students regarding the decisions the groups made. Encourage students to agree or disagree with the decisions and to state why.

Case Studies

1. A pediatrician lost his practice after his HIV antibody status was revealed in a local newspaper by a reporter. Should patients have the right to know the HIV antibody status of their health care providers? Should HIV-infected health care providers be allowed to practice? Have more people become infected from patient to health care worker or from health care worker to patient?

2. A group of health care providers at a medical facility indicate they want the option of not treating HIV disease. Should health care providers be required to treat people with HIV disease? What responsibility should health care providers have to educate themselves about HIV disease?

3. People with sexually transmitted diseases (STDs) have been sued for infecting sex partners with a disease. Should people with HIV disease have sex without notifying their partner? Does it make a difference depending on the STD? What responsibility do partners have in asking about the sexual history of a partner? What if the partner does not know that he or she is infected? Should laws require a person to disclose their HIV status to a sexual partner?

4. There is a confirmed case of a student with HIV disease who is living in one of the residence halls on campus. Upon learning this information, the student's roommate requests a room change, which was denied. The student appeals the denial and reveals that the roommate has HIV disease and states that s/he does

not feel comfortable living with his/her roommate. Should a student's request to change rooms in this situation be honored? If authorities know of a student with HIV disease living in a residence hall, should the roommate be notified? What rights should the student with HIV disease have regarding disclosing his/her status (i.e., to the school/university, roommate, etc.)?

5. You have a close friend who has HIV disease. Your friend does not practice safer sex. You know that he/she typically has a couple of sexual partners per year. This concerns you. How would you resolve this situation? How would your response differ if he/she was practicing safer sex every time? Should partners with HIV disease have sex without notifying their partners?

(SOURCE: Reginald Fennell, Ph.D., CHES, "Challenging Attitudes toward HIV/AIDS," *FLEducator* [Winter 1992/1993], 28–30. Reprinted with permission of ETR Associates, Santa Cruz, Calif. For information about this and other related materials, call 800-321-4407.)

You can develop case study descriptions from a variety of sources:

- *News stories.* Write brief summaries of current news articles, or duplicate actual newspaper accounts.
- *TV soap operas, dramas, and sit-coms.* Write summaries of television relationship situations.
- *Guest speakers.* Panel presenters and other guest speakers are sometimes asked to tell their stories (e.g., a person living with AIDS); use these personal histories in the same manner as a case study.

Here we describe two more case study and story activities.

1. "A Conversation about Sex," in *New Methods for Puberty Education,*[10] is a story dialogue between two girls used to introduce the lesson on female sexual response. The story is an interesting way of both presenting information and bringing up possible feelings and reactions to hearing this information.

2. In *9/10 F.L.A.S.H.,* the lesson "Touch and Abstinence"[11] uses four case studies to illustrate nurturing touch, affectionate touch, violent touch, and sexual touch. The activity proceeds to discussion and a quadrant exercise that bring up cultural and family differences and other issues around student-generated examples of the four types of touch.

Case studies and stories should be adapted to the culture, language, and learning level of students to be effective. The main reason for using this method is to help learners personalize needed information or concepts; this goal is lost if students cannot identify with the situation or characters.

ANONYMOUS STATEMENTS

Asking learners to make anonymous, written statements about a controversial issue allows the examination of the variety of feelings, values, and attitudes present in a group. Tension and interest can be high because students are hearing the real ideas of their peers. Care should be taken to assure anonymity and enforce ground rules, especially regarding acceptance of varying opinions and feelings.

The example in the box illustrates the steps of this method.

Choosing Condoms

Objectives
1. Participants will examine their own feelings and attitudes about the implications of using condoms.
2. Participants will become familiar with the wide variety of condoms available on the market.
3. Participants will evaluate different brands and types of condoms by conducting a "Condom Report."

Rationale: Although the AIDS crisis has led to the popularization of condoms, considerable resistance to their use remains. In fact, publicity about using condoms for "safer sex" (for protection against AIDS and other sexually transmitted diseases) has made some people fearful that to suggest using a condom is to suggest that one's partner or oneself is infected. In this lesson students will confront the issue of talking with a partner about condom use and will reflect on the impact attitudes may have on a couple's ability to protect themselves. In addition, when students examine and evaluate a variety of brands, condoms are demystified. Students overcome the common aversion to touching condoms, learn there are many different types of condoms (if one is not satisfactory, another can be tried), and become confident as consumers should they ever decide to use condoms for protection against disease or pregnancy.

Materials: Worksheets "Condom Reports" and "In Search of Condoms"; variety of different types of condoms in their packs; 3" x 5" file cards.

Note to the teacher: You may want to begin this lesson with a brief description of the proper use of the condom.

Procedure
1. Ask students to assess how attitudes about the condom have changed during the last year or so. (They may refer to increased media coverage, to the association of condoms with AIDS, etc.).
2. Distribute 3" x 5" cards to each student. Note that in spite of increased discussion about condoms, people still have many different feelings about using them. Ask students to write on the card how they imagine they would feel if they were involved in a relationship and prior to intercourse a partner took out a condom and suggested they use it. Explain that their responses are anonymous: however, they should put M for male or F for female on top of their card. (A note of caution: If only a few students of either gender are in the class, asking them to label their 3" X 5" cards by gender denies them anonymity; in that case, omit this step.)

3. Collect cards and read them out loud, stating whether male or female each time.

Discussion questions
   a. Note that in nationwide studies, both males and females reported that when a partner initiated condom use, they felt it demonstrated caring and they liked the person better for this. Ask students if their own responses were similar or different from the nationwide research.
   b. Note that many family planning clinics are advising women who use the pill and the diaphragm to also use condoms. Why is this so?
   c. In an age of AIDS and other sexually transmitted diseases, who are the only people who do not need to use condoms?
4. Distribute the worksheet "Condom Reports." Review the directions with the entire class. Divide students into small groups (five or fewer is best) and give each group a selection of at least three condoms (in their boxes) to evaluate.
5. Conclude the lesson by asking each group to report which condom received the highest rating in their group and why.

(SOURCE: Peggy Brick et al., *Teaching Safer Sex* [Hackensack, N.J.: Planned Parenthood of Greater Northern New Jersey, 1989], 35–38. Reprinted with permission. Cautionary note added by authors of this text.)

The first worksheet for this activity ("Condom Reports," not reprinted in this text) asks students to report an evaluation of condom packaging, describe features of the condom, describe the wrapping of individual condoms, and any other comments students would like to add. The second worksheet ("In Search of Condoms," also not reprinted here) asks students to report specific details of a trip to purchase condoms.

CHAPTER 11

Helping Learners Develop Skills and Practice What They Know

Thinking is easy, action is difficult; to act in accordance with one's thoughts is the most difficult thing in the world.

(Johann Wolfgang von Goethe)

In this chapter we address the behavioral domain: how to help learners practice knowledge and skills and apply them to their own problems, their real lives. Methods that help learners practice skills not only improve those skills, but also help change their attitudes regarding the efficacy of the skills (e.g., that a particular communication skill really works) and their belief in themselves (self efficacy—"I really can carry out this skill").

ROLE PLAY

Role play and other practice methods are perhaps the most important methods for sexuality education. Role play provides opportunity to practice skills and behaviors as well as to explore attitudes and feelings:

> Role play, more than any other in-class pedagogical technique, forces students to apply learning to life. Although the same dilemmas can be examined in writing assignments and in discussions, the problems tend to remain cognitive, often subject to glib and heady solutions. But when students act, emotions and complexities surface and the situation is experienced more fully. [1]

Role play provides practice for application of a key concept, information, or skills. For example, in a lesson on decision making about sexual behavior, there are several important interactions to role play:

- Negotiating decisions about sexual behavior and limits with one's partner.
- Discussing with one's parents (or another adult) the decision to have sex.
- Discussing contraception and/or STD prevention with one's partner.
- Discussing contraception or STD prevention with a health care provider.
- Refusing to participate in any sexual behavior; saying "no" while maintaining the relationship.

This method is quite varied. Learners can play out situations from case histories or videos, from group brainstorming, or from the results of problem-solving discussions (see following). Role plays can be entirely scripted, partially scripted or completely ad libbed or composed by the participants. Scripts can be written by the teacher, taken from a curriculum, or written or suggested by students.

Although role plays are generally verbal interactions, ask learners also to attend to concomitant nonverbal behaviors, such as facial expression, tone of voice, loudness, eye contact, and posture. For example, prior to verbal role plays, *Reducing the Risk*[2] has students do a nonverbal practice of refusal skills, including hand and arm gestures, full body posture, a strong voice, and a serious expression to demonstrate strength in refusals.

Role play can be done in front of the whole group or in small groups. Role plays can be spontaneous, informal, and short, with learners practicing only a sentence or two; for example, during a discussion on refusal skills, you might say, "How would you refuse a date? What would you say? Try it—practice saying the words." Or they can be tightly controlled and formalized, more of an exercise or specific activity than part of a discussion.

We suggest the following steps and variations for using role plays in the sexuality education classroom:

1. Make sure that students are acquainted, that they know each other's names; you may need to do some "get acquainted" activities.
2. Warm up learners' ability to pretend: for example, have pairs of students carry on a conversation using only gibberish, expressing teacher-suggested emotions (joy, anger, suspicion, sorrow); then have the same pairs enact teacher-suggested scenes in gibberish, for example, a policeman giving a ticket to someone who is parked illegally.[3]
3. Introduce and discuss the process and content of the role play activity; connect it to previous learnings and key concepts. If students have developed or written the role plays, realism and relevance are increased.
4. You may want to begin by showing role plays, for example, by older students, by teachers, by teacher and volunteer student, or on video. The *Human Sexuality: Values and Choices* curriculum,[4] for example, includes video segments of students doing role plays. Also, seeing a teen theater production (see Chapter 12) helps prepare students for role play.[5]
5. Describe and discuss the following roles:
   • The main *characters* in the situation being played.
   • *Coach.* Sometimes called an "alter ego," this person stands or sits at the shoulder of one of the role players and suggests strategies, statements, tone of voice, and so forth: "Try saying it louder." "Get assertive!" "Give him another idea of something to do instead." "Look her in the eyes." The educator may wish to demonstrate this "doubling" process, particularly when first introducing it to the group.
   • *Observers.* All other members of the group become observers, watching the process, thinking about how they would play the parts, giving feedback after

the role play is finished. Or you can formalize the observer role by posting or handing out follow-up discussion questions (see following for suggestions).

6. Encourage learners to discuss the case and the characters before role playing, looking at values, options and behavior. Characters should describe themselves in role; the teacher may need to ask specific questions: "Who are you?" "How old are you?" "What do you look like?" Players and audience also need to be able to visualize the scene in detail; the teacher may ask specific scene-setting questions about the time of day, surrounding objects, and so forth. However, be aware that many learners would rather talk *about* a situation than play it and may need an extra push to begin role playing.

7. Address students by their role names during role play. Encourage them to *be* the person they are playing, to feel the feelings, try the words, respond spontaneously. Encourage observers to refer to role players by their role names. To facilitate this process, have players wear name tags indicating the names of their characters. Then, when they remove the name tags, they can more easily separate from the role—in their own minds, as well as in the minds of observers.

8. Gently redirect a student who drops out of character during a role play ("Say that to your date").

9. In the middle of a role play, have characters reverse roles. The purpose of "role reversal" is to increase empathy, knowledge or understanding of the other (e.g., if Dana is playing herself and Nancy is playing Dana's mother, reverse roles shortly after beginning so that Nancy can see how Dana perceives her own mother; then Nancy will know how she should play the mother).

10. Insist that observers not distract players. Observers may want to identify with one player and feel what s/he is feeling, thinking of alternative responses and content issues. Observers can be filling out observation sheets during the role play. Possible questions are as follows:
    - How would you have played the part of _____ ?
    - What was effective?
    - What are some statements you would have made differently?
    - What suggestions would you make for changes in nonverbals, such as tone of voice, eye contact, loudness, posture, and so on?
    - What was the turning point?
    - Who was the dominant person?
    - How would the interaction be different if the characters were different races? Different genders? Different ages?

11. If several small group role plays are taking place concurrently, circulate among the groups, observing, coaching, answering questions, encouraging, giving feedback.

12. Do not allow scenes that seem to be going nowhere to continue; stop the group, discuss, provide direction, and continue if appropriate.

13. Follow role play with discussion: Let players discuss how they felt in their roles, what they would do or say differently; ask observers to give feedback and discuss their observation sheets; discuss how the role play situation relates

to real life; give students a chance to verbalize any insights and express feelings; help them generalize to other aspects of their lives. Discussion is also a time for positive reinforcement, not a time for judging each other.

14. Proceed to the next role play activity, reinforcing new skills and providing opportunity for new learning.

To reduce initial learner anxiety and provide a gradual skill-building process, role plays in the *Reducing the Risk* curriculum[6] progress from a fully scripted format to a series of partially scripted role plays, with learners at first writing the unscripted conclusion and then finally spontaneously ad libbing scene conclusions. The following example of a scripted role play from this curriculum (see the box) gives students practice on refusal skills. Observers use checklists (not reprinted here) on which they note whether players used appropriate and effective verbal and nonverbal skills. (*Note:* The teacher instructions reprinted here refer to this scripted role play as well as to a partially scripted role play that follows in the curriculum.)

Role Play in Small Groups

1. Explain to students that they will be working in small groups on role plays. In their group they will be rotating through various role plays. Each student will have the opportunity to read a script (scripted role), respond to a script (unscripted role) and watch (observer).

Pass out the role play "At a Party" (following). At their seats, give students no more than 5 minutes to write down what they might say in the role play to avoid unprotected sex when they have the unscripted part. They can use these responses to help prepare for the role play, although they should not just read when they do the role play. They should act as if this is a real scene and they have no script to rely on—they have to rely on themselves.

2. Have students divide into groups with a mixture of males and females. Students should bring their own role plays and ideas for responses to the group.

3. Make sure each student still has an "Observer Checklist" (not reprinted here). Instruct students to alternate within the group, reading the script and playing in the unscripted role. After a student reads the script, that student takes the unscripted role. Make sure each student has the chance to participate in both the scripted and the unscripted roles and to provide observer comments. The observer is the person who is next in order to read the script.

If the groups do not have equal numbers of boys and girls, then have them assume the other role so everyone has the opportunity to participate in both roles. If there is time to go around a second time, the script readers can make up the script or choose to ad lib and make up their own lines.

Note to the teacher: It is important to help groups "get going" with the role plays. It may be necessary for the teacher to designate who in each group will start the scripted and unscripted roles. Walk around and guide the role play process.

---

4. When groups are finished, have students return to the full group and discuss the experience. Explain that their comfort working like this in small groups will increase each day as the process is repeated throughout the unit.

"At a Party"

Setting the stage: You are at a party with someone you have gone out with a few times. The party is at somebody's home and the parents are gone. A lot of kids are getting high and some couples are leaving—maybe to have sex. You don't want to have sex and don't want to leave the party.

PERSON 1: Let's get out of here so we can talk—it's too crowded.

PERSON 2: Yes, it is crowded in here—but the porch is empty.

PERSON 1: I just want to be with you. This is our chance.

PERSON 2: I want to be with you, too, but the party's fun.

PERSON 1: C'mon, I just want to be alone with you.

PERSON 2: No, I like this party—I'm glad we came.

PERSON 1: I've been looking forward to this night with you—please don't spoil it.

PERSON 2: I hope the night won't be spoiled.

PERSON 1: If I'd known you'd be like this, I wouldn't have come here with you.

PERSON 2: I guess not, but I know we can have fun. Let's get something to eat in the kitchen.

PERSON 1: I guess I don't have much choice.

PERSON 2: Yes, I suppose so. But I'll give you the choice of the next movie we go to.

(SOURCE: Richard P. Barth, MSW, Ph.D., *Reducing the Risk* [Santa Cruz, Calif.: ETR Associates, 1993], 71 and 75. Reprinted with permission from ETR Associates. For information about this and other related materials, call 800-321-4407.)

In the following variation on the role play method (see the box), rather than playing a scene, students develop and then practice responses to the many excuses people give for not using condoms. This activity could be called a "rehearsal" method.

You Would (Use A Condom) If You Loved Me

Objectives
1. Participants will examine the many excuses people give for not protecting themselves from sexual transmission of disease.
2. Participants will practice initiating conversation with a partner about safer sex and responding to a partner's excuse for not practicing safer sex.

Rationale: AIDS education seldom addresses the difficulty many people have raising the issue of condoms or safer sex with a partner. In fact, talking about safer sex is difficult. If a person raises the issue, will the partner think she or he is infected? Or, think that the partner is infected? What does this imply about the past behaviors and relationships of each? To be effective, safer sex education must address the issue of communicating with a partner. This lesson encourages people to think about different ways they could talk with a partner and suggests that a partner who cares will be willing to act so as to prevent infection with disease.

Materials
- Video: "Condom Talk," available from Planned Parenthood of Bergen County, 575 Main Street, Hackensack, NJ 07601; $29.95 plus postage and handling.
- Ten pieces of newsprint; masking tape, magic markers.
- Pictures of couples talking romantically, cut from magazines and mounted on colored paper; one for every two participants.

Procedure
1. There is a lot of advice around the importance of using condoms to protect against sexually transmitted disease including AIDS. However, not much of this advice deals with the difficult issue of talking with a partner about condoms. Ask participants to brainstorm all of the things people say when they don't want to use a condom.
2. As they call out the things people say, list each one on the top of a separate piece of newsprint; then tape it to the wall.
3. Tell participants they are going to have a chance to write answers to each excuse. Demonstrate by reading one excuse, asking possible responses, and writing them on the newsprint. Then give participants 10 minutes to circulate around the room, writing their own answers.
4. When they are finished and seated, ask for volunteers to read each response.
5. Note that it may be as difficult for someone to initiate talk about using condoms as to respond to negative attitudes about them.
6. Show video, "Condom Talk." Discussion questions:
   a. How did you feel about the woman taking the initiative?
   b. How do you think her partner felt? Is this realistic?
   c. What does she mean in the final scene when she says, "I know some things we can do without condoms that are safe."
7. Tell the group they are going to have a chance to talk about condoms. Ask them to find partners (or use a method of chance selection) and give each pair one of the magazine pictures of couples. Explain that they will have 5 minutes to compose the first two sentences of the dialogue this couple is having about safer sex or using a condom.
8. When the pairs are ready, have them stand, one pair at a time, holding up their picture. Now they say to each other the dialogue they have composed.

(If you have time, the dialogues may be written on "balloons" of white paper, glued to the pictures, and posted on the wall.)

(SOURCE: Peggy Brick et al., *Teaching Safer Sex* [Hackensack, N.J.: Planned Parenthood of Greater Northern New Jersey, 1989], 39–40. Reprinted with permission.)

In a similar activity called "Stating One's Needs,"[7] students are given sample responses to pressure statements, practice saying them, and then discuss these responses and others they suggest:

- I don't feel comfortable doing this. Let's stop.
- I would like to be sexual with you, but I'm not ready for intercourse.
- Before we go any further, we need to talk about our sexual pasts.
- I want to talk about using protection first.
- I don't want to have sex at this point in my life.
- I really want to have intercourse with you, but I don't have any condoms, so can we do something else?
- No! Stop. This is not OK with me.

Students may react to role play activities with boredom, frustration, anger, or anxiety. Participants may have had previous bad experiences with this learning method or little experience with participatory methods in general. Performance anxiety may also be an inhibiting factor. A sense of trust, built over time with the group and individuals, is necessary for ease of facilitation and to maximize learning. This atmosphere of trust is most likely in a group where ground rules have been enforced over a period of time and the teacher has facilitated a variety of interactive processes. Role play must be free from threat; ground rules of not judging, ridiculing, or laughing at others should be enforced.

Through role play students can . . .

- Try out new skills without having to reveal personal private behaviors.
- Learn and practice new social skills in relative safety with feedback and suggestions from fellow learners.
- Develop increased self-understanding and awareness of their own feelings without necessarily revealing personal beliefs.
- Release negative feelings safely (e.g., hostility, anger) and then go on to explore other, more appropriate reactions and socially acceptable behaviors or solutions.
- Develop empathy for and insight into other people and situations.
- Increase group process skills, developing responsibility for contributing and working together cooperatively.
- Enhance learning about the subject matter of sexuality.[8]

SELF-TALK

Often called "self-instruction" or "inner speech," self-talk is going on in most people all the time. As a learning tool, coaching in self-instruction helps the learner develop and rehearse positive inner speech or visualize personal behavior or skills that will help him or her in some activity or problem. Self-instruction is used for a number of purposes,[9] all of which deal with current real-life situations rather than assumed roles:

1. To rehearse what one is going to say to someone during an anticipated encounter. For example, a teen could rehearse how to bring up going to a family planning clinic with his or her parents.
2. To rehearse what one is going to say to *oneself* to get through an anticipated situation. For example, one could prepare and then use an internal dialogue for self-instruction when tempted by drugs or alcohol.
3. To give oneself positive affirmations about some aspect of one's character.
4. To visualize oneself successfully doing a behavior (such as assertively meeting someone's eyes, or completing a homework assignment) or avoiding a behavior (such as taking a cigarette or a drink).

To help learners develop and rehearse self-instruction, ask them to relax (see "Guided Imagery" in Chapter 10) and then guide them through an imagining sequence. You can be more or less specific with the guided imagery. For example, in an open-ended imagery, learners imagine any situation during which they would have difficulty saying what they really felt. In a more specific imagery, learners imagine what they could say to themselves to stay assertive while negotiating with a partner.

After the guided imagery process, learners write down the imagined dialogue, practice it by themselves or with a trusted friend or helper, continue to imagine the visualization, and use it when needed. Or they learn to use specific phrases (e.g., positive self-affirmations) every day or during specific problematic situations.

For example, the *Human Sexuality: Values and Choices* curriculum[10] provides students with wallet cards listing values that are important for relationships: equality, self-control, promise keeping, responsibility, respect, honesty, and social justice. The reverse side of the card has some questions (e.g., "Is this a risky situation?") that can help a young person deliberately think through a situation at the moment.

The *Special Education F.L.A.S.H.*[11] curriculum includes an exercise in which students look in a mirror and say something they like about the person they see there, a self-affirmation type of self-talk used for enhancing self-esteem.

SKITS

A skit is a short play, preplanned around a theme or plot and generally involving more characters and more relationships than role plays. More learning takes place when students develop their own skits, within parameters set by the educator. Small groups can develop and produce skits that portray a number of situations needing practice: teens discussing sexuality with parents; two friends purchasing condoms in a drugstore; or a couple discussing their risk for AIDS and then separating to discuss their partners' reactions with best friends. Afterward, ask learners to stay in role while the rest of the group questions them.

In the illustration of this method (see box), groups of students discuss a variety of gender-related body care products and then develop skits that demonstrate and provide practice for purchasing such a product.

Buying Body Care Products

Objectives
1. The students will be able to discuss the use and selection of various body care products.
2. The students will be able to practice, through a role-play experience, the purchasing of a body care product.

Grades: 6–8
Time: 60 minutes
Materials: Examples of body care products placed on a display table in front of the classroom—e.g., acne medication, bras, tampons, sanitary pads, athletic supporters (jock straps), deodorant.
Rationale: As early adolescents begin to assume more responsibility for taking care of their own bodies, they need information and skills for selecting and purchasing body care products. For example, the purchasing of a first bra or athletic supporter involves acceptance of the need for that product, the knowledge of where it can be obtained, an understanding of what size and type is desirable, and finally, the comfort and skill for communicating one's own needs to others.

This lesson begins with a brief, informal lecture by the teacher about a variety of body care products. The teacher displays samples of the products to help students become familiar and more comfortable with them. Through discussion and role play activities, the students learn more about the products and examine the purchasing process in detail. By openly discussing these products, the lesson works toward helping the students understand that they are not alone in the desire for information about the use and selection of the products.

Procedure
1. Tell the students that today's session will involve a discussion about common products that people use in taking care of their bodies. Identify the products on the display table and write the name of each product on the board. Explain the function of each product.
   Bras. These are used by females as support for breasts. They can be purchased at department stores, women's specialty shops, and many other places. Some bras are made of stretchable material and one size fits all. Others are made to fit individual girls and women and have two sizes. One

size is the cup or breast measurement and the other measures the circumference of the upper torso. For a girl to get a general idea of her size, she would measure her own chest, by putting a tape measure around her breasts and back. Many females like to try on a bra before they buy it to make sure it fits.

Athletic supporters (jock straps). These are worn by men and boys to support their penis and testes during sports or other strenuous physical activities. They can be bought at sporting goods or department stores. They are made out of elastic material that stretches as a male moves. They come in various sizes. If a boy wants to purchase an athletic supporter he would find his size by measuring his own waist with a tape measure.

Acne Medications. These are creams, lotions, and ointments that are intended to help clear up pimples on a person's face. They often contain chemicals (retinoic acid, which is Vitamin A, or benzoyl peroxide), which help to degrease, peel, and degerm the skin. Some acne medications can be obtained in a supermarket or drugstore. For the stronger kinds of acne medications, a person needs a prescription from a doctor. A person who has a severe case of acne should ask a doctor for the kind of medication to use.

Tampons and sanitary pads. These are used by girls and women during their menstrual periods to absorb the menstrual flow. They can be purchased at drugstores, supermarkets, and other places. Tampons are inserted into the vagina. Pads are worn outside the body and usually have adhesive tape on one side that attaches securely to the underpants. There are many kinds of tampons and pads. They differ in thickness, absorbency, and mode of application. Information about the various qualities is usually provided on the packages. *Note*: Toxic shock syndrome (TSS) is a severe illness that is thought to be related to tampon use. It is advisable to obtain current information on the syndrome if you plan to discuss it in class. Contact the Food and Drug Administration or the Centers for Disease Control in Atlanta, Georgia, for the latest research information on toxic shock syndrome.

Deodorants. These products are used by people to stop or decrease perspiration or odor from under their arms. Deodorants are made of chemicals that either decrease the amount of perspiration or cover body odors with an artificial fragrance. Some deodorants do both. Some people find that some deodorants will cause an irritation or rash on their skin. Deodorants can be found in drugstores, supermarkets, and most convenience stores.

2. Discuss the products with the entire class. Discussion questions:
   * Which products would be used only by boys? Girls? Both?
   * Which product might require a doctor's prescription?
   * Which products might affect a person's health or safety? In what ways?
   * There are often many different brands of these products. What things might a person want to consider when deciding which brand to buy?
   * How do you think people feel when they go to stores to buy these types of products?
   * In buying any of these products, what assistance might a person need from a store employee?

3. Divide the class into same-sex groups of four or five students per group. Have each group choose a gender-appropriate product. More than one group may choose the same product.
4. Instruct the groups to create a role play (skit) about what it might be like to purchase their products at a store. Some things they might include in the role play would be (a) the type of store where the product might be found, (b) the reactions of store employees, (c) portrayal of the feelings the person buying the product might have, (d) how the person decides which brand to buy. Allow the groups 10–15 minutes to create their role plays.
5. Have the students act out their role plays, using the products as props. After all of the groups have performed, conduct a discussion on the experience with the entire class. Discussion questions:
   • How did the buyers feel about purchasing their products?
   • What problems did the buyers face in selecting their products?
   • What skills did the buyers use in making their purchase?
   • What did the store employees do to make the buyers more comfortable? Less comfortable?
   • What might a buyer do to make best use of a store employee?
   • Are there any other sources that might help a person decide which brand of product would be best to buy?
   • What did you learn from being in a (skit)?
     What did you learn from observing the (skits)?

(SOURCE: Carolyn Cooperman and Chuck Rhoades, *New Methods for Puberty Education* [Hackensack, N.J.: Planned Parenthood of Greater Northern New Jersey, 1992], 109–111. Reprinted with permission.)

PROBLEM SOLVING

During problem solving, learners consider a difficult, confusing situation, one with potential negative consequences, and break it into manageable pieces for the purpose of finding a solution or making a decision. Problem solving, in sexuality education, usually focuses on interpersonal relationships and involves the use of several methods, such as introspection, brainstorming, and role playing, and many skills, such as planning, rehearsing, and decision making.

Problem-solving exercises can take place in the whole group or small group, with learners striving for consensus about problem definition and solutions, or individually as an introspective assignment. Problems can be generated by the group, assigned as case histories by the educator, or be real, current issues or concerns of individuals.

Use ground rules to protect students' confidentiality and establish a comfortable learning situation. Instructions should give learners options for choosing problems that are safe for them to explore. Also, learners should be told ahead of time whether they will share any writing about real personal problems or whether they will be asked to discuss those problems with anyone, including the educator.

The *interpersonal* problem-solving model includes several steps. In the class-room or workshop, learners go through each step as a sort of rehearsal and to learn a process they can put to use in real life; learners can work through each step individually, in small groups, or in the whole group. In actual interpersonal problem solving, the first step is done by the individual as an introspection, and the remaining steps take place with the other person(s) involved.

As learners go through the model, they should consider some of the following questions: [12]

1. *Diagnosis.* Here the individual analyzes the problem from his or her own perspective:

- How do I define the problem?
- How do I think _____ would define the problem?
- Who has the problem?
- Who else is involved?
- How do I feel about it?
- What's in it for me to work on this problem?
- What do I have to lose or gain?
- How do I feel about the other person(s) involved?
- What will happen if the problem continues?
- What was the sequence of events that got me into this?
- When should I initiate discussion with the other person(s)?
- Where should I talk with that person?
- How can I start the conversation?
- How do I deal with my own embarrassment or other feelings?
- How do I deal with his/her reactions?
- Who can support me if I initiate problem solving with the other person?

2. *Initiation.* The second step is to initiate a process of clarifying the two perspectives of the situation, yours and that of the person with whom you have a problem. Both parties need to be able to hear and understand the other's view-point. Many people get stuck in this step, believing that if they listen they are expressing agreement with the other person. The learner can rehearse the initial discussion or confrontation with the other person(s) involved, considering the following:

- What can I say to get that person to listen to me?
- How can I listen to him/her?
- How will I know s/he really understands me?
- How will I know I understand him/her?

3. *Negotiation and resolution.* Many people jump to suggesting solutions before they clearly define the problem, before they listen to each other. In this step, solutions are brainstormed and then analyzed and rejected or accepted:

- What can I do to solve the problem?
- What do I want to ask the other person to do?
- How can I request changes?
- What can *we* do to solve the problem? What are all the possible ideas we each can contribute?
- How do I rank order the solutions, in terms of what I want to do?
- What am I willing to give up?
- What are the potential results of each solution?
- What is my prediction of whether I can carry out each solution?
- Why do I choose this particular solution?
- When will I carry it out?

As presented here, this is a complex problem-solving model. However, the basic parts of problem solving can be practiced without naming them, by asking learners to consider some key questions as they plan an interaction. An example of the use of this model, in simplified form, would be to ask learners to imagine discussing birth control with a partner, anticipating how they would feel during the discussion, considering when and where to initiate the conversation, what statements they would use to start, how to deal with their own embarrassment, and how to deal with their partner's reactions. This planning session could be followed by role playing.

Here is another idea for a problem-solving activity on relationship issues: divide learners into small groups; give each group a brief case history of a problem in an intimate relationship; ask groups to conduct a problem-solving process for their case (using steps and questions from the previous model). This is a sample list of problems:

Problem 1: One person in the relationship wants to have sex, the other person doesn't.

Problem 2: One person in the relationship is disliked and rejected by the other person's family.

Problem 3: One person in the relationship is very uncomfortable talking about feelings (or can't, or won't), and the other person really wants to talk about how they both feel.

Problem 4: One person in the relationship is always the one who pays for activities they do together and is really beginning to resent this.

Problem 5: One person in the relationship never gives gifts, remembers the other's birthday, Valentines Day, and so on; the other person is beginning to feel hurt.

Problem 6: One person in the relationship contracts an STD from the partner while under the assumption that they had a monogamous relationship.

Problem 7: One person in the relationship refuses to use condoms (to prevent pregnancy or STD); the other person is getting scared.

Here is a simpler problem-solving model, one that does not include the interpersonal component:

1. Define the problem; gather facts and ideas for alternatives.
2. Consider your options, listing the advantages, disadvantages, and possible outcomes of each.
3. Choose the alternative(s) you wish to pursue.
4. Make an action plan for carrying out your chosen alternative(s), listing steps and potential obstacles.
5. Carry out your plan.
6. Evaluate your decision and the actions you have accomplished.

In *New Methods for Puberty Education,* the lesson entitled "Problem Solving"[13] proposes such a simple problem-solving process for concrete problems, that is, personal body care problems that do not focus on relationships. Students list, critique, and imagine trying solutions to such problems as feeling too tall, being dissatisfied with too-oily hair, being embarrassed to buy sanitary pads, or getting an erection in class. The lesson recommends that the class set aside one day a week in family life education as "Problem Solving Day," using this problem-solving model on problems that gradually build in complexity and sensitivity.

SIMULATIONS

Simulations are, in effect, extended role plays. They also share elements of games (see Chapter 12) in the ways they involve learners, but generally are more serious. Simulations imitate conditions of real life, providing vicarious experiences in which learners practice interpersonal and/or intrapersonal skills and observe and analyze their own and others' feelings and behaviors.

Participants in simulations practice and experiment with a variety of skills, including listening, negotiating, decision making, abstract thinking, observing, confronting, problem solving, and expressing feelings. As learners become involved in the process, that is, as they imagine themselves in the "real-life" situation, opportunity for personalizing key concepts occurs. After the simulation is finished, be sure to conduct an analysis (or debriefing), giving learners the opportunity to share feelings, interpretations, and perceptions of their experiences, to analyze meanings and to project applications to real life.

For example, in Bellevue, Washington, a public school biology teacher collaborates with a Planned Parenthood educator to simulate a clinic visit[14] for his advanced biology class. The class goes to the clinic for one and one-half hours beginning at 7:30 A.M., before regular clinic hours. There the Planned Parenthood educator greets them, introduces herself, describes what it is like to work in family planning, discusses the goals of family-planning programs in general and Planned Parenthood in particular, and describes the wide range of services available.

Then students divide into groups of four and progress through the following stations:

1. In the waiting room students complete patient history forms and discuss the importance of knowing their families' and their own medical histories.
2. Other students look through a display of materials on the history of family planning.
3. At another table, students look at and handle all types of contraceptives.
4. In the clinic library, another group completes an assignment of locating materials in several categories, for example, materials on relationships, for young children, and so on.
5. In the lab, students perform pregnancy tests on urine samples taken from volunteer male students and positive samples obtained from the clinic. They also view slides of STDs, a rodent fetus, sperm, and eggs under the microscope.
6. Finally, in the exam room, the Planned Parenthood educator discusses why women might be nervous about pelvic exams. She also describes pelvic exam, Pap smear, and STD check procedures. She skillfully uses humor and an interactive manner and process to get students to volunteer to get on the exam table (male and female, fully clothed—no skirts) with their feet in the supports.

The biology teacher remains in the lab throughout the clinic visit, and the Planned Parenthood educator stays in the exam room; groups of students circulate independently through all other stations.

The worksheets used in the pregnancy test and pelvic exam portions of this simulation are provided in the box.

Pelvic Exam Worksheet

It can be very helpful to know when people need a pelvic exam and what happens during the exam. For information to help you with this section, you may wish to read the pamphlet "Your Pelvic Exam."
1. When and why is a pelvic exam recommended?
2. What happens before the exam?
3. To understand some of the feelings that some people have about and during this exam, you may take turns climbing up on the exam table while you work on this section. For our class exercise, of course, keep your clothes on, but you might imagine what it would be like with your clothes off! This exercise may be particularly helpful for the young men in the class, but everyone may try it. Follow the directions posted on the wall for you for correct use of the table and positioning for the exam.
4. What is a speculum? When and why is it used?
5. Why might the person being examined want to ask for a mirror if none were offered?
6. What is a Pap test? How is it done?
7. What happens during the bimanual exam?
8. What were some of the feelings you had while participating in the exam table exercise?

9. How do you think it affects people to know in advance what happens during the exam and to see and get on the exam table just for practice?
10. What questions might someone have that they might want to discuss with a clinician before, during, or after these exams?

Pregnancy Test Worksheet

It is now possible to tell through a urine test whether someone is pregnant. If you would like to conduct this test . . .

1. With a sample of urine, follow the laboratory directions placed on the counter for you.
2. Summarize the procedures; include a diagram if that is helpful to explain the steps.
3. How soon after someone has unprotected intercourse could conception occur?
4. How soon after conception could a urine test indicate a pregnancy?
5. What is in the urine that allows the test to tell if there is a pregnancy? (Hint: It is a hormone not otherwise there.)
6. How accurate are the test results of drugstore pregnancy "home test kits"? What are the chances of a false positive result? Of a false negative result? Why would someone have a lab test rather than a home test? Why would someone have a home test rather than a lab test?

Following the clinic visit, students write evaluative comments, which are sent to the Planned Parenthood educator; here are some actual comments.

One of my favorite things that we did was being able to see what goes on during a pelvic exam. I had always heard horror stories of how embarrassing and painful they were. . . . It was your explanation of what goes on during an exam that really set me straight and put my fears to rest. I now feel more comfortable going in to have a pap smear because the "unknown" is taken away from the whole situation.

I'm glad some guys got up there to see how it is!

I had never been to Planned Parenthood before and of course had heard all the untrue rumors said about it. Now that I have been there and seen the inside of the infamous "clinic" I see just how crazy those rumors are.

Here are two more examples of simulations.

1. The *Reducing the Risk* curriculum uses a simulation entitled "Months of the Year Risk Activity"[15] to help students "experience" and personalize the risk of pregnancy after unprotected intercourse. Students are told that a couple has a 1 in 12 chance of becoming pregnant each time they have unprotected intercourse and that almost everyone who continues to have unprotected intercourse will become pregnant within a year. Participants choose and record a number from 1 to 12; the facilitator draws a number from twelve slips numbered 1 to 12. Those with

the number drawn stand up; they are "pregnant" or have "gotten someone pregnant." The facilitator continues drawing until all numbers are drawn and all students are standing, "experiencing" the feeling of being pregnant. Variations are then played, where some abstain and some use birth control.

2. An AIDS simulation involving an entire high school of 1,400 students made the news in Seattle recently.[16] The simulation, called "The Seven-Year Promise," was organized by students for HIV/AIDS Awareness Week with help from a math teacher and a school nurse. Roles and risks were assigned to students according to probabilities based on the following statistics: (1) 90 percent of young people are sexually active by the time they're 24; and (2) 60 percent of high school seniors are sexually active and more than half of those don't use condoms. For simplification, organizers exaggerated risk by assuming that a student who had unprotected sex once with an HIV-positive partner was immediately infected, did not allow participants to change their behavior as they became more aware, and they didn't include other ways (besides sexual intercourse) of transmitting the virus. Based on their profiles, students drew "chips" throughout the day with information about hypothetical sexual partners. If a chip showed that the partner was HIV-positive and neither party used a condom, the student "got" HIV. The simulation lasted "seven years" in the one day. At the closing assembly ("the reunion"), students were asked to rise if they had contracted AIDS; half stood up. Herpes and chlamydia risks were also simulated, and informational and debriefing activities were included.

REAL-LIFE HOMEWORK

With "real-life" homework, learners practice skills in real situations; for example, they talk with parents about sexual issues; they visit or call a family-planning clinic for information; they go to a library and ask for material on gay and lesbian issues; or they go to a drugstore and locate and price condoms. Real-life homework is similar to the simulation method, but is done more independently. Such home-work is challenging and sometimes uncomfortable for learners; discomfort and resistance should be acknowledged and thoroughly discussed beforehand.[17]

The rewards from real assignments are great: learners not only practice and increase their social skills, they also increase their belief that they will be able to carry out skills and use community resources when needed.

Assigning such homework can be controversial in public school settings. To successfully implement such methods you must first lay groundwork for district, parent, and community acceptance. A deliberate process for establishing such a program is described in Barth, Middleton, and Wagman's article, "A Skill Building Approach to Preventing Teenage Pregnancy."[18]

During the following real-life homework activity (see box), students go into the community to locate, price, and describe various contraceptive methods.

Visit or Call a Clinic

1. Explain that many people—including adults—avoid going to a clinic or local doctor to discuss protection because they don't know what to expect. Besides learning what services are offered at local family planning clinics, this homework assignment asks students to rate their comfort level while at the clinic. Hand out the two-page homework and tell students they can complete the assignment in one of four ways:

a. They can visit a clinic, complete the homework, and describe the way to get to a clinic.

b. They can visit a clinic and complete the homework.

c. They can call a clinic, complete the homework, and describe the way to get to a clinic.

d. They can call a clinic and complete the homework.

Whichever version of the assignment students choose, they must all complete "Visit or Call a Clinic." For additional points, they may complete "The Way to the Clinic."

Pass out a local phone directory (or several) and have students find the clinic section in the yellow pages. Select two or three conveniently located clinics (or the clinics that have agreed to participate) from which they can choose. Have them choose in class so you can control the number of students contacting each clinic. (If there is only one clinic, consider the alternatives following).

Have the students write the name of their clinic in the space provided on the worksheet. If the clinics have given you information about the best times to answer questions or come in, share those with students. As a general rule, encourage them to visit the clinic in pairs, but discourage going in groups larger than three. Encourage students to go with their boyfriends or girlfriends, even those who aren't in the class. Tell students they should bring back some literature available from the clinic. This could be a pamphlet or a flier describing services. Remind them that clinics are professional places and that they should use their best behavior. Additionally, they should keep to themselves the names of anyone they see at the clinic.

2. Conduct a brainstorming session to generate some questions that can be used when visiting the clinic. If students are slow getting started, help them prepare to ask:

a. How much does a clinic visit cost?

b. What is the confidentiality policy?

c. What services are available?

d. How long does it take to get an appointment?

e. Do you have to want a method of protection now, or can you make an appointment for consultation only?

f. What happens during a typical appointment and how long does it take?

g. Does the clinic also offer HIV antibody testing? If so, how is the test done (anonymous or confidential)? How are results verified and recorded? How much does the test cost? Is pre- and post-test counseling offered?

Worksheet: "The Way to the Clinic"

Complete the following questions for bus or train route from school to the clinic:

1. Which bus did you catch? Name or number of bus: _____
2. Where do you get on the bus?
3. Do you need a transfer?
4. What are the transfers?
5. Where do you get off?
6. About how far did you have to walk from the last bus to the clinic?

For car, bike, or walking route, describe the way from your house or the school to the clinic. Give all street names and freeway numbers. Try to remember and write down other landmarks (like a fast-food restaurant or a park) that cue you where to turn (you may attach a map and mark the route).

(SOURCE: Richard P. Barth, MSW, Ph.D., *Reducing the Risk* [Santa Cruz, Calif.: ETR Associates, 1993], 119–120, 125. Reprinted with permission from ETR Associates. For information about this and other related materials, call 1-800-321-4407.)

CHAPTER 12

Multipurpose Methods

The sexuality education methods we describe in this chapter are so complex, so varied, and so versatile that they cannot be categorized, even arbitrarily, by learning domain. We describe how brainstorming, for example, can be used for a variety of purposes throughout lessons and curricula. We also apply the principles of effective sexuality education to the use of peer educators, teen theater, debate, guest speakers, and games. And we give ideas for activities that utilize kinesthetic learning processes.

BRAINSTORMING

Brainstorming is a process for spontaneously generating ideas or information about a topic. When teachers use brainstorming, they acknowledge that learners bring with them considerable content for sexuality lessons. Use brainstorming for a variety of purposes:

- As a warm-up to focus individuals and the group on the topic and/or concept of the lesson.
- To assess learner needs, interests, knowledge, and misinformation (for example, begin a session on HIV by asking learners to list the ways HIV can be transmitted; use the list to begin a presentation by elaborating on some responses and correcting others).
- To generate expression of feelings, values, attitudes, and beliefs (for example, ask learners to brainstorm desirable characteristics of a long-term relationship, or how they would feel if a best friend told them s/he had AIDS).
- To generate solutions to problems (see examples in Chapter 11).
- To generate appropriate verbal and nonverbal behavior for practice and application (for example, ask learners to list effective responses to pressure lines).

Use brainstorming activities at any time during a lesson, to begin a session, or as part of a complex sequence of activities. Precede a brainstorm with individual introspective activities, such as focus writing, or use it to summarize a lesson.

We recommend the following steps for facilitating this method in sexuality education and training sessions; included are suggestions for varying the process:

1. Attempt to foster an open, accepting atmosphere by briefly stating the rules of brainstorming:
   - All input is valid.
   - Participants should not censor, edit, or criticize their own or others' comments—they should "suspend critical judgment."
   - Quantity is important; say "I want to get as many ideas on the board as possible; then we will step back and take a look at them."
   - Suggest that if they don't know the word, try for the idea, and you or others can help them with wording; reserve the right to translate slang into "correct" language.

2. Introduce the topic or question for brainstorming. Take care to be clear in the phrasing of your question. Wait for several responses before you "coach" them by suggesting other ways of viewing the topic; too much initial input by the facilitator may limit or narrow learner thought processes.

3. Suspend your own critical judgment of participant responses. Even a subtle editing of ideas can squelch enthusiasm and shut down shy people. You may be tempted to simplify, categorize, and summarize as you write; try instead to record abbreviated key words of all responses. If responses are too long and rambling, ask the respondent to "give me the key word." Do not change words: for example, don't write "caring" when the participant said "affectionate" or say that the idea is already recorded because someone else already said "caring." If participants use different words, they are expressing a different thought or feeling. Aim for precision in distilling just enough of the person's ideas in as much of his or her own language as possible. *And do it quickly.*

4. Listen for *intent* as well as *content* of participant input; paraphrase responses to be sure you have correctly heard learner contributions.

5. Abbreviate. Drop ends of words, use acronyms and initials, leave out vowels (if quicker for you—it takes practice), don't worry about correct spelling. Remember, participants heard the words and need only brief cues to remind them what was said.

6. Take care in asking another person to record for you; that person may not be able to write quickly or legibly and controls the content of what is written. With large or particularly verbal groups, you might want to use a skilled assistant to help you record. Decide on the process for working together ahead of time, for example, each of you writing every other comment on two separate flip charts. Keep eye contact with your fellow recorder, and use prearranged signals regarding who writes what. Unless this is done smoothly, the recording process may detract from the brainstorm. Cofacilitators may decide to have one person (the fastest writer) record and the other facilitate.

7. Late in the brainstorm, add comments of your own. Wait for participants,

though; they have not thought about the topic as long or as thoroughly as you have. Your input can stifle theirs, and can even turn the brainstorm into a competition between you and participants. But do add key elements; for example, when brainstorming a list of "kinds or types of relationships," and participants have listed "best friend," "parents," "teacher-student," "sibling," "grandparent-grandchild," and "husband-wife," use the opportunity to add "same gender lovers or partners," "foster parent–foster child," etc.

8. If participants get caught up in discussion of some points, keep the brainstorming process moving by reiterating the question.

9. As input slows, stimulate input by suggesting any unexplored viewpoint: "How about people from X community?" or "What about environmental factors?" Build on ideas of other brainstormers. If a comment is unclear, ask the person to "Say more about that" or "Can you elaborate?"

10. Do not let a brainstorm drag on too long, in an attempt to get all possible responses posted; this results in redundancy and loss of learner attention and group momentum.

When it seems there will be no more input, or when your brainstorming time is concluded, the information generated can be processed, categorized, or analyzed in a number of ways:

- Use selected criteria for *prioritizing* the topics listed; for example, prioritize by student interest, or by most common to least common.
- Ask the group to "apply critical judgment" to the list: "Which responses are incorrect?" "How can the information be categorized?" "Which items can be eliminated?" "What decisions need to be made?" Or ask students to categorize the results into groupings, such as *myths, beliefs, facts,* and *feelings* — or *cause* and *effect.*
- Begin your follow-up presentation by correcting learner misinformation and myths reflected in the brainstorm content. Draw the connection between learner concepts, feelings, information, and ideas and the key concepts of your lesson.

The key concept for the following example of a brainstorm activity (see box) is "distortion," specifically distortion of communication.

The Arc of Distortion

This activity provides a simple conceptual model of miscommunication for teen and adult groups. The "arc" is the number of degrees of angle that the direction of communication is bent, or distorted, off the intended direction—a graphic representation of a math concept. Facilitate this brainstorm process as follows.

1. Introduce the situation: "Person A has been in a relationship with Person B for a few months; Person A wishes to communicate something directly to Person B but there are many factors that can interfere with direct communication."

2. Draw a horizontal line on your board, flip chart, or overhead projector representing the direction of intended communication between Person A and Person B (see illustration). Note that we call the characters "A" and "B" rather than "Ann" and "Bob," keeping the situation gender neutral; this allows learners to imagine the relationship as either heterosexual or gay or lesbian. You can make this point explicit or leave it unsaid.

3. Draw a line at an angle from Person A, in the direction that the communication actually travels, missing Person B (see illustration).

4. Within this angle (the "arc of distortion"), brainstorm and record all the factors that can cause this distortion of communication. Several times during the brainstorm restate the question in different terms to help learners see different perspectives, for example, "What are some differences between people that can cause miscommunication or misunderstanding?" "What factors in the environment can interfere?" Responses that learners list typically include race, education, language, gender, age, noise, illness, emotions, sexual attraction, smells, and so forth.

5. Follow the brainstorm with activities that make use of the information generated.

Here are two more ideas for brainstorming activities.

1. The lesson "Words Hurt," from *When I'm Grown: Life Planning Education for Grades 3 & 4,*[1] includes a brainstorm of names children call each other. Typical responses include words that are intellectual and social putdowns, and homophobic or racial slurs. Children then identify feelings they have when they

THE ARC OF DISTORTION

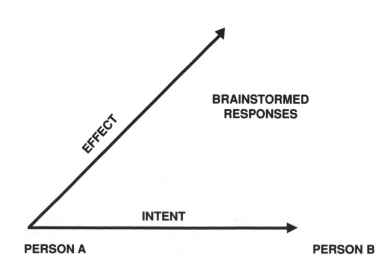

BRAINSTORMED RESPONSES

EFFECT

INTENT

PERSON A   PERSON B

hear the words; we also suggest that you ask students to try to identify the feelings of those who are *targets* of such words.

2. A variation on the typical brainstorming session (during which the teacher stands in front of the group and records responses) is to set up several stations, each with an easel and felt pens, and have learners circulate and record their own responses. For example, in a lesson on gender, set up stations for brainstorming the advantages of being male, the disadvantages of being male, the advantages of being female, and the disadvantages of being female.

Brainstorming allows low-risk sharing for all individuals. Silent participants often find themselves spontaneously contributing to a brainstorm, and this method is an opportunity to help everyone feel included and that their opinions are valued. Brainstorming helps learners see that others have similar ideas ("I'm not the only one!"), and, conversely, that not everyone thinks alike or knows the same things. They also begin to see each other as resources.

By asking questions, the educator introduces topics, concepts and ideas and stimulates thinking. Brainstorming is basically a questioning process. We caution sexuality educators, however, that some types of questions and ways of asking, whether in a brainstorming session or a general discussion, should not be used: do not ask questions about a learner's personal sexual behavior or experiences (e.g., "How many of you have ever had an STD?"); do not use accusatory questions that imply error on the part of the learner (e.g., "why" questions, such as, "Why didn't you use birth control?" asked of a group of pregnant teens); and do not condescend to learners by asking values and belief questions for which you believe you already have the only right answer. Asking for facts is an appropriate way of evaluating knowledge; but asking leading *values* questions (e.g., "What is the *only* way to avoid an STD?" with the expected answer, "By having sex only in a monogamous marriage") devalues student input, beliefs, and cultural differences and implies a strong negative judgment of those who believe or act differently. If all you want is agreement, don't ask.

When this method is used inappropriately (e.g., to ask blaming questions, or questions for which only you know all the answers), individuals may feel alienated from the group or insulted by the facilitator. Many individuals will risk what they perceive to be unusual ideas or minority opinions only if they trust the group and the facilitator. Recognize and validate input of all group members.

GUEST SPEAKERS AND PANELS

Guest speakers and panel presentations are best used when the guest's expertise and credibility in a particular area are greater than the host educator's, when a different perspective is needed or when the charisma and personal life history of the speaker(s) would increase learner interest. Many AIDS education programs today use panels of persons with HIV to help learners see the relevance of prevention in their lives and to begin bridging the gap between "them" and "us."

When planning for the use of guest speakers or panels, first ascertain your organization's or school district's policies and procedures for the use of guest speakers. Make sure the content and process of the speaker's agenda fits the goals, concepts, and content of your curriculum. Solicit speakers whose reputation is sound, or whom you have seen speak. Find out as much as you can about your guest (see the box).

What a Classroom Educator Should Know about a Guest Speaker in a Sexuality Education Class

Before inviting a guest into the classroom, a teacher should try to find out the following information about a speaker and his/her sponsoring agency:

1. *About the agency.* What is their organizational philosophy? What is their reputation in the community and with schools in particular? What experience do they have providing sexuality or HIV education in schools? How well trained are their educators?
2. *About the speaker.* What training has s/he had in sexuality education content and methods? What is the speaker's experience in working with students like yours? What is his/her preferred teaching style? What is the speaker's reputation as a teacher? How will s/he want to be introduced? Is there any information about the speaker that you should not share with learners (e.g., HIV status)?
3. *About the planned presentation.* What teaching methods will be used for this presentation? What kind of support will be needed? How will the presentation fit with your ongoing curriculum? What suggestions does the speaker have for follow-up?
4. *About materials to be used.* Will materials be age appropriate and meet school expectations regarding, for example, explicitness? Will you have an opportunity to preview the materials, films, or anything else that will be used?

Prior to guests' planned visits, preview their materials, agendas, handouts, and videos. Give your guests as much planning time and information as possible: be sure they know the characteristics of your group, their needs, interests and special circumstances, and environmental factors that may affect their presentations (interruptions, amount of time, available equipment, seating arrangements, etc.). Work with your guests to plan their learning design, making sure they know the context of their presentation in your curriculum.

On the day of the presentation, greet and introduce your guest(s) in a manner that shows learners your respect and enthusiasm for the speaker's presence. Reiterate class ground rules and include your guest's input. Remain with the group throughout the guest's presentation: if you are a teacher in a public school, you are legally liable and will be held accountable for whatever happens during the session; you can facilitate problem solving if a disturbance or emergency takes place; furthermore, you need to know what was presented, what questions were raised, and what discussion took place in order to plan a follow-up to the session. Last, ask your guests for suggestions for follow-up.

Suggestions for the Guest Speaker

Ascertain your organization's guidelines for accepting speaking engagements in schools or other organizations. Consider whether or not your goals and priorities and the mission of your organization are compatible with those of your host. Do a needs assessment (see Chapter 6) with your host; find out as much as possible about the learners with whom you will be working and any environmental factors that may affect your learning design. Assure that someone in authority will remain with your group during your session. Ask if there will be any parents or other guests in the classroom. When you arrive, add to your host's introduction and to class ground rules, if necessary.

PEER EDUCATION

Because social norms have such a strong influence on adolescent behavior, peer education is one of the most effective and important means of sexuality and HIV education today. Peer-led teaching can be very powerful, especially for adolescents. Teens report that other teens are the primary sources of their information about sexuality, whether or not that information is correct.[2] Why not make it correct? If every group of teens had key members who were trained to deal with the sexual questions and concerns of their peers, who had the information and skills to positively influence their friends' life skills, there would probably be far less sexual risk taking. The rationale for peer education programs is well stated in Advocates for Youth's *Peer to Peer* manual:

> Teens exist in an environment where most of their information, attitudes and behaviors are profoundly affected by their peers. Young adults frequently have a wonderful peer communication network and can be very effective at exchanging correct information and positive support. . . . Through peer education, both the peer educator and the recipient of the information benefit. . . . Training teenagers to educate other youth creates expertise and establishes resource people within peer groups. Frequently, youth educators can become positive community role models, resource people and special advocates for their peers.[3]

A variety of activities are conducted by peer educator programs. Some provide cofacilitators to work with professional educators in school sexuality education programs. For example, one of the key elements of the *Postponing Sexual Involvement*[4] curriculum is the use of trained teen leaders who work with adults to conduct the curriculum. Some programs conduct teen theater productions. Some peer educators do parent/child puberty education sessions. Others work with teens one-on-one or in support groups, advocate for condom distribution, produce videos and write for newspapers, write informational brochures, work on phone hotlines, provide referrals, or act as individual advocates.

Many successful peer sexuality and HIV education programs are found in school districts; others are part of county health departments, youth-serving community organizations, Planned Parenthoods and other family planning organizations, universities, and school-based health centers.

Successful managers are respected and trusted by the teens involved. They do careful planning, setting criteria for peer educator recruitment; they work collaboratively with other organizations, businesses, parents, and schools; and they regularly evaluate their programs. Here are some specific guidelines for managing an effective program:

- Allow the teens to make many of the decisions in the program, including who is recruited, what the application looks like, what activities are undertaken, and so on.
- Help teens utilize a variety of skills, including writing for school and city newspapers, working one-on-one with friends, making referrals, mediating conflicts, facilitating support groups, speaking to classes, or presenting teen theater.
- Recruit teens who are members of target population groups and who bring with them a variety of life experiences. Ideally, each should have leadership qualities. Care should be taken to recruit nontraditional leaders, including members of disenfranchised, high-risk groups.[5]
- Train teen educators in the sexuality content they need for working with their peers, including information about HIV and STDs, contraception, sexual abuse, harassment, physical abuse, substance abuse, homophobia, racism, safer sex, gender roles and stereotypes, self-esteem, and so forth.
- Train peer educators in the skills of communication, interaction, speaking, education, acting, mediation, counseling, facilitation, and other skills or techniques they may need to conduct the program's activities.
- Provide incentives for participants, such as stipends, free clinic services, food, retreats, and other desirable opportunities.

The following manuals provide further guidelines and resources for peer education.

1. *Peer to Peer: Youth Preventing HIV Infection Together*[6] summarizes steps for developing and implementing a peer education program, including recruitment, community organizing, involvement of parents, training, educational techniques for peer educators, and evaluation. The manual also reviews fourteen successful peer education programs.

2. *Peer Education . . . a little help from your friends . . .*[7] describes the program developed by Planned Parenthood Centers of West Michigan. It includes information on developing a program, sample application forms and other paper work, teaching tips, and a 40-hour training course design.

Teen theater is thought by some to be the ultimate peer education. Its strength lies in the power of social norm setting; however, used by itself, theater is a passive method. It may entertain, inform, evoke emotions, raise issues, raise awareness, dispel myths and misinformation. But unless the teens in the theater troupe interact with the audience, the effect for many students may be no more than the effect of an interesting video with teen actors.

For the teens involved in producing teen theater, the impact can be tremendous. The best teen theaters set up a process wherein troupe members study sexual issues, brainstorm problems they might want to depict on stage, select several, and work in groups to develop and write their own skits. Then they work to develop the scene, the characters, and the conflict or dilemma to be presented. Besides learning acting skills, students in such programs gain self-confidence, learn about relationships and sexual issues, clarify their own values, and increase communication with their parents.

The most effective teen theater is improvisational and *interactive* with the audience, that is, it presents unresolved dilemmas and sets the stage for audience participation. It presents learners with a dilemma and gets them working on solutions, exploring alternatives, resolving conflicts, articulating values and beliefs, and, ultimately, trying role play themselves. When used in this way, teen theater does more than inform and increase comfort with sexual topics; it also models and increases comfort with role play, an important life skills practice method. A colleague describes her experiences using teen theater in this manner:

> Our local Teen Life Theater has been a valuable resource in helping students consider alternative ways of responding to personal crises. Members of the Teen Life troupe portray dilemmas common to adolescents and then let the audience challenge their behavior while they remain "in character." Students tend to identify with some of the characters; and as they watch the scenes, they struggle to find solutions they think are satisfactory. These theater techniques give self-insight, provide new options and demonstrate effective problem solving, at the same time showing students how they can experiment with alternative behaviors for themselves through role play.[8]

The following two examples of teen theater projects are built on this interactive concept.

1. With the *Hope is Vital* program,[9] a dramatic laboratory is set up where young people can safely and honestly look at difficult issues, values, choices, and consequences regarding sexuality. In a one- or two-week residency, this program trains ten to twenty high school, middle school, or college students to use a combination of theater, discussion, informational sessions, and role play in workshops for youth in their communities. The program focuses on HIV/AIDS awareness and explores concepts of self-esteem, choice, and communication skills.

2. The S.T.A.R. Theater troupe of the AIDS and Adolescents Prevention and Treatment Program[10] of Mount Sinai Adolescent Health Center in New York City writes its own role plays. Audience members interact with the troupe, ques-

tioning the behavior decisions of in-character actors and discussing the situations and people portrayed.

In the community, teen theater can be an important tool for raising awareness about teen concerns and problems among parents and other adults. Some communities form coalitions of youth-serving organizations to provide funding, direction, and training for a teen theater project.

KINESTHETIC AND SENSORY METHODS

Methods that involve touch and movement are particularly important for kinesthetic learners; others with predominantly visual or aural learning styles will benefit both from seeing a concept visually represented by movement and from experiencing learning with their bodies. There are other advantages to using methods beyond "sit and talk": the group is energized, everyone gets involved, and lessons are more varied.

Consider the following when trying to develop kinesthetic activities: What is the concept you are trying to teach? How can it be visualized? What concrete learning activities involving body movement or sensory exercises can you develop that will help students understand—perhaps even feel—the concept? Use your imagination to create kinesthetic representations of facts and concepts. Remember, learners must understand the concept of *symbol* before they can assimilate a symbolic kinesthetic experience; for example, younger students doing the "STD Handshake" activity (see description in Chapter 4) may take the exercise literally and assume STDs are transmitted by shaking hands.

Since this method is so varied and valuable, we describe several examples. In the first lesson (see box), students have fun while gaining understanding of the concepts of *conformity* and *individuality*.

Conformity and Individuality

Objectives
1. The students will be able to define the terms "conformity" and "individuality."
2. The students will be able to identify evidence of conformity and individuality in how people present themselves to others.

Grades: 6–8

Time: 40 minutes

Rationale: Early adolescents have a need to conform to group standards in dress and behavior. This conformity is important developmentally in that it provides a sense of stability at a time of rapid body changes. For example, a student who feels abnormal or awkward because he is taller than his peers finds reassurance by dressing and acting like his friends. Conformity also serves to help students learn about the needs of others through the close bonding of the peer group.

At the same time, it is important for students to appreciate their uniqueness as individuals. This lesson attempts to help students explore how conformity and

---

individuality operate in their lives, without attempting to undermine the importance of either.

Procedure

1. Select a large, open classroom area or gymnasium where students can move about freely. Gather the class into a large group standing close together with their arms at their sides. Tell the students that to participate in this activity, they must stand and move in coordination with the rest of the group. They are all part of a giant being, known as "The Clump."

2. Direct the Clump's movements accordingly:
   - Clump, take ten short steps to the left.
   - Take ten short steps to the right.
   - Move around the room in one large circle.
   - Take three hops forward.
   - Sway to the left. Sway to the right.
   - Walk on your tiptoes to the front of the room.
   - Squat down and move to the center of the room.
   - Clump, decide on your next move.

3. Have the students separate from the Clump. Tell the class that when they were in the Clump, they all moved the same way and did the same things. Now they are going to take a look at how people do things differently.

4. Ask the students to see if they can do the following:
   - Wiggle their ears.
   - Raise one eyebrow.
   - Fold their tongues.
   - Bend the first joint of their index fingers.
   - Pat their heads and rub their stomachs at the same time.
   - Demonstrate a unique capability of their own.

5. Ask the students to describe their reactions to moving as a group and moving as individuals. Drawing from the two experiences, have the students create definitions of the terms "Conformity" and "Individuality."

6. Apply the concepts of conformity and individuality to personal appearance. Write on the board the following headlines:
   - Ways that people look unique.
   - Ways that people make themselves look similar to others.

   Have students brainstorm examples under both categories; review the lists.

Discussion Questions
- How did it feel to be part of the Clump?
- How did it feel to display your special ability?
- In what ways do teachers conform to each other? Businessmen? Fashion models? Athletes? Kids your age?
- What are the advantages and disadvantages of wearing a uniform at school?
- When detectives solve crimes, what kinds of individual differences can be used as evidence?
- How might parents be able to tell triplets apart?

- In what ways can adopted children resemble other members of their family? How might they differ?
- How do you appear to be different from other members of your family? How are you similar?

(SOURCE: Carolyn Cooperman and Chuck Rhoades, *New Methods for Puberty Education* [Hackensack, N.J.: Planned Parenthood of Greater Northern New Jersey, 1992], 129–131.)

An activity about sexual orientation from *11/12 F.L.A.S.H*[11] helps learners gain understanding of how it feels to grow up being different. Students are given colored paper with simple line drawings of the symbols used by the Nazis in the Holocaust, stars on yellow paper, triangles on pink paper, and the like. They are also given scissors with which to cut out the symbols; unknown to participants, the scissors are all for left-handed persons. While learners are trying to cut, the facilitator reads aloud a monologue called "Southpaw: An Allegory" about someone who has strong feelings and intense experiences from growing up left-handed. While they hear the story, they experience the feeling of being "different-handed." This activity is debriefed in a number of ways, and other activities follow to help learners understand the experience of growing up gay, lesbian, or bisexual in a society in which such people are feared and hated. This activity is useful in adult workshops on diversity as well as in lessons with high school students.

The activity, "A Scientific Experiment: The Properties of Condoms," in *When I'm Grown: Life Planning Education for Grades 5 & 6*,[12] sets up stations at which groups of students test different aspects of condoms—for leakage, tendency to break, ability to stretch, and sense of touch through the rubber. For the latter test we suggest that the teacher have students experience touch through the condom at the tip of the finger, not just on the back of the hand—since finger tips have a concentration of nerve endings, as does the penis.

New Methods for Puberty Education[13] describes a series of activities in which learners build their own three-dimensional models of sexual and reproductive anatomy, thereby providing concrete learning experiences for exploring many complex concepts.

In an activity called "The Family," groups of students design and build models symbolizing a family. Various family relationships or dynamics can be represented, such as power (or authority, control), alignments and boundaries. Various objects can be used to build the models, such as Tinker Toys or chairs. Mature learners in small groups can use their own bodies to build the model and include movement to represent change in dynamics.

"Egg and Sperm" is a fun warm-up exercise for demonstrating the concepts of ejaculation and fertilization. At the command "Go!" the group races through a narrow opening (i.e., the cervix), such as a doorway or an opening in chairs set up for that purpose, then surrounds the "egg," a person standing inside a circle of chairs. The first "sperm" to get through the circle impregnates the egg. Vary this a second time with a barrier set up across the opening of the "cervix" to demonstrate "barrier" contraceptive methods.

GAMES

Games are usually thought of as forms of play, amusement, competition, diversion, or entertainment. In sexuality education, games are more than just fun. They are used as warm-up activities, to increase comfort with a sexuality topic, to open discussion of opinions and values, to teach empathy and understanding, to review information, to practice skills (such as negotiation and conflict resolution), and to evaluate (see Chapter 13). We provide several examples to give a sense of the variety and inventiveness of games for sexuality education. Our first example, "Safer Sex Auction" (see box), is used with "Safer Sex Mixer" (not reprinted here) in *Teaching Safer Sex*.

Safer Sex Auction

Objectives: (1) Participants will examine their values, attitudes, and assumptions regarding AIDS and safer sex; (2) participants will feel more comfortable discussing issues of safer sex.

Rationale: This lesson combines two classic sex education strategies—the mixer and the auction. Together these activities reduce anxiety and encourage vigorous discussion about a variety of issues concerning safer sex. In both exercises participants make decisions that reveal their own values and priorities.

Procedure: Pass out the worksheet "Safer Sex Auction" (following). Read directions and give participants 5 minutes to decide how they would like to bid. Begin bidding; move quickly to determine who gets each item. Remind participants that if they do not get an item, they can put their money toward another item not yet auctioned. After bidding is complete, discuss; discussion questions:

a. Did you bid to protect yourself or to protect others?
b. What do your selections show about what is important to you?
c. If you won the item you most valued, what would the result be?
d. Did you learn anything from doing this exercise? If so, what?

Worksheet: Safer Sex Auction

You have $1,000 to spend at this auction. Put the amount you plan to bid on the line next to each item. As the auction proceeds and you spend some of your money, or lose out on the items you hoped to purchase, revise your plan on the second and third lines.

1. An inoculation that will make you permanently immune to any sexually transmitted disease, including AIDS.
2. An uninfected, loyal, and trustworthy life partner.
3. The ability to change the unsafe sexual behavior of American teens.
4. The power to institute comprehensive sexuality education, K–12, in the nation's schools.
5. Invent a cure for herpes.

6. End homophobia—people's fear of homosexuality.
7. Write a book that would make you famous for describing healthy sexual development through the lifespan.
8. Make 5 million dollars inventing and marketing "The Comfy Condom."
9. Be certain no one you know will die of AIDS.
10. Teach workshops to help people feel good about their sexuality.
11. A magic ring that tells you whether someone is infected with a sexually transmitted disease.
12. A chance to talk honestly with adults you respect about sex.
13. An endless supply of free condoms for you and your friends.
14. Outlaw all sexual intercourse outside of marriage.
15. Require that everyone carry a card telling their HIV status.

(SOURCE: Peggy Brick et al., *Teaching Safer Sex* [Hackensack, N.J.: Planned Parenthood of Greater Northern New Jersey, 1989], 21 and 23. Reprinted with permission.)

We have enjoyed the following team form of "Sexuality Pictionary" (see box) as a hilarious warm-up with adult groups; with appropriate choice of concepts (or words for objects or behaviors) it also can be used with adolescents or children.

Sexuality Pictionary

1. Participants are divided into groups of five or six; each group is given a sheet of flip chart paper and a felt marker.
2. One person in each group is chosen as the first "player"; each person will have a turn, since you will play six or more rounds.
3. The "player" from each group goes to the game facilitator and is given a card with that round's concept written on it. All groups get the same concept. Concepts are more difficult to draw than objects or behaviors and could include contraception, friendship, choice, transmission, love, intimacy, and so on.
4. The player then runs back to his or her group and attempts to draw or diagram the concept so that members of the group can guess it. The player cannot give verbal clues, or use words or numbers in his or her drawing.
5. The first group to guess the concept wins that round. Prizes can be given to the group that wins the most number of rounds.

The *Talk Listen Care Kit*[14] is a set of materials designed to improve communication about sex and other sensitive topics among parents and children ages 4–12. The kit includes the "TLC Game" in which participants draw a "situation" card, read it aloud and give their opinions. Situation cards describe dilemmas and incidents that may cause conflict in the family, such as one in which a mother finds her daughter's birth control pills and confronts her; the daughter feels she can't trust her mother; the mother feels she can't trust her daughter. Players describe what they think about the situation.

Judy Drolet, in "Games People Play,"[15] describes activities in which students develop games based on popular TV game shows. Teams prepare sets of questions on selected health education topics and use them to play "Jeopardy," "Family Feud," "Tic Tack Know," etc.

DEBATE

A debate is a formal discussion of differing sides of an issue. In sexuality education, use debate as a teaching method to explore viewpoints about public policy and laws relating to sexuality. For example, in a mock debate before a "city council" (i.e., the teacher), groups of high school or college students could role play a variety of "community representatives" giving their viewpoints on what is pornography and what kinds of materials should be censored. Here are some possible roles:

- A conservative Christian, who believes pornography is sinful and that nudity and anything to do with sex should be censored; this person is particularly concerned about the impact of pornography on children.
- A radical feminist, who believes pornography is misogynistic, inherently violent and exploitative of women, and should therefore be banned.
- A sex industry worker, who believes that pornography is like any business— some regulation is to be expected (e.g., no sale to minors), but censorship is antidemocratic and antibusiness.
- A health department worker, who believes violent pornography is bad but is concerned that important sexuality and HIV education materials (e.g., breast self-exam teaching videos, brochures illustrating effective use of condoms, etc.) would be censored under proposed antipornography laws.
- A First Amendment advocate, who doesn't particularly like pornography but is opposed to any form of censorship; this person believes that consenting adults should have the freedom to decide whether or not to use or see any materials.

Volunteer role players in this activity need not choose a role based on their own views, but one they feel they could represent effectively. Once all initial statements are heard, "community representatives" are given the opportunity to respond to each other. Be sure to establish and enforce rules for this debate, for example, time limits for initial statements and for responses. Close the debate with a discussion on definitions of pornography and the difficulties diverse groups may have in coming to agreement on what constitutes pornography.

The Washington State Office of Superintendent of Public Instruction has published a Social Studies Supplement to their *KNOW AIDS* Prevention Curriculum,[16] which includes a debate lesson for analyzing the impact of the HIV epidemic on social issues. This debate activity follows the National Forensic League rules; suggested topics include the following:

- Gay rights
- Mandatory testing
- Mandatory reporting of HIV-positive persons
- Quarantine of HIV-positive persons
- Free needles to I.V. drug users
- School attendance of HIV-positive persons
- Condom distribution in the schools
- Homosexuality: Choice or life-style

Unfortunately, use of some of these topics in a competitive debate process could break many of the important ground rules for teaching about sexuality and HIV (see Chapter 3) and may be counter to a pluralistic sexuality education ethic—acceptance of diversity. For example, when debating "gay rights," individuals in the class may feel personally attacked because of the fervor of the presenters of the "negative" case, even though all sides of the issue are aired. Many of these topics, particularly the ones that could remotely apply to a person in the class (e.g., "Homosexuality: Choice or Life-Style") are better considered with other methods than debate. On the other hand, debating a policy issue, such as "condom distribution in the schools," may be a productive way of presenting a wide variety of opinions and a considerable amount of important information.

CHAPTER 13

Evaluating Learners, Educators, and Programs

Evaluation is useful for learner and educator growth and for documenting and improving programs. Although often intimidating to learners and distasteful to educators, evaluations should be viewed as guideposts and learning tools, not as causes for self-denigration or congratulation. All of us, whether learners or educators, can grow in knowledge and skills, and all education programs can be improved. In this chapter we offer some ideas and perspective on evaluating sexuality education programs, learners and teachers.

Whether you are a classroom teacher or a community educator doing sexuality or HIV education or training, you have many reasons for evaluating:

- To help learners assess their own learning.
- To help learners review the information, concepts or messages that were covered in the lesson or course, and to reinforce what they learned.
- To assess learner understanding and retention, whether for grading purposes or to give them feedback.
- To document the effectiveness of your education efforts and give you data for revision of the program.
- To give you data for developing the next lessons or sessions that need to take place with this particular group.
- To empower students by taking and utilizing their feedback.
- To produce data for justification of your program with your supervisors or administrators, funding sources, supporters, opponents, the media, legislators, or the community at large.
- To give you information and feedback needed to improve your skills.

Evaluation is taking place on an informal level all the time as you observe groups and individuals. We have discussed many methods for this kind of informal assessment, including brainstorming, anonymous questions, role play and many other activities during which learners reveal their knowledge, needs, interests, lack of information, misinformation, attitudes, feelings, reactions, or skills. Informal, ongoing assessment or observation is one kind of *formative* evaluation, that is, evaluation that allows you to assess as you go. It helps you "form" and reform your program.

Sexuality educators also should use *formal,* formative evaluation methods, that is, specific tools for checking periodically on student and program progress. Finally, use *summative* evaluation, that is, formal and informal evaluative activities at the end of the learning experience for closure, for further crystallization of learner knowledge, as a documentation of learning, and as a projection about future events and processes.

We have described many sexuality education methods that can be used for formal evaluation. Introspective methods, including journals (see Chapter 8), can help learners evaluate themselves; journal writing assignments can even focus on personal behavioral goal setting, helping students articulate, plan, and get motivated for carrying out changes in behavior. Anonymous questions (see Chapter 9) help to evaluate student needs for information and desires to discuss particular values. Surveys and polls (also Chapter 9) assess learner attitudes. Completion of a variety of assignments, including reading, worksheets, task groups, field trips (see Chapter 9), and real-life homework (see Chapter 10) can be documented in portfolios (see following) for a cumulative evaluation. And finally, participation in a variety of practice activities, including role play, skits, simulations (see Chapter 11), peer education, and teen theater (see Chapter 12) help the learner and educator assess skills.

Classroom teachers sometimes must evaluate learners for grading purposes. Remember that grades by themselves are an inadequate method of assessing student performance, much less for giving feedback for future growth—especially in sexuality education. If you must grade, there are problems with whatever criteria you use. Grading on attendance alone is an arbitrary measurement and implies that exposure to information equates with absorption and subsequent use. Grading based on participation presumes that you have accurate, objective observation abilities, violates the ground rule that learners may participate at their own level or style, and assumes those with quiet learning styles are learning less than more vocal learners. Grading on completion of activities or assignments may be somewhat less arbitrary and more objective.

In this chapter we offer methods for evaluation of learners and learner self-evaluation, ways for learners to give feedback on your performance, and methods by which learners can give feedback on the content and processes of your program. Finally, we describe methods with which you can document your program. We do not discuss outcome evaluation, for example, whether your program affects pregnancy rates or reduction in incidence of risky behaviors; outcome evaluation falls more within the realm of research and is beyond the scope of this text.

EVALUATIVE GAMES

Games are a valuable, fun means of reviewing and crystallizing cognitive learning from a sexuality education unit. Though the process is more for learner self-evaluation and review, the educator also can get a sense of the group's overall grasp of information.

"Myth Busters" is one example of an evaluative game (see the box). In this activity, students not only "bust" myths about HIV and AIDS by stating factual and more complete information, they also counter the myths by role playing, thereby reviewing skills and information.

Myth Busters

This activity is used as a mid-unit review or end-of-unit review. Questions should be adapted to reflect the scope of your program. Also, determine a point system and plan how to control or deal with noise.

Procedure

1. "Myths" are written on small pieces of paper and placed inside balloons, which are then blown up.
2. Divide students into two relay teams.
3. Designate two students as "decision makers" to be at the front, facing the relay teams; they will decide whether the students in the relay team have "busted the myth" accurately (the instructor can be consulted).
4. Distribute one balloon to each student (have extra ones available).
5. On a signal, the first student in line breaks his/her balloon, reads the myth on the piece of paper out loud, and then "busts" that myth by stating factual information to the decision maker. If the decision maker feels the student has adequately responded, the student will "tag" the next person in line, and the process is repeated. Students who don't answer adequately will get another balloon and go to the end of the line to try again.
6. When students have successfully "busted" their myths, they take their seats. The first team totally seated will receive X number of points.
7. The team that was not seated first now has the opportunity to score some extra points by role playing. Students may choose one of the myths, and role play the situation to again "bust the myth" written on the piece of paper.
8. Students will have X minutes to decide who in their group will role play the situation. No individual is allowed to do more than one role play. Monitor the length of role plays (e.g., 3 minutes maximum).
9. The instructor and/or class can decide whether the role play "busted the myth" or not. Vary the process by discussing the role play or letting the other team "add-on" to opponents' role play.

Examples of "Myth Buster" Statements

(Basic messages: HIV/AIDS is preventable; you can do things to protect yourself; you can and do make a difference.)

1. A negative HIV antibody test means a person is immune from HIV.
2. Donating blood is a risky activity for HIV infection.
3. Latex condoms (when used properly) are not effective in reducing risk.
4. Anyone who has anal sex will get infected with HIV.
5. Sharing needles to use steroids or for a tattoo is not risky.
6. People under age 18 need parent permission to get an HIV antibody test.
7. Getting "high" or drunk isn't risky as long as you don't "shoot up."
8. An HIV-positive woman who's pregnant can't transmit HIV to her fetus or newborn unless she is very sick.
9. Most people with AIDS were infected when they were in their 30s.
10. Withdrawal is 100 percent effective in preventing HIV.
11. "Safer sex" means "no sex."
12. If someone gets infected with HIV, it will show up on a blood test within a few days.
13. Latex condoms or barriers won't reduce someone's risk for HIV if they're having oral sex.
14. Two people who are HIV infected don't need to practice safer sex together.

(SOURCE: Suzanne Hidde, Region 6 AIDSNET, Olympia, Wash., 1994; unpublished; printed with permission.)

Another example of an evaluative game is "Facts Bingo"[1] in *When I'm Grown: Life Planning Education for Grades 5 & 6.* Instead of numbers, the squares on the bingo cards have phrases such as "respect and understanding" or "latex condoms." The instructor calls out definitions, such as "qualities that good friends exhibit" or "a thin rubber covering that fits over the penis and prevents the exchange of semen and HIV or other viruses," and students mark the appropriate box to cover rows, columns, or diagonals on their cards.

TESTS

Some sexuality education curricula include a number of evaluative tests. *9/10 F.L.A.S.H.,*[2] for example, has an extensive pre-test and a correlated post-test covering all the major units of the curriculum, including the reproductive system, puberty and adolescence, sexual exploitation, pregnancy, birth control, STDs, and sexual health care. The boxed example from the curriculum takes the form of a crossword puzzle.

Across

1. It's a good idea for teens to talk with their _____ about birth control, if they can.

6. An operation to keep someone from ever having more children is called _____ . (Some people call it "getting your tubes tied.")

7. _____ is birth control that comes in a can. It looks like shaving cream, but it kills sperm.

10. Not all touch includes _____ . . . and even sexual touch doesn't have to include intercourse.

11. A _____ or "rubber" is worn over the penis. It keeps the sperm away from the egg. It also protects both people from germs.

13. Not having intercourse around the time the woman releases an egg is called " _____ awareness," or "natural family planning." People can't guess at it, though. Without months of careful study, there is no "safe" time.

15. Two methods have important safety risks. These are the pill and

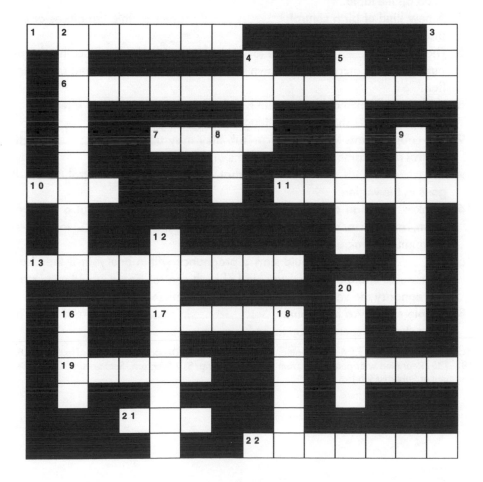

the _____ . For most people, though, even these two methods are safer than having a baby.

17. Hormones the woman can take by mouth, to keep from releasing any eggs, are called birth control _____ .

19. There are some kinds of birth control that people can get in a drug _____ , without seeing a doctor. These are: condom, sponge, foam, and film.

20. If a couple is too embarrassed to _____ about birth control, they might be happier waiting to share sexual touch.

21. People of any _____ can get birth control in most states.

22. Each family and each religion has its own _____ about birth control. Now is a good time to talk about them.

Down

2. _____ is the only 100 percent perfect birth control. (It means saying "no.")

3. People _____ start a pregnancy the first time they have intercourse. They _____ even start one without intercourse, if sperm are ejaculated on the labia.

4. A new kind of birth control, _____ , comes in little flat pieces of gel that kill sperm.

5. The intra- _____ device (or I.U.D) is a small plastic object the doctor puts inside the uterus. It cuts down the chances of fertilization and implantation.

8. Withdrawal (pulling the penis out before ejaculation) is not very effective . . . but works better than using nothing at _____ .

9. If a couple wants to be extra careful, they may use _____ of birth control at the same time (like condoms and foam).

12. The _____ is a rubber cup that is used with birth control cream. It goes in the vagina.

14. It takes less than a _____ to put a condom on, or put a sponge, foam, or film in. It can also take less than a _____ to start a pregnancy. Think about it.

16. _____ people would start a pregnancy within one year if they had intercourse and did not use any kind of birth control. Some would even start a pregnancy the very first time they had intercourse.

18. People can buy a little round _____ in most drug stores. It is full of foam that kills sperm for up to 24 hours.

(SOURCE: Beth Reis, *7/8 F.L.A.S.H.* [Seattle: Seattle–King County Department of Public Health, 1988], 183–185. Reprinted with permission from Family Planning/STD Program, Seattle–King County Department of Public Health.)

Narrative Worksheets and Opinion Questionnaires

Narrative worksheets do more than measure recall by asking learners to "fill in the blanks." Some worksheets allow learners to respond creatively, to record feelings as well as knowledge.

One such creative approach is used in *New Methods for Puberty Education* in "Fran and Fred: Two Stories about Growing Up."[3] Students complete two stories, one about a girl who is having her first menstrual period, and one about a boy who has his first wet dream. Not only do blanks in the stories ask for factual information, but the students also get a chance to ask questions and express feelings in a safe, comfortable format: they put words into the mouths of the characters of the stories, for example, by suggesting one thing that embarrassed Fran about her period, or by suggesting a question that Fred might have. Students then read their stories aloud and discuss others' stories. This process allows for informational review, evaluation of knowledge, expression in the affective domain, increased understanding of others, and continued learning.

We discussed questionnaires as an introspective method in Chapter 8. Educators also can use questionnaires on feelings, values, attitudes, and opinions for learner self-assessment. You probably should never grade such questionnaires against a set standard; use them instead to help learners assess their own growth and set goals. Also use questionnaires to help learners project future behavior, or project themselves into hypothetical situations (see the questionnaire examples in Chapter 8).

Portfolios

Portfolios document accomplishment of tasks and completion of assignments. Learners have a sense of accomplishment and get a total picture of the sexuality education unit as they accumulate concrete evidence of the activities in which they have participated. Portfolios can include anything that was done on paper, such as introspective questionnaires, journal writing, notes on presentations, tests, written reports, letters, completed worksheets, summaries of class surveys, documentation of completed field trips, or questions generated for interviewing guests. Portfolios may also include nonwritten documentation, such as photographic essays, sculpture or other art, audio tapes, video tapes, collages, slide presentations—the possibilities are limitless.

One of our colleagues uses an extensive portfolio process[4] for all units of her high school health classes. Students are required to complete projects for each unit and include the completed project or documentation of a completed process (such as a visit to a clinic) in the portfolio. These are sample projects for the unit on relationships and parenthood:

- A poster of a family tree, with a two-page summary of the student's family history.

- A financial plan for having a baby, including a list of resources for information.
- A self-help book on dating tips, including a bibliography of sources.
- Documentation of volunteering for a minimum of 4 hours at a day care center.
- Documentation of a visit to a family planning clinic, including a summary of personal feelings about the visit.
- A report on the problems of drug-affected babies, including interviews with clinicians who work with such infants.
- A report on fetal alcohol syndrome, including an interview with a clinician.
- A report on divorce in the U.S., with discussion of reasons and effects.

LEARNER DECLARATIONS: "I LEARNED" STATEMENTS

The educator begins the process of learner declarations by posing a variety of stem sentences so that students can declare whatever was significant for them in the lesson, unit, workshop, or program: "I was surprised that . . ."; "As a result of this activity, I will . . ."; "I was upset that . . ."; "I wonder if . . ."; "One thing I intend to do differently is . . ."; or "I predict that . . ." Then give learners a few minutes to rehearse, either on paper with a focus writing process, or by silent thinking. Finally, learners share their sentence completions in a "round robin" process.

This method provides opportunities for declaration of behavioral growth, reaction in the affective domain, or declaration of cognitive learning. Students can predict a future personal plan of action; such declarations are, in effect, rehearsals, or "self-talk." They can articulate feelings, values, beliefs or opinions, thereby making those learnings more "real." They can list facts or concepts that were new to them, thereby reviewing or reinforcing learning. Students also benefit by hearing the diversity of responses. The process provides you, the educator or facilitator, feedback about the effect of the activity or lesson.

The effectiveness of a learner declaration process depends on the comfort level in the group. If participants have worked together for some time and have developed a sense of group trust, declarations will have more depth. Remember to reiterate ground rules, especially "no put-downs" and "anyone has the right to pass," and remind learners that this is not the time for program or teacher evaluation.

In a variation of the public declaration process, an activity from *Reducing the Risk*[5] asks students to write "I learned" statements at the end of a unit on abstinence and avoiding unprotected sexual activity. To protect confidentiality, written responses are kept private and are not publicly declared. The teacher can check to see that statements are written, without reading them. In this way, students may be more complete or personal about what they declare to themselves because they are assured privacy.

NARRATIVE SELF-EVALUATIONS

As a starting point for learners to write narrative evaluations, provide a series of open-ended questions or stem sentences, like those listed previously in Learner

Declarations, or pose specific, content-focused questions. The resulting personal declarations of learning are longer than "I learned" statements and are a valuable tool for both the learner and the educator. Using this method reinforces the notion that students are responsible for and uniquely qualified to assess or evaluate their own learning. Self-evaluations provide the teacher with a valuable perspective she or he otherwise might never know and are especially helpful with students who are more reflective and passive, who don't "learn by talking" in class but have learned nonetheless.

OBSERVATION AND FEEDBACK

A good teacher always observes his or her students, and frequently gives feedback based on observation. Educators often ask for feedback from learners as well. Furthermore, educators often are observed and given formal feedback by colleagues, either supervisors or peers. Here we define behavioral feedback and suggest a set of guidelines for giving it.

"Feedback" is communication that helps another person consider changing his or her behavior or becoming more effective in the use of skills. Feedback also gives information about the effect one has on others. For example, following a student role play, the teacher and other observers can give feedback on the apparent effect of one player's body language on the other player's responses.

Here are some guidelines for giving useful, effective feedback.

1. *Plan your feedback.* Plan the content and amount: find out what kind of feedback the receiver wants or needs to hear, and prioritize if there's too much for the receiver to hear without feeling overwhelmed. Plan the process: the receiver could give himself or herself feedback first, then other members of the group could give their reactions; or, give positive feedback first, then feedback on behaviors that could be more effective. Also plan for timing, who else is involved, location, privacy, etc.

2. *Be "descriptive" rather than "evaluative."* By describing your own perception—what you saw, heard, and/or felt—you leave the receiver of your feedback free to use it as s/he sees fit. If you avoid evaluative language ("You did very poorly on that exercise"; "That was a no-brainer"), you reduce the chance that the receiver will react defensively or feel hurt or angry.

3. *Be specific rather than general.* Describe specific, observable behaviors, including nonverbal body language, mannerisms, use of language (quote the person), tone of voice, etc. Don't use general adjectives (i.e., "dominating," "amazing," "delightful," "angry," "boring") except as a description of your reaction followed by specific behavior descriptions: "I began to get a bit bored when you . . ."; "I was delighted by your use of the term . . ."; "You were very effective with the audience when you turned that question back to them"; "You really looked angry when you role played . . ." What did the person you were observing do? What did the person look like? How did he or she sound? What specific reactions did you observe in the people s/he was trying to affect?

4. *Consider the needs of the receiver of feedback.* Feedback should come from

motivation to help, not hurt. Pay attention to the receiver's ability to hear and use what you say. Carefully gauge how much feedback you give, when you give it, what you say, and how you say it. Listen to the receiver to perceive that person's reactions, feelings, and the other influences on him/her at that time (tiredness, illness, etc.). Feedback can be destructive when it serves only your own needs and you fail to consider the needs of the person on the receiving end.

5. *Direct feedback only toward behavior that can be changed or modified.* When people are reminded of personal characteristics over which they have no control, they feel frustration and tend to resist other feedback.

6. *Use thoughtful timing when giving feedback.* Give feedback at the earliest opportunity after the given behavior, depending, of course, on the receiver's readiness to hear it, on support available from others, and so on. If necessary, spread your feedback out over a period of time.

7. *Check the receiver's perception of your feedback* to ensure clear communication. One way of doing this is to have the receiver try to rephrase or summarize the feedback.

8. *Check the accuracy of your feedback* by discussing and listening to the feedback of other observers (in group settings).

9. *Model the feedback process* and discuss these guidelines with learners to help them learn this important communication skill, for example, when giving feedback following role-play activities.

Try using these guidelines whether you are giving feedback to participants of a practice activity, to a student in an individual student-teacher conference, to another teacher you are training, or when soliciting formal feedback for yourself.

Educators who facilitate or coordinate teen councils, peer educators, teen theaters, and other extensive, ongoing sexuality education projects are often in the position of giving behavioral feedback to learners, whether the feedback is built into the program or is asked for in the form of letters of recommendation for students applying to colleges or other programs. Occasionally learners ask trusted teachers for extensive feedback; care should be taken that such feedback not fall into the realm of counseling.

You may be in the position of giving feedback to other sexuality educators, particularly if you do training. The Association for Sexuality Education and Training has developed a set of skills criteria (please see Appendix B) for evaluating and giving feedback to sexuality educators and trainers.

PROGRAM AND TEACHER EVALUATION: FEEDBACK FORMS AND REACTION SHEETS

To obtain reactions to the content, processes, or materials of your program, lesson, workshop, or curriculum, use a variety of forms or worksheets to gather qualitative and/or quantitative information. Generally, you will find out more about participant reaction if you ask for narrative responses to questions or stem sentences, but rating scales are easy for participants to use and the results are easy to summarize. Gather data anonymously or invite learners to give their names if they want you to respond privately to a particular concern or question. Use feedback processes intermittently, for feedback on specific activities or lessons, or at the end for general evaluation of the entire program.

You can ask for several kinds of information:

- The opinion of participants regarding to what extent the objectives of the program were accomplished.
- How participants reacted to specific activities.
- What they think they learned or gained (see Learner Declarations).
- Feedback on your skills (i.e., your ability to stay on task, engage everyone, respond to participants, etc.; see the Educator Trainer Assessment Tool in Appendix B for sample criteria).
- What learners think they will do with the information or skills gained.
- Their emotional responses, for example, what they liked or disliked about the program, or feelings about specific topics.
- Background or demographic information about participants, for example, age, gender, race or ethnicity, or grade in school.

The primary intent of reaction and feedback sheets is to give you information for improving your program. However, some of the possible benefits for participants are that they have an opportunity to articulate feelings and values, they may do some "self-talk" or rehearsal, and they may feel empowered by giving input.

In Chapter 9 we reprinted a lesson from *New Methods for Puberty Education* centered on "Owning a Family Life Education Book"; in the box is the evaluation form students complete at the end of that lesson.

Book Evaluation Form

1. Did anyone comment about your owning a family life education book? What did they say?
2. State three things you liked about this book.
3. State three things you did not like about this book.
4. Describe the condition of your book. Check one of the following:
   - Looks good as new
   - Is slightly worn
   - Is badly damaged

   State some reasons why your book is in this condition.
5. Would you recommend this book to a friend? Why or why not?

(SOURCE: Carolyn Cooperman and Chuck Rhoades, *New Methods for Puberty Education* [Hackensack, N.J.: Planned Parenthood of Greater Northern New Jersey, 1992], II:4:B.)

Here are more narrative evaluation questions for use on feedback forms:

- What aspects of this (course/workshop) were most useful or valuable to you? Why?

- What aspects were least useful or valuable? Why?
- In general, how would you evaluate the effectiveness of the facilitator? You may address preparation, group facilitation, provision of resources, timing and pacing, addressing group or individual goals or needs, and the like.
- What suggestions can you give for improvement of future (courses/workshops)?
- What will you do as a result of this session?
- What are some major issues or concerns that came up for you?
- Any additional comments?

PROGRAM AND TEACHER EVALUATION: ANONYMOUS NOTES

Asking learners to write anonymous notes is only slightly different in effect from feedback forms. This method is somewhat more like journal writing, allowing opportunity for learner self-talk or rehearsal. Learners also may be more honest and will open up a bit more. [6]

Human Sexuality: Values and Choices [7] uses a course evaluation format that asks students to write the instructor an anonymous letter telling what they thought about the course. Students are asked to include comments about what they liked and why, what they would change, and what things they learned that will help them now or in the future.

PROGRAM AND TEACHER EVALUATION: PROGRAM DOCUMENTATION

Program documentation is an important process for self-evaluation and program planning and is sometimes needed to satisfy funding sources, supervisors, and other decision makers. Whether you are a classroom sexuality educator or a community educator, you should keep a record of your programs. Documentation can include some or all of the following data:

- A record of needs assessment information.
- What you did, that is, a record of the course objectives, curriculum, agenda, lesson plans, and/or learning designs.
- Your budget and funding sources.
- The date(s) of the program, and its length or duration.
- Whom you taught, that is, the number of learners and some demographic data about them, including perhaps age or grade, gender, and ethnicity or race; a list of participants.
- Any field notes or logs.
- Any required administrative forms, such as permission slips.
- A compilation of feedback and written evaluations.
- A record of the satisfaction of your host or sponsoring organization; any thank you letters.
- Ideas for future revisions.

CONCLUSION

In Part I, our objective was to shed some light on guiding principles and compelling issues in effective sexuality and HIV education. In Part II, we examined specific teaching methods and how they can be used to construct effective lessons and workshops in sexuality education. In the appendixes to this text, we list our references, index the activities we described, and suggest numerous resources for curricula, learning activities, topical bibliographies, student materials, professional journals, associations and training, and other information important to sexuality educators.

Resources for Evaluating Sexuality and HIV Education Materials and Curricula

The following resources are valuable for evaluating sexuality education programs; please see Appendix C for addresses of publishers:

1. *Guidelines for Comprehensive Sexuality Education: Kindergarten–12th Grade,* SIECUS, 1991.
2. *Unfinished Business: A SIECUS Assessment of State Sexuality Education Programs,* SIECUS, 1993.
3. *Criteria for Evaluating an AIDS Curriculum,* National Coalition of Advocates for Students, 1992.
4. *HIV/AIDS Audiovisual Resources: A SIECUS Guide to Selecting, Evaluating and Using AVRs,* SIECUS, 1991.

In addition, the following criteria for evaluating sexuality education materials are excerpted and adapted from *ASSET*'s *Sexuality Curriculum and Materials Review Packet;* the complete packet includes forms and directions for evaluation processes and is available from *ASSET (Association for Sexuality Education and Training),* P.O. Box 668, Oak Harbor, WA 98277, 206-675-2439.

High-quality curricula . . .

1. *Are sequential,* kindergarten through grade 12. They provide knowledge and skills that build logically on earlier learning.
2. *Are educationally sound in form.* They reflect what is known about intellectual and academic development (including reading level and reasoning ability), visual appeal (print size, illustrations, layout), and learning style (with interactive, varied teaching methods that will be effective for kinesthetic, visual, and aural learners, right and left-brain thinkers).
3. *Are age appropriate in content.* They reflect what is known about child and adolescent psychosocial and sexual development, behavior and experience.

They should be anticipatory (e.g., learning about puberty should begin at least a year before young people begin puberty, by age 8 at the latest).

4. *Are medically, scientifically and legally accurate.* They contain demonstrable facts. Hypotheses and theories are identified as such, and emphasized only if shared by most experts in a field.

5. *Are comprehensive.* Taking number 3 (preceding) into account, they cover, in the course of thirteen years' schooling sexual anatomy and physiology, sexual health and safety, and sexual aspects of social and emotional health.

6. *Teach relatively universal values.* Specifically, they . . .
   a. Encourage and enhance family communication.
   b. Are tasteful and tactful.
   c. Are respectful of learners, not condescending or patronizing.
   d. Promote intimacy, tenderness, caring, and honesty within all relationships (parent-child, friends, boyfriend-girlfriend, spouses).
   e. Foster thoughtful, sober decisions about sex, taking care not to foster fear about sex, nor to foster casual flippant sexual decision making.
   f. Encourage students to abstain from sexual intercourse, taking care not to express a laissez-faire, casual attitude toward teen sexual activity, nor to express a punitive or degrading attitude toward nonvirgin teens.
   g. Encourage risk-reduction for teens who do have sex (or who will in the next ten years), without condoning their choice, and taking care not to convey a punitive attitude toward these students, nor to suggest that condoms (for HIV and STD protection) or any contraceptives are 100 percent safe, easy "excuses" for casual sex.
   h. Foster healthy, positive body image, taking care not to promote the attitude that bodies are unclean or embarrassing, nor to infer that modesty or a desire for privacy are unimportant or juvenile.
   i. Express respect for diverse family constellations, teaching that healthy families are those that support their members' physical and emotional well-being, taking care not to assume homogeneity of family constellation nor to characterize any one family pattern as the only model of "normalcy," nor to disparage the nuclear family as outmoded.

7. *Address controversial issues* (as opposed to avoiding them). When they do, they take care to . . .
   a. Clearly distinguish facts from beliefs or values.
   b. Even-handedly, sensitively describe a full range of community values.
   c. Encourage students to find out the beliefs of their families and faiths.
   d. Teach respect for all families and individuals, taking care not to promote any one value position.
   e. Dispel sex role stereotyping (substituting accurate information), promoting respect for both males and females and their abilities, taking care not to express judgment of those who do not choose traditional roles, nor to denigrate those who do choose traditional roles.
   f. Dispel sexual orientation stereotyping (substituting accurate information)

and support the self-esteem of gay and lesbian students, without sanctioning their becoming sexually active, and taking care not to assume that all students or families are heterosexual, nor to encourage homosexual experimentation.

g. Discourage teen parenting, and convey the medical, legal, and sociological facts, taking care not to express a laissez-faire, casual attitude toward teen parenting, nor to convey a punitive or degrading attitude toward teen parents.

h. Respect differing beliefs about premarital sex (for adults), taking care to convey the risks involved in casual or brief sexual relationships, without implying that premarital sex is wrong or sinful, nor suggesting that it is good or acceptable.

i. Respect differing beliefs about contraception and abortion, conveying the medical, legal, and sociological facts, without suggesting that everyone should use either or that they are risk free, always easy or right, nor suggesting that nobody should use them, or that they are dangerous, always difficult, or wrong.

j. Respect differing beliefs about masturbation, artificial insemination, in vitro fertilization, conveying the medical, legal, and sociological facts about each, without expressing judgment of people who engage in or partake of each, nor expressing judgment of those who choose not to.

8. *Are "teacher friendly."* They are well organized, clear, self-contained, and affordable.

Evaluating Sexuality Educators and Trainers

The following set of criteria for evaluating sexuality educators and trainers of sexuality educators was developed for *The Northwest Institute for Community Health Educators (NICHE)* by *The Association for Sexuality Education and Training (ASSET)* and *The Center for Health Training (TCHT)*. Written by Joan Helmich, Beth Reis, Maureen Considine and Kelly Riggle-Hower, it includes suggestions for use in a variety of assessment processes.

EDUCATOR TRAINER ASSESSMENT TOOL (ETAT)

Introduction

The Educator Trainer Assessment Tool was originally developed for use at the Northwest Institute for Community Health Educators, a skill-based residential training event for sexuality and HIV educators. It is meant as an assessment of trainers (those who provide continuing education to professional sexuality educators), but most of the skills, behaviors, and philosophies expressed or implied apply to sexuality educators (those who provide direct classroom or community education) as well. For example, the desired behavior "provides an emotionally safe learning environment for every learner" (#1 in the Ethics section) is an appropriate assessment criterion whether the learners are a group of sexuality educators or a classroom of ninth graders. On the other hand, "encourages the group to analyze his/her choice of teaching methods" (#11 in the Methodology section) is not applicable to the evaluation or assessment of a K–12 teacher.

This tool is meant to be used during an observation of an actual training or education session. However, it could also be used as a list of criteria for self-assessment and improvement, for interviewing and hiring new community or classroom sexuality educators, or for writing job descriptions and evaluating staff. Please see our suggestions for using the Educator Trainer Assessment Tool.

The first four sections of the criteria—setting the stage, methodology, delivery, and content—are presented as a somewhat chronological approach to a training session. We also have included a section for co-trainers and team teachers and sections on philosophy, attitude, and ethics. Don't be overwhelmed with the number of criteria; we have tried to cover all aspects of sexuality education and training but realize that each trainer will find only a few criteria from each section relevant. Also, each criterion is a goal; no educator meets all criteria all the time, and each one can be approached with a different style.

Overall, this Educator Trainer Assessment Tool espouses an approach to sexuality training and education that is democratic and pluralistic. We believe that, to be effective, sexuality training and education must . . .

- Provide a positive, comprehensive, and honest perspective of human sexuality.
- Respect cultural pluralism and promote universal values.
- Respect and empower students.
- Utilize a variety of teaching methods to address the diversity of learning styles among learners.
- Address all three learning domains: cognitive, affective and behavioral.
- Be taught by willing, comfortable and well-trained teachers.
- Promote lifelong learning about sexuality.

Suggestions for Using the Educator Trainer Assessment Tool

The Educator Trainer Assessment Tool (ETAT) can be used in a variety of ways with several levels of formality.

1. *Brief self-assessment.* To use the ETAT as a self-assessment, read over the criteria, note those items that describe your strengths and those that indicate needed improvement. You might want to make an action plan for receiving feedback and increasing your skills.

2. *Observing mentors.* The ETAT can be used by new or experienced educators and trainers to analyze the skills of admired experts. Choose a few criteria prior to observing this person and analyze his/her behaviors. Or, review the criteria after observing the expert and analyze those that made the training or education effective.

3. *Formal self-assessment.* A more extensive self-assessment could include the following steps:

a. Videotape yourself doing a teaching or training session.
b. Review the criteria and select those you wish to assess.
c. View the videotape with those criteria in mind; you may want to rate yourself on each criterion and write notes about ways you could improve.
d. Videotape yourself again (and on a regular basis) to assess changes in style, technique, and skill.

4. *Hiring new educators/trainers.* To use the tool for hiring new staff, you may want to review the criteria and choose those that reflect important factors you wish to assess, have applicants do mock presentations, and rate or rank them on each of the chosen criteria. Or you could more simply discuss important criteria in an interview, asking them to rate themselves.

5. *Staff evaluation.* Part or all of the ETAT can be used to evaluate staff. The staff to be evaluated could do either a brief or a formal self-assessment (above) and then discuss it with his/her supervisor. Or the supervisor could do a formal observation and assessment (see below) of the staff member's actual performance in a training or education session.

6. *Formal assessment.* During a more formal assessment, the trainer chooses criteria on which he or she wishes feedback and discusses those criteria with one or more observers. S/he is then observed (and possibly videotaped) performing an actual training or education session. Then the educator or trainer and observers discuss their observations and possibly review and analyze the video of the session. This is the process used at NICHE; more complete instructions for formal assessment follow.

Formal Assessment: Instructions for Trainers to be Observed

Before an observation. Choose one or more observers. If you have a co-trainer, each of you may choose one observer; then the four of you can debrief together. Look through the criteria for assessing your skills as a trainer. Circle the numbers of two or three behaviors about which you would particularly appreciate feedback. You may circle the same numbers for each observer or different ones for different observers. Then give each observer a copy.

After being observed. Debrief as soon as possible after the session. The following format seems to work well:

A. You, as the trainer-being-observed, begin by giving yourself feedback. Using the criteria as a guide . . .
   1. Describe what you liked best about what you did, what you're the most proud of.
   2. Describe what you would do differently if you had it to do again or what you will do differently next time.
   3. Let your observer(s) know if there are specific criteria with which you are already struggling and about which you'd prefer not to hear feedback or get advice at this time.
B. Co-trainers give one another feedback.
C. Invite your observers to give their feedback. Try accepting complimentary feedback without having to make self-deprecating retorts. And try hearing critical input for what it is: your colleagues' feelings and ideas, from their own cultural and personal perspectives, about how you might do an even better job.
D. Gather the written feedback from your observers for future reference.

E. Do whatever closure you would like. That may include reiterating what you are most proud of having done, or describing the one thing you heard that you most want to work on, or simply acknowledging that you will think about the feedback without making any commitments.

Formal Assessment: Instructions for Observers

During the observation. Jot down feedback that is behavioral and specific. Note factors with which you are impressed and phrases you want permission to "borrow," as well as behaviors you think might be improved. Remember that the process is for your own learning just as much as it is for that of the person you're observing.

Giving feedback. Using the criteria as a guide . . .

1. Be descriptive rather than evaluative. Describe your own perceptions—what you saw, heard, and/or felt.
2. Be specific rather than general. Describe specific observable behaviors, including nonverbal body language, mannerisms, use of language (quote the person), tone of voice.
3. Consider the needs of the trainer receiving your feedback, paying attention to his/her ability to hear and use what you say. In other words, a few crucial comments may go a long way; don't feel you need to say everything you noticed.
4. Direct feedback only toward factors that s/he could change, those over which s/he has control.
5. Check the accuracy of your perceptions with other observers, if you are debriefing as a group.
6. Compliment the trainer with the same specificity and ownership with which you critique.

CRITERIA FOR EXCELLENCE IN SEXUALITY EDUCATION AND TRAINING

Setting the stage. The educator/trainer . . .

1. Assesses group and individual needs verbally (actively listening) and/or in writing.
2. Establishes credibility with the group.
3. Describes his or her intentions or objectives for a particular session, relating them to the group's perceived needs.
4. Outlines agenda for the session (verbally or in writing).
5. Establishes ground rules and/or reiterates them as needed, modeling and promoting protection of confidentiality, demonstrating consideration for others' feelings, and acknowledging occasions when he/she may have unintentionally broken a ground rule or offended someone.
6. Acknowledges in advance possible feelings or differences of opinion that a session may generate.

7. Arranges the physical environment in a way that meets the needs of the audience.

Methodology. The educator/trainer . . .
1. Uses teaching methods appropriate to the objectives of the session.
2. Uses a variety of methods to address the needs of visual, auditory, and kinesthetic learners (e.g., props, colors, music, storytelling, movement).
3. Uses lecture only when an increase in knowledge is the primary purpose of a segment and, even then, judiciously.
4. Uses interactive methods.
5. Uses audiovisual equipment skillfully and judiciously.
6. Uses the resources of the group, allowing and encouraging group members the opportunity to influence each other.
7. Enriches his/her teaching by judiciously drawing appropriate relevant examples from personal experience (as a parent, teacher, consumer, nurse, therapist, partner, adoptee, administrator, diabetic, etc.).
8. Adapts prepackaged curricula to his/her own teaching style and the needs of a particular group of learners.
9. Incorporates new knowledge and evolving perspectives into one's interpretation of a curriculum.
10. Encourages the group to analyze his/her word choices.
11. Encourages the group to analyze his/her choice of teaching methods.

Delivery. The educator/trainer . . .
1. Is clear and unambiguous when explaining complex ideas.
2. Is concise, repeating him/herself only when audience cues indicate a need; avoids tangents.
3. Is straightforward and matter-of-fact when necessary.
4. Is serious, empathetic, and even sobering, when appropriate.
5. Smiles and uses enhancing and tasteful humor when appropriate, but never at anyone's expense.
6. States instructions slowly, clearly, and one at a time.
7. Demonstrates verbal skills, speaking loudly enough, with varied tones and without verbal tics ("um," "uh").
8. Moves around, uses hands, and otherwise provides visual variety.
9. Maintains a balance of control and spontaneity.
10. Makes appropriate interventions and/or revises plans as necessary (e.g., asking for feedback, suggesting an unscheduled stretch).
11. Begins and ends on time.
12. Paces the session comfortably and avoids communicating his/her own anxiety about the time.
13. Presents in an organized, logical fashion, making the organization and logic clear to the group.
14. Refers to previous relevant messages and to issues that will be addressed in greater detail later.

15. Provides rational transitions between parts of the session and meaningful closure at the end.
16. Demonstrates reasonable comfort with the subject and with his/her role as educator or trainer.
17. Communicates the expectation that learners are capable of performing a new skill.
18. Provides useful feedback to learners.

Content. The educator/trainer . . .
1. Provides complete, accurate information.
2. Makes handouts organized, readable, useful, relevant, and reproducible.
3. Makes visuals (transparencies, flip charts) organized, readable, and visually appealing.
4. Provides content appropriate for the particular audience.
5. Defines new, vague, or technical terminology and avoids acronyms and jargon.
6. Identifies slang as such (without judgment, except when a term is derogatory) and translates to standard or medical terminology.
7. Distinguishes between crucial points to remember and background information, emphasizing and prioritizing key concepts.

Teamwork. The educator/trainer . . .
1. Gives useful, concrete feedback (both complimentary and critically constructive) to learners and co-trainer(s).
2. Gives feedback respectfully, in a timely way, and in private (or as previously negotiated).
3. Asks for and handles feedback from others graciously and uses it constructively.
4. Asks for colleagues' assistance when faced with a question or situation he/she isn't prepared to handle.
5. Offers appropriate assistance and input during co-trainers' pieces (respectfully, on task, cognizant of time constraints, and without interfering with learners' opportunities to contribute).
6. Negotiates with co-trainer(s) in a respectful way about whether or how to rearrange the schedule.
7. Problem-solves with co-trainer(s) as needed regarding group process.
8. Shares in team responsibilities prior to and during training.

Philosophy and attitude. The educator/trainer . . .
1. Communicates respect for and enjoyment of children and adolescents.
2. Communicates respect for and enjoyment of adult learners.
3. Encourages positive working relationships and open communication among teachers, family, religious leaders, health care providers, and school administrators.
4. Communicates respect, through language and tone, for diverse individuals and avoids generalizations about them (people of both genders and of various ages, races, ethnicities, family constellations, religious and political persua-

sions, sexual orientations, socioeconomic classes, and physical and mental abilities—for example, avoiding antireligious or anticonservative comments).

5. Uses examples from groups (listed in number 4) so that no learner is consistently rendered invisible by omission.

6. Makes very clear that he/she is not making assumptions about learners' sexual history or their current behavior, values, orientations, and so on, and, in fact, welcomes the probable presence of diversity within the group.

7. Speaks for him/herself, from his/her own life experience (not for all members of an identity group, e.g., women, Catholics, whites, people with disabilities) and never expects others to represent a whole group either.

8. Dresses in a professional, credible, and appropriate manner.

9. Communicates genuine support for abstinence from oral, anal, and vaginal intercourse.

10. Communicates genuine support for informed choice in all health behavior and health care decisions.

11. Communicates reverence for and appreciation of the human body and its capacities.

12. Communicates reasoned confidence in the efficacy of sexuality education, without defensiveness.

13. Takes obvious pleasure in teaching and facilitating.

Ethics: The educator/trainer . . .

1. Provides an emotionally safe learning environment for every learner.

2. Ensures that learners are exposed to a broad range of beliefs, in a fair and respectful way.

3. Accurately represents his/her capabilities, education, training, and experience (and the limits thereof), apologizing for mistakes and faux pas, and modeling that it is OK to say "I don't know."

4. Expresses research findings honestly and without distortion.

5. Makes every effort to acknowledge the author/originator of activities, songs, materials, and studies.

6. Opposes the use of deception, intimidation, fear, shame, guilt, or censorship in the name of "education."

7. Addresses controversial issues but distinguishes unambiguously among personal opinions and values, agency/district opinions and values, and those that are generally accepted as universal.

8. Attempts to recognize and acknowledge his/her own cultural assumptions.

9. Acknowledges and follows pertinent sexuality education laws and policies.

Resource Organizations

This list is a selection of those organizations of interest to professionals working in the field of sexuality education. The organizations publish or distribute materials (including journals, newsletters, curricula, teaching guides, textbooks, pamphlets, videos, etc.), provide training and/or hold major conferences, act as clearinghouses, and conduct research. All are regional or national in scope; we do not list statewide or local organizations. We include organizational names, addresses, phone numbers (when available) and titles of journals (when known).

AIDS Education and Training Center
  for Southern California
University of Southern California
1420 San Pablo St., B207
Los Angeles, CA 90033
213-342-1846

AIDS Education and Training Center
  for Texas and Oklahoma
The University of Texas
1200 Herman Pressler St.
POB 20186
Houston, TX 77225

Advocates for Youth (was CPO: Center
  for Population Options)
1025 Vermont Ave., NW
Washington, DC 20005
202-347-5700

The Alan Guttmacher Institute
Family Planning Perspectives

120 Wall St.
New York, NY 10005
212-248-1111

American Alliance for Health, PE, Recreation and Dance (AAHPERD)
1900 Association Dr.
Reston, VA 22091
703-476-3400

American Association of Sex Educators, Counselors and Therapists
  (AASECT)
435 N. Michigan Ave., Suite 1717
Chicago, Illinois 60611-4067
312-644-0828

American College Health Association
1300 Piccard Dr., Suite 200
Rockville, MD 20850
301-963-1100

American Foundation for AIDS Research (AmFAR)
1515 Broadway, Suite 3601
New York, NY 10036
212-719-0033

American Home Economics Association
2010 Massachusetts Ave., NW
Washington, DC 20036-1028

American Journal of Health Promotion
1812 S. Rochester Rd., Suite 200
Rochester Hills, MI 48307-3532

American Public Health Association
The Nation's Health
1015 15th St., NW
Washington, DC 20005
202-789-5600

American School Health Association
Journal of School Health
7263 State Route 43
Box 708
Kent, Ohio 44240
216-678-1601

American Social Health Association
STD News
(also operates AIDS & STD hotlines)
Dept. NSL
PO Box 13827
Research Triangle Park, NC 27709
800-783-9877

The Annual Workshop on Sexuality
PO Box 447
Fayetteville, NY 13066-2226

Association for Advancement of Health Education
Journal of Health Education
1900 Association Dr.
Reston, VA 22091
703-476-3437

Association for Childhood Education International
3615 Wisconsin Ave., NW
Washington, DC 20016

Association of Reproductive Health Professionals
Health and Sexuality
2401 Pennsylvania Ave., NW
Washington, DC 20037-3826
202-466-3825

Association for Sexuality Education and Training (ASSET)
PO Box 668
Oak Harbor, WA 98277
206-675-2439

Association of Supervision and Curriculum Development
1250 N. Pitt St.
Alexandria, VA 22314
703-549-9110

Baltimore STD Prevention/Training Center
303 E. Fayette St., 5th Floor
Baltimore, MD 21202
410-396-4448

Birmingham STD Prevention/Training Center
1400 6th Ave., S., Room 102
Birmingham, AL 35202
205-930-1196

Carnegie Council on Adolescent Development
2400 N St., NW, 6th Floor
Washington, DC 20037
202-429-7979

Carnegie Council on Children
437 Madison Ave.
New York, NY 10022

The Centers for Disease Control and
Prevention
Division of Adolescent School Health
MS K-31
1600 Clifton Rd.
Atlanta, GA 30333
404-488-5372

Center for Early Adolescence
The University of North Carolina at
Chapel Hill—D-2
Carr Mill Town Center, Suite 223
Carrboro, NC 27510

The Center for Family Life Education
575 Main St.
Hackensack, NJ 07601
201-489-1265

The Center for Health Training
South West Institute for Community
Health Educators (SWICHE)
421 East 6th St., Suite 202
Austin, TX 78701
512-474-2166

The Center for Health Training
Western Region Institute for Community Health Educators (WRICHE)
2229 Lombard St.
San Francisco, CA 94123
415-929-9100

The Center for Health Training
Northwest Institute for Community
Health Educators (NICHE)
1809 Seventh Ave., Suite 400
Seattle, WA 98101-1313
206-447-9538

Chicago STD Prevention/Training
Center
1306 S. Michigan Ave.
Chicago, IL 60605
313-747-0116

Child Study Association of America
853 Broadway
New York, NY 10010

Child Welfare League of America, Inc.
(CWLA)
CWLA Publications
440 First St., NW, Suite 310
Washington, DC 20001-2085
202-638-2952

Children's Aid Society
Bernice and Milton Stern National
Training Center for Adolescent Sexuality and Family Life Education
350 E. 88th St.
New York, NY 10128
212-976-9716

Children's Defense Fund
25 E St., NW
Washington, DC 20001
202-628-8787

Cicatelli Associates, Inc.
North Atlantic Training Institute for
Community Health Educators
(NATICHE)
505 8th Ave., Suite 1801
New York, NY 10018
212-629-3321

Cincinnati STD Prevention/Training
Center
3101 Burnet Ave.
Cincinnati, OH 45229
513-357-7324

Dallas STD Prevention/Training
Center
1939 Amelia Court
Dallas, TX 75235
214-920-7984

Delta Region AIDS Education and
Training Center

Louisiana State University
1542 Tulane Ave.
New Orleans, LA 70112
504-568-3855

Denver STD Prevention/Training
   Center
Colorado Dept. of Health
DCEED STD A3
4300 Cherry Creek Dr., S.
Denver, CO 80222-2723
303-692-2723

Development Systems, Inc.
921 West 44th St.
Kansas City, MO 64111-2542
816-471-4484

District of Columbia AIDS Education
   and Training Center
2212 Georgia Ave., NW
Washington, DC 20060
202-806-4002

ETR Associates/Network Publications
Family Life Educator
PO Box 1830
Santa Cruz, CA 95061
408-438-4060

East Central AIDS Education and
   Training Center
The Ohio State University
Department of Family Medicine
1314 Kinnear Rd., Area 300
Columbus, Ohio 432212
614-292-1400

Emory AIDS Training Network
Emory University
735 Gatewood Rd., NE
Atlanta, Georgia 30322
404-727-2929

Equity Institute
6400 Hollis St., Suite 15
Emeryville, CA 94608

Family Planning Council of Southeast-
   ern Pennsylvania
260 S. Broad St., Suite 1900
Philadelphia, PA 19102
215-985-2604

Florida AIDS Education and Training
   Center
University of Miami
PO Box 016960 (D-90)
Miami, FL 33101
305-585-7836

Gay and Lesbian Curriculum and Staff
   Development Project
Harvard University
210 Longfellow Hall
Cambridge, MA 02138
617-495-3441

Gay and Lesbian School Teacher Network
c/o ISAM
222 Forbes Rd., Suite 105
Braintree, MA 02184
617-849-3080

Gay Men's Health Crisis
129 West 20th St.
New York, NY 10011
212-337-1950

Girl Scouts of the United States of
   America
420 5th Ave.
New York, NY 10018-2702
1800-223-0624

Girls Incorporated
441 W. Michigan St.
Indianapolis, IN 46202
317-634-7546

Guelph Conference and Training Institute on Sexuality
Office of Continuing Education
University of Guelph
159 Johnston Hall
Guelph, Ontario, Canada N1G 2W1
519-767-5000

Health Care Education and Training
Great Lakes Institute for Community Health Educators (GLICHE)
2346 S. Lynhurst Dr., Suite 504
Indianapolis, IN 46241
317-247-9008

Hetrick Martin Institute
401 West St.
New York, NY 10014
212-633-8920

Institute for Advanced Study of Human Sexuality
1523 Franklin St.
San Francisco, CA 94109
415-928-1133

Institute for Family Research and Education
Syracuse University
760 Ostrom Ave.
Syracuse, NY 13210

International Society for AIDS Education
AIDS Education and Prevention
University of South Carolina
Executive Office, School of Public Health
Columbia, SC 29208
803-777-4845

International Planned Parenthood Federation
People and the Planet
c/o Planet 21
Distribution Unit

60 Twisden Rd.
London NW5 1DN, UK

JSI Research and Training Institute
210 Lincoln St., 6th Floor
Boston, MA 02111
617-482-9485

JSI Research and Training Institute
1738 Wynkoop St., Suite 201
Denver, CO 80202
303-293-2405

The Jacobs Institute of Women's Health
Women's Health Issues
409 12th St., SW
Washington, DC 20024-2188
202-863-4990

Johns Hopkins University
The Population Report
Population Information Program
527 St. Paul Place
Baltimore, MD 21202

Kinsey Institute for Research in Sex, Gender and Reproduction
Indiana University
Morrison 416
Bloomington, Indiana 47401

Mid-Atlantic AIDS Education and Training Center
Medical College of Virginia
PO Box 159, MCV Station
Richmond, VA 23298-0159
804-371-2447

Midwest AIDS Training and Education Center
University of Illinois at Chicago
808 S. Wood St. (M/C779)
Chicago, IL 60612
312-996-1373

Mountain Plains Regional AIDS Education and Training Center
University of Colorado
4200 E. Ninth Ave., Box A-096
Denver, CO 80262
303-355-1301

National Adolescent Health Resource Center
The University of Minnesota
Division of General Pediatrics and Adolescent Health
1313 Fifth St., SW, Suite 205
Minneapolis, MN 55414
612-627-4488

National Advocacy Coalition on Youth and Sexual Orientation
1025 Vermont Ave., NW, Suite 200
Washington, DC 20005
202-783-4165, ex. 49

National AIDS Clearinghouse
PO Box 6003
Rockville, MD 20849-6003
800-458-5231

National Audubon Society
Population Crisis Committee
666 Pennsylvania Ave., SE
Washington, DC 20003

National Center for Education in Maternal and Child Health
2000 15th St., N., Suite 701
Arlington VA 22201-2617
703-524-7802

National Children's Advocacy Center
106 Lincoln St.
Huntsville, AL 35801
205-533-5437

National Coalition for Advocates for Students

100 Boylston St., Suite 737
Boston, MA 02116-4610
617-357-8507

National Coalition for Sex Equity in Education
1 Redwood Dr.
Clinton, NJ 08809
908-735-5405

National Council of Churches
Commission on Family Ministries and Human Sexuality
475 Riverside Dr.
New York, NY 10115

National Family Planning and Reproductive Health Association (NFPRHA)
122 C St., NW, Suite 380
Washington, DC 20001-2109
202-628-3535

National Gay and Lesbian Health Foundation
PO Box 65472
Washington, DC 20035
202-797-3708

National Maternal and Child Health Clearinghouse (NMCHC)
8201 Greensboro Dr., Suite 600
McLean VA 22102
703-821-8955, X254 or X265

National Minority AIDS Council
300 Eye Street, NE, Suite 400
Washington, DC 20002-4389
202-544-1076

National Native American AIDS Prevention Center
3515 Grand Ave., Suite 100
Oakland, CA 94610
510-444-2051

National Organization on Adolescent
  Pregnancy, Parenting and Prevention
4421A East West Highway
Bethesda, MD 20814
301-913-0378

Network for Family Life Education
Family Life MATTERS
Rutgers, The State University
Building 4086, Livingston Campus
New Brunswick, NJ 08903-5062
908-445-7929

New England AIDS Education and
  Training Center
University of Massachusetts
55 Lake Ave., N.
Worcester, MA 01655
508-856-3255

New Jersey AIDS Education and Training Center
University of Medicine and Dentistry
Office of Continuing Education
30 Bergen St., ADMC #710
Newark, NJ 07107-3000
201-982-3690

New York University
Human Sexuality Program
54 South Building
New York, NY 10003
212-598-3925

New York/Virgin Islands AIDS Education and Training Center
Columbia University School of Public
  Health
600 W. 168th St.
New York, NY 10032
212-305-3616

Newark STD Prevention/Training
  Center

110 Williams St.
Newark, NJ 07102
201-648-2631

Northwest AIDS Education and Training Center
University of Washington
1001 Broadway, Suite 217
Mail Stop ZH-20
Seattle, WA 98122
206-720-4250

NOVA Research Company
4720 Montgomery Lane, Suite 210
Bethesda, MD 20814
301-986-1891

Pennsylvania AIDS Education and
  Training Center
University of Pittsburgh
Graduate School of Public Health
130 DeSoto St., Room A425
Pittsburgh, PA 15261

Planned Parenthood Federation of
  America
Link Line
Education Department
810 Seventh Ave.
New York, NY 10019
212-541-7800

The Population Council
Studies in Family Planning
One Dag Hammarskjold Plaza
New York, NY 10017
212-339-0500

Puerto Rico AIDS Education and
  Training Center
University of Puerto Rico
Medical Sciences Campus
GPO 36-5067 Room 745A
Rio Piedras, PR 00936-5067
809-759-6528

San Francisco STD Prevention/Training Center
1360 Mission St., Suite 401
San Francisco, CA 94103-2609
415-554-9630

San Francisco AIDS Foundation
PO Box 426182
San Francisco, CA 94142
415-861-3391

San Juan STD Prevention/Training Center
CLETS—Training Center Division
PO Box 71423
San Juan, PR 00936-1423
809-765-1010

Search Institute
SOURCE Newsletter
122 W. Franklin Ave., Suite 525
Minneapolis, MN 55404

Sexuality Information and Education Council of the US (SIECUS)
SIECUS Report
130 W. 42nd St., Suite 350
New York, NY 10036
212-819-9770

Society for Adolescent Medicine
Journal of Adolescent Health Care
Elsevier Science Publishing, Inc.
655 Ave. of the Americas
New York, NY 10010

Society for Public Health Education (SOPHE)

2001 Addison, Suite 220
Berkeley, CA 94704
510-644-9242

Tampa STD Prevention/Training Center
1112 E. Kennedy Blvd.
Tampa, FL 33602
813-272-6326

Teaching Tolerance
400 Washington Ave.
Montgomery, NC 36104

UN Population Fund
220 E. 42nd St.
New York, NY 10017

University of Pennsylvania
Human Sexuality Education
Graduate School of Education
3700 Walnut St.
Philadelphia, PA 19104
215-243-6455

Western AIDS Education and Training Center
University of California—Davis
5110 E. Clinton Way, Suite 115
Davis, CA 93727-2098
209-252-2851

ZPG Population Education Program
1400 16th St. NW, Suite 320
Washington, DC 20036
202-332-2200

Index of Activities Described in Teaching about Sexuality

This index lists all the activities used as examples in this text. Activities that are reprinted, fully or in part, are indicated with an asterisk; the full source is given in the text and briefly noted here, unless the activity was developed by Helmich or Hedgepeth. Activities listed without asterisks are described (not reprinted) within the narrative and complete sources are given in the endnotes.

We have indexed the activities by topic to further facilitate your use of them in your programs. However, these activities were chosen not because they are the best way of teaching the topic to any particular group, but as excellent examples or interesting variations of the sexuality education *method* or *principle* being described. This text in no way represents an exhaustive review of sexuality education teaching materials and curricula, though we did try to use a mix of activities for a variety of topics, for all age groups, and from a number of sources. Space limitations made it impossible for us to reprint or describe many excellent examples. We would suggest that you review materials available locally to you with the review criteria in Appendix A; also keep in mind the principles of effective sexuality education described in Part I. For materials known around the United States, see the bibliography in Appendix E for recommendations, and see the list of organizations in Appendix C for further resources.

ANATOMY AND PHYSIOLOGY

- *"Draw the Body Parts" (Chapter 3)
- "Egg and Sperm" (Chapter 12)

BODY IMAGE

- Stem sentence samples (Chapter 8)
- "Picture Survey," *New Methods for Puberty Education,* 145 (Chapter 8)

COMMUNICATION

- "Personal Styles" Quadrant (Chapter 10)
- *"Arc of Distortion" (Chapter 12)

CONDOMS

- "A Scientific Experiment: The Properties of Condoms," *When I'm Grown: Life Planning Education for Grades 5 & 6*, 156–158 (Chapter 12)

CONTRACEPTION

- "Contraception from Many Angles" (Chapter 2)
- *"Contraceptive Counseling Role Play" (Chapter 4)
- Stem sentence samples (Chapter 8)
- Brief knowledge assessment (Chapter 9)
- *"Birth Control Worksheet," *7/8 F.L.A.S.H.*, 183–185 (Chapter 13)

DECISION MAKING

- Topics for role play (Chapter 11)

ENVIRONMENT AND POPULATION

- *"Earth: The Apple of Our Eye," *For Earth's Sake: Lessons in Population and Environment* (Chapter 9)

FAMILY RELATIONSHIPS

- "The Family" (Chapter 12)

GENDER ROLES AND STEREOTYPES

- *"Balancing the Gender Scales" (Chapter 2)
- *"A Workshop on Gender" (Chapter 6)
- Gender differences stem sentence samples (Chapter 8)
- "Girls and Boys," *When I'm Grown: Life Planning Education for Grades 3 & 4*, 25 (Chapter 8)
- "Media Messages," *New Methods for Puberty Education*, 148 (Chapter 8)
- *"Questions for Discussion: Female Roles" and "Questions for Discussion: Male Roles," *Postponing Sexual Involvement: An Educational Series for Young Teens*, 27–28 (Chapter 10)
- *"Girls and Boys," *When I'm Grown: Life Planning Education for Grades 3 & 4*, 25 (Chapter 10)

- *"Gender Roles," *11/12 F.L.A.S.H.,* 37 (Chapter 10)
- Gender advantages & disadvantages brainstorm (Chapter 12)

GETTING ACQUAINTED

- "Getting to Know You" (Chapter 3)
- "Blatant Lies," Kelly Riggle-Hower (Chapter 3)
- "Quick Introductions in a One-Time Experience" (Chapter 3)

HIV/AIDS

- "HIV/STD Transmission Web" (Chapter 4)
- *"A Friend Discloses" (Chapter 8)
- *"Challenging Attitudes toward HIV/AIDS," *FLEducator* (Winter 1992/1993), 28–30 (Chapter 10)
- *"Choosing Condoms," *Teaching Safer Sex,* 35–38 (Chapter 10)
- High School AIDS Simulation, unpublished (reported in *Seattle Times,* May 5, 1994 (Chapter 11)
- *"Safer Sex Auction," *Teaching Safer Sex,* 21 & 23 (Chapter 12)
- *"Myth Busters," Suzanne Hidde (Chapter 13)

LOVE

- Stem sentence samples (Chapter 8)

MISCELLANEOUS AND MULTIPURPOSE

- *"Anonymous Questions," *9/10 F.L.A.S.H.,* 5 (Chapter 9)
- *"Values Question Protocol," *11/12 F.L.A.S.H.,* vi–vii (Chapter 9)
- *"Owning a Family Life Education Book," *New Methods for Puberty Education,* 41–43, plus Assignment Sheet II:4:A (Chapter 9)
- "Parent Survey," *Postponing Sexual Involvement: An Educational Series for Parents of Preteens* (Chapter 9)
- "Individual Field Trip," *9/10 F.L.A.S.H.,* 15 (Chapter 9)
- Miscellaneous questions for dyad/triad discussion (Chapter 10)
- "Professionals as Resources," *New Methods for Puberty Education,* 123–127 (Chapter 10)
- Miscellaneous continuum topics (Chapter 10)
- Miscellaneous forced choice topics (Chapter 10)
- Clinic visit simulation (including worksheets), Paul Witt and Gail Stringer, unpublished (Chapter 11)
- *"Visit or Call a Clinic," *Reducing the Risk,* 119–120, 125 (Chapter 11)
- Debate on pornography and censorship (Chapter 12)
- *"Book Evaluation Form," *New Methods for Puberty Education,* II:4:B (Chapter 13)

- "First Knowledge of Sex" Survey, Peggy Brick (Chapter 9)
- "Mixed Messages," *Teaching Safer Sex,* 17 (Chapter 10)
- "Touch and Abstinence," *9/10 F.L.A.S.H.,* 26–27 (Chapter 10)
- *"Sexuality Pictionary" (Chapter 12)
- "TLC Game," *Talk Listen Care Kit* (Chapter 12)

STDs

- "STD Handshake" (Chapter 4)
- *"Graffiti Sheets," The Clarity Collective's *Taught Not Caught: Self Esteem in Education,* 168 (Chapter 7)
- Stem sentence variations for "Graffiti Sheets," Gail Stringer (Chapter 7)
- Recommendations for use of STD slides, Gail Stringer (Chapter 9)
- "Continuum of Probabilities," *Teaching Safer Sex,* 1–3 (Chapter 10)

TEEN SEX: RISKY BEHAVIOR, REFUSAL SKILLS, ABSTINENCE, ETC.

- "Thrill Seekers," *Entering Adulthood: Coping with Sexual Pressures* (Chapter 8)
- "Talk to Your Parents," *Reducing the Risk,* 55–56 (Chapter 10)
- "Setting Limits on Physical Affection," *Postponing Sexual Involvement: An Educational Series for Young Teens,* 45–46 (Chapter 10)
- *"Role Play in Small Groups," *Reducing the Risk,* 71 and 75 (Chapter 11)
- *"You Would (Use a Condom) If You Loved Me," *Teaching Safer Sex,* 39–40 (Chapter 11)
- "Stating One's Needs," David Vaughan (Chapter 11)
- Wallet cards, *Human Sexuality: Values and Choices* (Chapter 11)
- "Months of the Year Risk Activity," *Reducing the Risk,* 13 (Chapter 11)

TOLERANCE (RACE, LANGUAGE, FAMILY CONFIGURATION, SEXUAL ORIENTATION, ETC.)

- *"Heterosexuals in an Alien World" (Chapter 3)
- "When Race Is the Issue," *FLEducator* (Spring, 1993), 26–28 (Chapter 10)
- "Adult Households," *When I'm Grown: Life Planning Education for Grades 5 & 6,* 51 (Chapter 10)
- "Words Hurt," *When I'm Grown: Life Planning Education for Grades 3 & 4,* 26 (Chapter 12)
- Sexual orientation activity, *11/12 F.L.A.S.H.,* 79–81 (Chapter 12)

VIOLENCE, ANGER

- "Where Does Violence Come From," *Life Planning Education: A Youth Development Program* (Chapter 8)

Notes to Chapter 1

1. Pat Donovan, *Risk and Responsibility: Teaching Sex Education in America's Schools Today*" (New York and Washington, D.C.: The Alan Guttmacher Institute, 1989).
2. Debra Haffner, comment made as a guest on "ABC Nightline: 'What'll We Tell the Kids?' " February 17, 1995.
3. Douglas Kirby, *Sexuality Education: An Evaluation of Programs and Their Effects. An Executive Summary. Final Report to the U.S. Department of Health and Human Services* (Santa Cruz, Calif.: Network Publications, 1984).
4. Evonne Hedgepeth, "Sexuality Comfort: Its Measurement and Relationship to Other Variables in Sexuality Education." Diss., University Microfilms, 1988.
5. Kirby, *Sexuality Education.*
6. *Ibid.*
7. Douglas Kirby, Lynn Short, Janet Collins, Deborah Rugg, Lloyd Kolbe, Marion Howard, Brent Miller, Freya Sonenstein, and Laurie S. Zabin, "School-Based Program to Reduce Sexual Risk Behaviors: A Review of Effectiveness," *Public Health Reports,* Volume 109, Number 3 (May–June 1994): 339–359.
8. Kirby, *Sexuality Education.*
9. Planned Parenthood Federation of America, Inc., "Sexuality Education Can Make a Difference," Reference Sheet #1 (undated).
10. *Ibid.*
11. Douglas Kirby, Richard P. Barth, Nancy Leland, and Joyce V. Fetro, "Reducing the Risk: Impact of a New Curriculum on Sexual Risk-Taking," *Family Planning Perspectives,* Volume 23, Number 6 (November/December 1991): 352–263.
12. E. Brann, L. Edwards, T. Calicott, E. Story, P. Berg, J. Mahoney, J. Stine, and A. Hixson, "Strategies for the Prevention of Pregnancy in Adolescents," *Advances in Planned Parenthood* (1979). Cited in Douglas Kirby, *Sexuality Education,* 13.
13. L. Zabin, R. Street, and J. Hardy, "Research and Evaluation in a University, Clinic and School-Based Adolescent Pregnancy Prevention Program," paper delivered to the American Public Health Association meetings, Dallas, 1983; cited in Kirby, *Sexuality Education.*
14. Leighton C. Ku, Freya L. Sonenstein, and Joseph J. Pleck, "The Association of AIDS

Education and Sex Education with Sexual Behavior and Condom Use among Teenage Men," *Family Planning Perspectives*, Volume 24, Number 3 (May/June 1992): 100–106.

15. World Health Organization, *Global AIDSNEWS: The Newsletter of the World Health Organization Global Programme on AIDS*, Number 4 (1993): 1–2.

16. Ku et al., "The Association of AIDS Education," 1992.

17. Advocates for Youth (formerly, Center for Population Options), "Adolescent Sexuality, Pregnancy and Parenthood," Fact Sheet (May 1990).

18. Gallup Poll cited in "The Case for Sexuality Education," *Planned Parenthood Review*, Volume 2, Number 3 (Fall 1982): 10.

19. Donovan, *Risk and Responsibility*.

20. Sharon J. Alexander, "Improving Sex Education Programs for Adolescents: Parents' Views," *Family Relations*, Volume 33, Number 2 (1984): 251–257.

21. John Leo, "Sex and Schools," *Time* (November 24, 1986): 54–63.

22. Gallup Poll, September 1987.

23. Peter Scales, "Arguments against Sex Education: Facts Versus Fiction," *Children Today* (September/October 1981): 22–25.

24. National Coalition in Support of Sexuality Education (NCSSE), list provided by SIECUS, 1995.

25. The United States Conference of Mayors, *AIDS Information Exchange*, Volume 8, Number 4 (September 1991): 2.

26. Pamela M. Wilson, "Forming a Partnership between Parents and Sexuality Educators," *SIECUS Report* (February/March 1994): 1–5.

27. David C. Marini and Richard Fopeano, "Sexuality Education: What It Is and What It Isn't," paper presented at the Annual Meeting of the American School Health Association, Phoenix, Ariz., October 1982, 1–12.

28. Advocates for Youth, "Parent-Child Communication about Sexuality" (June 1990).

29. Barbara Huberman, presentation at the Annual Washington State Council on Family Planning/Association for Sexuality Education and Training, Bellevue, Wash., September 1993.

30. Karen H. Bonnell and Larry M. Caillouet, "Patterns and Communication Barriers between Teenagers and Parents about Sex-Related Topics," paper presented at the Annual Meeting of the Central States Communication Association, Chicago, April 11–14, 1991.

31. Alan Guttmacher Institute (AGI), *Sex and America's Teenagers* (New York and Washington, D.C., 1994).

32. Stanley Elam, "The Second Gallup/Phi Delta Kappa Poll of Teachers' Attitudes toward the Public Schools," *Phi Delta Kappan* (June 1989): 785–796.

33. J. Norman and M. Harris, *The Private Life of the American Teenager* (New York: Rawson Wade, 1981).

34. Michael Young and Rod Roth, "Attitudes of School Officials toward Sex Education Programs: A Discriminant Analysis" ERIC Document #223543 (1982).

35. Germaine Maslach and Graham Kerr, "Tailoring Sex Education Programs to Adolescents: A Strategy for the Primary Prevention of Unwanted Adolescent Pregnancies," *Adolescence*, Volume 18, Number 70 (Summer 1983): 449–456.

36. Jim Clay, "Youth and HIV: 'It Can't Happen to Me,' " *Hand-in-Hand Newsletter of Oregon's HIV Care Community* (June 1994): 1–3.

37. National Education Association (NEA), *And Justice for All* (Washington, D.C.: Executive Committee Study Group Reports on Ethnic Minority, 1987). Cited in Judith Scheer, *HIV Prevention Education for Teachers of Elementary and Middle School Grades*

(Santa Cruz, Calif.: Association for the Advancement of Health Education and ETR Associates, 1992).

38. Centers for Disease Control and Prevention, "National Youth Risk Behavior Survey," 1990.

39. Dr. Paul Gebhard, cited in Bennett L. Singer and David Deschamps, eds., *Gay and Lesbian Stats: A Pocket Guide of Facts and Figures* (New York: The New Press, 1994), 8. Also in this source (pp. 9–12) are a brief review, comparison, and critique of nineteen studies on gay/lesbian prevalence in the general population.

40. U.S. Department of Commerce, *Statistical Abstracts of the United States*, 114th ed. (September 1994): 857.

41. District of Columbia Commission on Domestic Partnership Benefits for D.C. Government Employees, Final Report and Recommendations, 7. Cited in Elizabeth Murphy, "Understanding the Domestic Partner Dilemma: Perspectives of Employer and the Insurer," Research Report for the City of West Hollywood, California (1983).

42. G. William Sheek, *A Nation for Families: Family Life Education in Public Schools* (American Home Economics Life Association, 1984).

43. AGI, *Sex and America's Teenagers*.

44. Ira L. Reiss, "Sexual Pluralism: Ending America's Sexual Crisis," *SIECUS Report*, Volume 19, Number 3 (1991): 5–9.

45. Advocates for Youth, "Adolescent Males and Teen Pregnancy" (May 1990).

46. Debra Haffner, speech given at Family Life Education Conference, Tenafly, N.J., October 27, 1988; cited in *Teaching Safer Sex*, p. v.

47. AGI, *Sex and America's Teenagers*.

48. Centers for Disease Control and Prevention, HIV/AIDS Prevention, "The Facts about Young Adults, Sexual Behavior, and Sexually Transmitted Diseases," Fact Sheet (undated); also, CDCP, 1990 National Youth Risk Behavior Survey.

49. Debra Haffner, ed., *Facing Facts: Sexual Health for America's Adolescents* (New York: SIECUS and the National Commission on Adolescent Sexual Health, 1995).

50. Advocates for Youth (AFY), "Adolescents and Condoms," Fact Sheet (October 1991).

51. AFY, "Adolescent Contraceptive Use," Fact Sheet (June 1990).

52. AFY, "Adolescents and Condoms" (1991).

53. Arnold H. Grossman, "HIV and At-Risk Youth: The Myth of Invulnerability," *Parks and Recreation*, Volume 26, Number 11 (November 1991): 52–55.

54. AFY, "Adolescents and Sexually Transmitted Diseases," Fact Sheet (July 1990).

55. AFY, "Adolescent Contraceptive Use" (June 1990).

56. AFY, "Adolescent Sexuality, Pregnancy and Parenthood" (May 1990).

57. Nancy Peterfreund and Karen Moe, "Seattle School District 1993 Teen Health Survey: Report on Findings" (Health Curriculum Office, Seattle School District, March 1994).

58. Denise D. Preston, Margaret Jehu Shaw, and Edward J. Zielinski, "Teachers Make a Difference. The Effects of AIDS Education Programs in Three Rural School Districts of Western Pennsylvania," *EDRS Research Report* (1988).

59. Candace A. Croft and Linda Asmussen, "Perceptions of Mothers, Youth and Educators: A Path toward Detente Regarding Sexuality Education," *Family Relations*, Volume 41, Number 4 (October 1992): 452–459.

60. Douglas Kirby, "School-Based Programs to Reduce Sexual Risk-Taking Behaviors," *Journal of School Health*, Volume 62, Number 7 (September 1992): 283.

61. William A. Firestone, "The Content and Context of Sexuality Education: An Exploratory Study in One State," *Family Planning Perspectives*, Volume 26, Number 3 (May/June 1994): 125–131.

62. Peterfreund and Moe, "Seattle Teen Health Survey" (1994).

63. Harris/Scholastic Research, *Hostile Hallways: The AAUW Survey on Sexual Harassment in America's Schools* (Washington, D.C.: American Association of University Women Educational Foundation, 1993).

64. Subhuti Dharmananda, "Child Abuse & HIV: An On-going Legacy," *Hand-in-Hand: Newsletter of Oregon's HIV Care Community* (November 1994): 5, 11.

65. Debra Boyer and David Fine, "Sexual Abuse as a Factor in Adolescent Pregnancy and Child Maltreatment," *Family Planning Perspectives,* Volume 24, Number 1 (January/February 1992): 4–12.

66. James Cassese, "The Invisible Bridge: Child Sexual Abuse and the Risk of HIV Infection in Adulthood," *SIECUS Report,* Volume 21, Number 4 (April/May 1993): 1–7.

67. Marianne Whatley and Bonnie Trudell, "Sexual Abuse Prevention and Sexuality Education: Interconnecting Issues," *Theory into Practice,* Volume 28, Number 3 (Summer 1989): 177–182.

68. Anke Ehrhardt, "Trends in Sexual Behavior and the HIV Pandemic," *American Journal of Public Health,* Volume 82, Number 11 (November 1992): 1459–1461.

69. Maria Natera, in *HIV Prevention for Teachers of Elementary and Middle Schools* (Reston, Va.: Association for the Advancement of Health Education and ETR Associates, 1992), 42.

70. Mike Males, "Schools, Society and 'Teen' Pregnancy," *Phi Delta Kappan* (March 1993): 566–568.

71. Haffner, ed., *Facing Facts.*

72. Males, "Schools, Society and 'Teen' Pregnancy."

73. Sheryl P. Bowen and Paula Michal-Johnson, "A Rhetorical Perspective for HIV Education with Black Urban Adolescents," *Communication Research,* Volume 17, Number 6 (December 1990): 848–866.

74. James T. Sears, "Helping Students Understand and Accept Sexual Diversity," *Educational Leadership,* Volume 49, Number 1 (September 1984): 54–56.

75. Alcohol, Drug Abuse, and Mental Health Administration, "Report of the Secretary's Task Force on Youth Suicide. Volume 3: Preventions and Interventions in Youth Suicide." DHHS Publication Number (ADM) 89–1623 (Washington, D.C.: U.S. Government Printing Office, 1989).

76. Cassese, "The Invisible Bridge."

77. Alan Rose, "AIDS: The Second Wave," and Donald L. Weston, "We Need to Feel Good Enough about Ourselves . . . ," *Hand-in-Hand: Newsletter of Oregon's HIV Care Community* (November 1994): 1, 10.

78. AFY, "Media and Adolescent Sexuality," Fact Sheet (August 1991).

79. AGI, *Sex and America's Teenagers.*

80. Faye Wattleton, "American Teens: Sexually Active, Sexually Illiterate," *Curriculum Review* (January/February 1988): 16–17.

81. Teen participants on a show about the impact of talk shows, "The Oprah Winfrey Show," June 1995. See also Debra Haffner, "Talk Show Chaos," *SIECUS Report,* Volume 23, Number 5 (June/July 1995): 16–17, for commentary on the misinformation provided by talk shows.

82. AFY, "Media and Adolescent Sexuality" (August 1991).

83. AGI, *Sex and America's Teenagers.*

84. Roper/Starch International, "Teens Talk About Sex: Adolescent Sexuality in the 90s. A Survey of High School Students" (New York: SIECUS, 1994).

85. Phyllis Gingiss and Richard Hamilton, "Teacher Perspectives after Implementing a Human Sexuality Education Program," *Journal of School Health*, Volume 59, Number 10 (December 1989): 427–431.

86. Barbara A. Rienzo and Steve M. Dorman, "Ten Consequences of the AIDS Crisis for the Health Education Profession," *Journal of School Health*, Volume 58, Number 8 (October 1988): 335–337.

87. William L. Yarber and K. A. Pavese, "School Personnel Estimates of Community Support for Sex Education," *Journal of Sex Education and Therapy*, Volume 10, Number 21 (1984).

88. Donovan, *Risk and Responsibility*.

89. SIECUS, preliminary analysis of data collected from college course catalogs to be published in fall of 1995. Contact SIECUS at 212-819-9770 for more information.

90. Barbara A. Rienzo, "The Status of Sex Education: An Overview and Recommendations," *Phi Delta Kappan*, Volume 63 (1981).

91. Donovan, *Risk and Responsibility*.

92. *Ibid.*

93. Donald C. Iverson and W. James Popham, "Combatting AIDS on the Front Lines," *The School Administrator*, Volume 49, Number 8 (September 1992): 22–23 and 26–27.

94. Donovan, *Risk and Responsibility*.

95. Leon Eisenberg, cited in Ehrhardt, "Trends in Sexual Behavior."

96. Ehrhardt, "Trends in Sexual Behavior."

97. Donovan, *Risk and Responsibility*.

98. Ehrhardt, "Trends in Sexual Behavior."

Notes to Chapter 2

1. William Yarber, "While We Stood By . . . The Limiting of Sexual Information to Our Youth," *Journal of Health Education*, Volume 23, Number 6 (September/October 1992): 326–335.

2. Douglas Kirby and Judith Alter, "The Experts Rate Important Features and Outcomes of Sex Education Programs," *Journal of School Health* (1980): 497–502.

3. Kathryn Rindskopf, "A Perilous Paradox: The Contraceptive Behavior of College Students," *Journal of the American College Health Association*, Volume 30, Number 3 (December 1981): 113–118.

4. Mary F. Schmidt and David McKirnan, "Affective Factors Which Influence Learning Sexually Transmitted Diseases," Education Document #250–298 (1992).

5. William A. Fisher, "All Together Now: An Integrated Approach to Preventing Adolescent Pregnancy and STD/HIV Infection," *SIECUS Report*, Volume 18, Number 4 (April/May 1990): 1–11.

6. Schmidt and McKirnan, "Affective Factors."

7. J. Stiff, M. McCormack, E. Zook, T. Stein, and R. Henry, "Learning about AIDS and HIV Transmission in College-Age Students," *Communication Research*, Volume 17, Number 6 (December 1990): 743–758.

8. William A. Fisher, "Predicting Contraceptive Behavior among University Men: The Roles of Emotions and Behavioral Intentions," *Journal of Applied Social Psychology*, Volume 14 (1984): 104–123.

9. Patti O. Britton, Diane deMauro, and Alan E. Gambrell, "HIV/AIDS Education: SIECUS Study on HIV/AIDS Education for Schools Finds States Make Progress but

Work Remains," *SIECUS Report,* Volume 21, Number 1 (October/November 1992): 1–8.

10. Susan Griffin, *Pornography and Silence: Culture's Revenge against Nature* (New York: Harper and Row, 1981).

11. Susan Shurberg Klein, "Sex Education and Gender Equity," *Educational Leadership,* Volume 45, Number 6 (March 1988): 69–75.

12. Myriam Miedzian, *Boys Will Be Boys: Breaking the Link between Masculinity and Violence* (New York: Doubleday, 1991).

13. Peter Scales, "The Changing Context of Sexuality Education: Paradigms and Challenges for Alternative Futures," *Family Relations,* Volume 35 (April 1986): 265–274.

14. Anke Ehrhardt, "Trends in Sexual Behavior and the HIV Pandemic," *American Journal of Public Health,* Volume 82, Number 11 (November 1992): 1459–1461.

15. Ira Reiss, "Sexual Pluralism: Ending America's Sexual Crisis," *SIECUS Report,* Volume 19, Number 3 (1991): 5–9.

16. Britton et al., "HIV/AIDS Education: SIECUS Study."

17. Jacqueline D. Forrest and Jane Silverman, "What Public School Teachers Teach about Preventing Pregnancy, AIDS and Sexually Transmitted Diseases," *Family Planning Perspectives,* Volume 21, Number 2 (March/April 1989): 65–72.

18. Michelle Fine, "The Missing Discourse of Female Desire," *Harvard Educational Review,* Volume 58, Number 1 (February 1988): 29–53.

19. Susan S. Klein, "The Issue: Sex Equity and Sexuality in Education," *Peabody Journal of Education,* Volume 64, Number 4 (Summer 1987; published 1989): 1–12.

20. Marianne Whatley, "Goals for Sex-Equitable Sexuality Education," *Peabody Journal of Education,* Volume 64, Number 4 (Summer 1987; published 1989): 59–70.

21. Pat Donovan, *Risk and Responsibility: Teaching Sex Education in America's Schools Today* (New York and Washington, D. C.: The Alan Guttmacher Institute, 1989).

22. Robert Selverstone, "Sexuality Education Can Strengthen Democracy," *Educational Leadership,* Volume 49, Number 1 (September 1991): 58–60.

23. C. L. Perry, "Prevention of Alcohol Use and Abuse in Adolescence: Teacher vs. Peer-Led Intervention." *Crisis,* Volume 10 (1989): 52–61.

24. L. Wagner, *Peer Teaching: Historical Perspectives* (Westport, Conn.: Greenwich Press, 1982).

25. Reiss, "Sexual Pluralism."

26. Ira Reiss, *An End to Shame: Shaping the Next Sexual Revolution* (Buffalo, N.Y.: Prometheus, 1990).

27. Wendy Martyna, "What Does 'He' Mean—Use of the Generic Masculine," *Journal of Communication,* Volume 28, Number 1 (Winter 1978): 131–138.

28. Elizabeth G. Calamidas, "Reaching Youth about AIDS: Challenges Confronting Health Educators," *Health Values,* Volume 15, Number 6 (November/December 1991): 55–61.

29. Gary W. Dowsett, "Working-Class Gay Communities and HIV Prevention," *FOCUS: A Guide to AIDS Research and Counseling,* Volume 9, Number 3 (February 1994): 1–4.

30. Calamidas, "Reaching Youth about AIDS."

31. John B. Jemmott, III, Loretta Sweet Jemmott, and Geoffrey T. Fong, "Reductions in HIV Risk-Associated Sexual Behaviors among Black Male Adolescents: Effects of an AIDS Prevention Intervention," *American Journal of Public Health,* Volume 82, Number 3 (March 1992): 372–377.

32. H. McCloskey and A. Brill, *Dimensions of Tolerance: What Americans Believe about Civil Liberties* (New York, N.Y.: Russell Sage Publication, 1983).

33. Sol Gordon, "From Where I Sit," *Family Life Educator,* Volume 10, Number 2 (1991/1992): 12–13.

34. Sol Gordon, "The Case for a Moral Sex Education in the Schools," *Journal of School Health,* Volume 51 (1981): 214–218.

35. Bernice McCarthy, *The 4MAT System: Teaching to Learning Styles with Right/Left Mode Technique*s (Oakbrook, Ill.: Excel, 1980/1981).

36. James W. Keefe, *Learning Style Theory and Practice* (Reston, Va.: National Association of Secondary School Principals, 1987).

37. M. Maxine Hammonds and Jerelyn B. Schultz, "Sexuality Education Instructional Techniques: Teacher Usage and Student Preference," *Journal of School Health,* Volume 54, Number 7 (August 1984): 235–238.

38. Edgar Dale, *Audio-Visual Methods in Teaching* (New York: Dryden Press, 1969).

39. Mary Field Belenky, Blythe McVicker Clinchy, Nancy Rule Goldberger, and Jill Mattuck Tarule, *Women's Ways of Knowing: The Development of Self, Voice and Mind* (New York: Basic Books, 1986).

40. Jo Durden-Smith and Diane deSimone, *Sex and the Brain* (New York: Warner Books, 1983).

41. Martyna, "What Does 'He' Mean?"

42. Deborah Tannen, *You Just Don't Understand: Men and Women in Conversation* (New York: Ballentine Books, 1991).

43. American Association of University Women, *Executive Summary of The AAUW Report: How Schools Shortchange Girls* (Washington, D.C.: AAUW, 1992).

44. Raphaela Best, *We've All Got Scars: What Boys and Girls Learn in Elementary School* (Bloomington: Indiana University Press, 1983).

45. AAUW, *How Schools Shortchange Girls.*

46. Myra and David Sadker, "Sexism in the Schoolroom of the '80's," *Psychology Today* (March 1985): 54–57.

47. Tannen, *You Just Don't Understand.*

48. Douglas Kirby, Richard P. Barth, Nancy Leland, and Joyce V. Fetro, "Reducing the Risk: Impact of a New Curriculum on Sexual Risk-Taking," *Family Planning Perspectives,* Volume 23, Number 6 (November/December 1991): 253–263.

49. Douglas Kirby, *Sexuality Education: An Evaluation of Programs and Their Effects: An Executive Summary* (Santa Cruz, Calif.: Network Publications, 1984).

50. Kirby et al., "Reducing the Risk."

51. Ronald Moglia, "Sexuality Education in Higher Education in the USA: Analysis and Implications," *Sexual and Marital Therapy,* Volume 9, Number 2 (1994): 181–191.

52. Douglas Kirby, Lynn Short, Janet Collins, Deborah Rugg, Lloyd Kolbe, Marion Howard, Brent Miller, Freya Sonenstein, and Laurie S. Zabin, "School-Based Programs to Reduce Sexual Risk Behaviors: A Review of Effectiveness," *Public Health Reports,* Volume 109, Number 3 (May/June 1994): 339–359.

53. Douglas Kirby, "Research on Effectiveness of Sex Education Programs," *Theory into Practice,* Volume 28, Number 3 (Summer 1989): 191–197.

54. Helen P. Koo, George H. Dunteman, Cindee George, Yvonne Green, and Murray Vincent, "Reducing Adolescent Pregnancy through School- and Community-Based Intervention: Denmark, South Carolina, Revisited," *Family Planning Perspectives,* Volume 26, Number 5 (September/October 1994): 206–217.

55. M. L. Vincent, A. F. Clearie, and M. D. Schlucter, "Reducing Adolescent Pregnancy through School and Community-Based Education," *Journal of the American Medical Association,* Volume 257, Number 24 (1987): 3382–3386.

56. Sol Gordon and Joseph Fay, "Moral Sexuality Education and Democratic Values," *Theory into Practice,* Volume 28, Number 3 (Summer 1989): 211–216.

57. G. Thomas Baer and Walter S. Foster, "Teacher Preparation: What Graduates Tell Us," ERIC Document #103402 (1974).

58. Ione Ryan and Patricia C. Dunn, "Sex Education from the Prospective Teacher's View Poses a Dilemma," *The Journal of School Health,* Volume 49 (1979): 573–575.

59. B. A. Rienzo, "The Status of Sex Education: An Overview and Recommendations," *Phi Delta Kappan,* Volume 63 (1981): 192–193.

60. Howard E. Munson, "What Teachers Think They Need to Be Sexuality Educators," *Health Education,* Volume 7, Number 2 (1976): 31–40.

61. Donovan, *Risk and Responsibility.*

62. SIECUS, preliminary data on a review of college catalog course descriptions, to be published in fall of 1995. Contact SIECUS at 1-212-819-9770 for more information.

63. Hammonds and Schultz, "Sexuality Education Instructional Techniques."

64. Dennis Thompson, "Sex Education Curricula in Teacher Education Institutions: A Survey," *Journal of Research and Development in Education,* Volume 16, Number 2 (1983): 44.

65. Carol Flaherty and Peggy B. Smith, "Teacher Training for Sex Education," *Journal of School Health,* Volume 51, Number 4 (1981).

66. SIECUS, preliminary data on a review of college catalog course descriptions, 1995.

Notes to Chapter 3

1. Robert Selverstone, "Sexuality Education Can Strengthen Democracy," *Educational Leadership,* Volume 49, Number 3 (September 1991): 58–60.

2. S. Vosko and R. Hiemstra, "The Adult Learning Environment: Importance of Physical Features," *International Journal of Lifelong Education,* Volume 7, Number 3 (July–September 1988): 185–195.

3. Evonne Hedgepeth, "Sexuality Comfort: Its Measurement, and Relationship to Other Variables in Sexuality Education," Ph.D. diss., University Microfilms, 1988.

4. William A. Fisher, "All Together Now: An Integrated Approach to Preventing Adolescent Pregnancy and STD/HIV Infection," *SIECUS Report,* Volume 18, Number 4 (April/May 1990): 1–11.

5. Douglas Kirby, *Sexuality Education: An Evaluation of Programs and Their Effects: An Executive Summary* (Santa Cruz, Calif.: Network Publications, 1984).

6. Fisher, "All Together Now."

7. Daniel Klein, Philip A. Belcastro, and Robert S. Gold, "Sex Education Program Outcomes: Student and Alumni Perceptions." Paper presented at the National Convention of the American Alliance for Health, Physical Education, Recreation and Dance (Minneapolis, Minn., April 9, 1983).

8. Fisher, "All Together Now."

9. Richard Hamilton and Phyllis Levenson-Gingiss, "The Relationship of Teacher Attitudes to Course Implementation and Student Responses," *Teaching and Teacher Education,* Volume 9, Number 2 (1993): 193–204.

10. Evonne Hedgepeth, unpublished report on teenage focus group discussions, conducted for the HIV Prevention Section of the Office of the Superintendent for Public Instruction, Washington State (February 1993).

11. Wendy Martyna, "What Does 'He' Mean — Use of the Generic Masculine," *Journal of Communication,* Volume 28, Number 1 (Winter 1978): 131–138.

12. Mary Crawford and Margo MacLeod, "Gender in the College Classroom: An Assessment of the 'Chilly Climate' for Women," *Sex Roles: A Journal of Research,* Volume 23, Numbers 3–4 (August 1990): 101–122.

13. Richard P. Barth, *Reducing the Risk: Building Skills to Prevent Pregnancy, STD & HIV,* 2d ed. (Santa Cruz, Calif.: ETR Associates, 1993).

14. Fisher, "All Together Now."

15. J. Stiff, M. McCormack, E. Zook, T. Stein, and R. Henry, "Learning about AIDS and HIV Transmission in College-Age Students," *Communication Research,* Volume 17, Number 6 (December 1990): 743–758.

16. Megan Monson, "What Is the Student's Role in Education about Sexuality?" *PTA Today* (December/January 1981/82): 23–24.

17. Carolyn Cooperman and Chuck Rhoades, *New Methods for Puberty Education* (Hackensack, N.J.: Planned Parenthood of Greater Northern New Jersey, 1992).

18. Peter Aggleton, "Priorities for School-Based HIV and AIDS Education," paper given at the 7th International Conference on AIDS Education, Chicago, November 1993, 2.

19. Judith Scheer, *HIV Prevention for Teachers of Elementary Education and Middle School Grades* (Reston, Va.: Association for the Advancement of Health Education, with ETR Associates, 1992).

20. Alfie Kohn, *No Contest: The Case against Competition* (Boston: Houghton Mifflin, 1992).

21. American Association of University Women, *The AAUW Report: How Schools Shortchange Girls: Executive Summary* (Washington, D.C.: AAUW, 1991).

22. David W. Johnson and Roger T. Johnson, *Learning Together and Alone: Cooperative, Competitive and Individualistic Learning* (Englewood Cliff, N.J.: Prentice Hall, 1975).

23. The only exception to this general principle is in tasks such as rote decoding and correcting, in which cooperation is equally effective with competitive or individualized work.

24. Kohn, *No Contest.*

25. Johnson and Johnson, *Learning Together and Alone.*

26. National Coalition of Advocates for Students, *Criteria for Evaluating an AIDS Curriculum* (Boston: NCAS, 1992).

27. Vosko and Hiemstra, "The Adult Learning Environment."

28. *Ibid.*

29. I. Altman, *Human Behavior and Environment: Advances in Theory and Research* (New York: Plenum Publishing, 1977). Cited in Vosko and Hiemstra, "The Adult Learning Environment."

30. Ironically, the actress who played June Cleaver was herself a working mom, who spent more time with her screen children than with her own! (Source: *Oprah Winfrey Show,* April 1995.)

31. H. Thomas Hurt, Michael D. Scott, and James C. McCroskey, *Communication in the Classroom* (Reading, Mass.: Addison-Wesley, 1976).

Notes to Chapter 4

1. Seth C. Kalichman and Tricia L. Hunter, "The Disclosure of Celebrity HIV Infection: Its Effects on Public Attitudes," *American Journal of Public Health,* Volume 82, Number 10 (October 1992).

2. "Sexual Risk Behaviors of STD Clinic Patients before and after Earvin 'Magic' Johnson's HIV-Infection Announcement—Maryland, 1991–1992," *Morbidity and Mortality Weekly Report,* Volume 42, Number 3 (January 29, 1993): 45–49.

3. "Sea change": a striking change, often for the better (Webster's Unabridged Dictionary, 1989).

4. A. D. Taylor, "Prevention after Magic," *FOCUS* (February 1993): 5–6.

5. V. S. Freimuth, T. Edgar, and S. L. Hammond, "College Students' Awareness and Interpretation of the AIDS Risk," *Science, Technology and Human Values,* Volume 12 (1987): 37–40.

6. Q. Thurman and K. Franklin. "AIDS and College Health: Knowledge, Threat and Prevention at a Northeastern University," *Journal of American College Health,* Volume 38 (1990): 179–184.

7. S. M. Kegels, N. Adler, and C. Irwin, "Sexually Active Adolescents and Condoms: Changes in One Year in Knowledge, Attitudes and Use," *American Journal of Public Health,* Volume 75 (1988): 460–461.

8. Estelle Weinstein, Efrem Rosen, and Joan Atwood, "Adolescents' Knowledge of AIDS and Behavior Change: Implications for Education," *Journal of Health Education,* Volume 22, Number 5 (September/October 1991): 313–318.

9. Douglas Kirby, "Sexuality Education: It Can Reduce Unprotected Intercourse," SIECUS Report (December 1992/January 1993): 19–24.

10. Elizabeth G. Calamidas, "AIDS and STD Education: What's Really Happening in Our Schools?" *Journal of Sex Education and Therapy,* Volume 16, Number 1 (1990): 54–63.

11. Rose E. Ray and Dwight R. Kirkpatrick, "Two Time Formats for Teaching Human Sexuality," *Teaching of Psychology,* Volume 10, Number 2 (April 1983): 84–88.

12. Douglas Kirby, Lynn Short, Janet Collins, Deborah Rugg, Lloyd Kolbe, Marion Howard, Brent Miller, Freya Sonenstein, and Laurie S. Zabin, "School-Based Programs to Reduce Sexual Risk Behaviors: A Review of Effectiveness," *Public Health Reports,* Volume 109, Number 3 (May/June 1994): 339–359.

13. Kirby, "Sexuality Education Can Reduce Unprotected Intercourse."

14. Douglas Kirby, *Sexuality Education: An Evaluation of Programs and Their Effects: An Executive Summary* (Santa Cruz, Calif.: Network Publications, 1984).

15. Kirby, "Sexuality Education Can Reduce Unprotected Intercourse."

16. Kirby et al., "School-Based Programs," 1994.

17. *Ibid.*

18. *Ibid.*

19. For a detailed review of Piaget's theory, see Ruth M. Beard, *An Outline of Piaget's Developmental Psychology for Students and Teachers* (New York: Basic Books, 1969), and Hans G. Furth, *Piaget for Teachers* (Englewood Cliffs, N.J.: Prentice Hall, 1970).

20. More accurately stated, Piaget distinguished between two "ways of knowing," acknowledging that "knowledge" has no existence separate from the individual learner. Other writers have expanded on this notion, hypothesizing many diverse "ways of knowing" based on the cultural, perceptual, gender, and other differences in learners (e.g., Belenky et al. 1986; Hale-Benson 1982; Samples 1987; McCarthy 1980/81.)

21. Hans G. Furth, *Piaget for Teachers* (Englewood Cliffs, N.J.: Prentice Hall, 1970).

22. Benjamin Samuel Bloom, *Taxonomy of Educational Objectives: The Classification of Educational Goals* (New York: Longman Publishing, 1984).

23. Richard P. Barth, *Reducing the Risk: Building Skills to Prevent Pregnancy, STD & HIV,* 2d ed. (Santa Cruz, Calif.: ETR Associates, 1993): 13–15.

24. David Fine et al. "Idaho State Department of Maternal and Child Health HIV/AIDS Knowledge, Attitudes and Behavior Survey" (Seattle: The Center for Health Training, unpublished data, 1990).

25. Susan Thornton and Jose Catalan, "Preventing the Sexual Spread of HIV Infection— What Have We Learned?" *International Journal of STD & AIDS*, Volume 4 (November/December 1993): 311–316.

26. Douglas Kirby, keynote address on effective sexuality education, Washington Alliance Concerned with School-Age Parents, Fall Conference, Bellevue, Wash., October 1993).

27. Beverlie Conant Sloane and Christine G. Zimmer, "The Power of Peer Health Education," *Journal of American College Health*, Volume 41 (May 1993): 241–245.

28. Maria Natera in Scheer, *HIV Prevention Education*, 39.

29. Sheryl P. Bowen and Paula Michal-Johnson, "A Rhetorical Perspective for HIV Education with Black Urban Adolescents," *Communication Research*, Volume 17, Number 6 (December 1990): 848–866.

30. Germaine Maslach and Graham Kerr, "Tailoring Sex Education Programs to Adolescents: A Strategy for the Primary Prevention of Unwanted Adolescent Pregnancies," *Adolescence*, Volume 18, Number 70 (Summer 1983): 449–456.

31. Elizabeth G. Calamidas, "Reaching Youth about AIDS: Challenges Confronting Health Educators," *Health Values*, Volume 15, Number 6 (November/December 1991): 55–60.

32. J. Liebman, "Research and Education in Outreach Efforts to IV Drug Users and Prostitutes," paper presented at the Eastern Communication Association Conference, Philadelphia, April 1990.

33. Sandra McClennen, "Sexuality and Students with Mental Retardation," *Teaching Exceptional Children* (Summer 1988): 59–61.

34. Greg M. Romaneck and Robert Kuehl, "Sex Education for Students with High-Incidence Special Needs," *Teaching Exceptional Children* (Fall 1992): 22–24.

35. David Van Biema, "AIDS," *Time* (April 4, 1994): 76–77.

36. Bowen and Michal-Johnson, "A Rhetorical Perspective."

37. Patrick McLaurin and Ivan Juzang, "Reaching the Hip-Hop Generation," *FOCUS: A Guide to AIDS Research and Counseling*, Volume 8, Number 3 (February 1993): 1–4.

38. Calamidas, "Reaching Youth about AIDS."

39. Amado M. Padilla and Traci L. Baird, "Mexican-American Adolescent Sexuality and Sexual Knowledge: An Exploratory Study," *Hispanic Journal of Behavioral Sciences*, Volume 13, Number 1 (February 1991): 95–104.

40. James J. Ponzetti, Jr., and Rose Ann Abrahamson, "The Need for Cultural Awareness in Native American Sex Education," *Canadian Journal of Native Education*, Volume 17, Number 1 (1990): 60–67.

41. G. Cajetan Luna, "AIDS and Native Youth," paper presented at the Canadian Conference on AIDS and Related Issues in the Native Community, Vancouver, British Columbia, Canada, April 12–14, 1989.

42. Bowen and Michal-Johnson, "A Rhetorical Perspective."

43. J. H. Price, S. M. Desmond, C. Hallinan, et al., "College Students' Perceived Risk and Seriousness of AIDS," *Health Education*, Volume 19, Number 4 (1988): 16–20.

44. Katie Roiphe, *The Morning After: Sex, Fear and Feminism on Campus* (Boston: Little, Brown and Company, 1993).

45. Anke Ehrhardt, "Trends in Sexual Behavior and the HIV Pandemic," *American Journal of Public Health*, Volume 82, Number 11 (November 1992): 1459–1461.

46. R. B. Hays, S. M. Kegeles, and T. J. Coates, "High HIV Risk-Taking among Young Gay Men," *AIDS,* Volume 4 (1990): 901–907.

47. M. L. Ekstrand and T. J. Coates, "Maintenance of Safer Sex Behaviours and Predictors of Risky Sex: The San Francisco Gay Men's Health Study," *American Journal of Public Health,* Volume 80 (1990): 973–978.

48. J. A. Kelly, J. S. Lawrence, T. L. Brasfield, A. Lemke, T. Amidei, and R. E. Roffman, "Psychological Factors That Predict AIDS High Risk versus AIDS Precautionary Behavior," *Journal of Consulting and Clinical Psychology,* Volume 58 (1990): 117–120.

49. L. McKusick, W. Hortsman, T. J. Coates, "AIDS and the Sexual Behavior Reported by Gay Men in San Francisco," *American Journal of Public Health,* Volume 75 (1985): 493–496.

50. Thornton and Catalan, "Preventing the Sexual Spread of HIV Infection."

51. Joseph A. Catania, Susan M. Kegeles, and Thomas J. Coates, "Toward an Understanding of Risk Behavior: An AIDS Risk Reduction Model (ARRM)," *Health Education Quarterly,* Volume 17, Number 1 (Spring 1990): 53–72.

52. Judith Scheer, *HIV Prevention for Teachers of Elementary and Middle School Grades* (Santa Cruz, Calif.: Association for the Advancement of Health Education, with ETR Associates, Inc., 1992).

53. Peggy Brick et al., *Teaching Safer Sex* (Hackensack, N.J.: The Center for Family Life Education, Planned Parenthood of Greater Northern New Jersey, 1989): 1–12.

54. K. H. Choi, R. Rickman, and J. A. Catania, "What Do U.S. Heterosexual Adults Believe about Condoms?" *New England Journal of Medicine,* Volume 331 (1994): 406–407.

55. Tim Melchert and Kent F. Burnett, "Attitudes, Knowledge, and Sexual Behavior of High-Risk Adolescents: Implications for Counseling and Sexuality Education," *Journal of Counseling and Development,* Volume 68, Number 3 (January/February 1990): 293–298.

56. Robert A. Hatcher, James Trussell, Felicia Stewart, Gary K. Stewart, Deborah Kowal, Felicia Guest, Willard Cates, Jr., and Michael S. Policar, *Contraceptive Technology,* 16th rev. ed. (New York: Irvington Publishers, 1994).

57. Seattle–King County Department of Public Health, "Special Report on Condom Effectiveness," *Focus on School Health,* Volume 3 (November 1992): 4. Report on a literature review of studies on condom effectiveness in preventing HIV transmission.

58. I. deVincenzi, for the European Study on Heterosexual Transmission for HIV, "A Longitudinal Study of Human Immunodeficiency Virus Transmission by Heterosexual Partners," *New England Journal of Medicine* (1994): 331 and 341–346.

59. Seattle–King County, "Special Report."

60. Center for Disease Control and Prevention, "Talking Points & Supporting Data: MMWR on the Effectiveness of Condoms," undated handout.

61. David Silven, "Behavioral Theories and Relapse," *FOCUS: A Guide to AIDS Research and Counseling,* Volume 8, Number 2 (January 1993): 136.

62. Raphaela Best, *We've All Got Scars: What Boys and Girls Learn in Elementary School* (Bloomington: Indiana University Press, 1983).

63. Debra Boyer and David Fine, "Sexual Abuse as a Factor in Adolescent Pregnancy and Child Mistreatment," *Family Planning Perspectives,* Volume 24, Number 1 (January/February 1992): 4–12.

64. Subhuti Dharmananda, "Child Abuse & HIV: An Ongoing Legacy," *Hand-in-Hand, Newsletter for Oregon's HIV Care Community* (November 1994): 5–6.

65. David Fine and Debra Boyer, "Abuse Dimensions of Teen Contraception and STD Prevention," preliminary findings for a Service Delivery grant funded by Office of Population Affairs, awarded to the Center for Health Training (Seattle, 1992–1995).

66. S. N. Feidman, W. D. Mosher, and S. O. Aral, "Women with Multiple Sexual Partners: U.S. 1988," *American Journal of Public Health,* Volume 82, Number 10 (1992): 1388–1393.

67. I. E. Swenson, "A Profile of Young Adolescents Attending a Teen Family Planning Clinic," *Adolescence,* Volume 27, Number 107 (1992): 647–654.

68. James Cassese, "The Invisible Bridge: Child Sexual Abuse and the Risk of HIV Infection in Adulthood," *SIECUS Report,* Volume 21, Number 4 (April/May 1993): 5.

69. Catania et al., "Towards an Understanding of Risk Behavior."

70. Joe Klein, "Learning How to Say No: Clinton's New Teen-Pregnancy Program will Counsel Abstinence," *Newsweek* (June 13, 1994): 29.

71. J. A. Kelly, J. S. Lawrence, and Y. E. Diaz, "HIV Risk-Behavior Reduction Following Intervention with Key Opinion Leaders of a Population: An Experimental Community Level Analysis," *American Journal of Public Health,* Volume 81, Number 2 (1991): 168–171.

72. C. Nathanson and M. Becker, "Family and Peer Influence on Obtaining a Method of Contraception," *Journal of Marriage and the Family,* Volume 48 (1986): 513–525.

73. Wayne Blankenship. "Relapse Prevention Interventions," *FOCUS: A Guide to AIDS Research and Counseling,* Volume 8, Number 2 (January 1993): 5–6.

74. S. M. Adib, J. G. Joseph, D. G. Ostrow, et al., "Predictors of Relapse in Sexual Practices among Homosexual Men," *AIDS Education and Prevention,* Volume 3, Number 4 (1991): 293–304.

75. Catania et al., "Towards an Understanding of Risk Behavior."

76. Donald C. Iverson and W. James Popham, "Combatting AIDS on the Front Lines," *The School Administrator,* Volume 49, Number 8 (September 1992): 22–23 and 26–27.

77. Diane M. Grimley, Ralph J. DiClemente, James O. Prochaska, and Gabrielle E. Prochaska, "Preventing Adolescent Pregnancy, STD and HIV: A Promising New Approach," *Family Life Educator* (Spring 1995): 7–15.

78. R. J. DiClemente and J. D. Fisher, "Social Influence Factors as Predictors of Condom Use in a Predominantly Minority Population" (1994), cited in Grimley et al., "Preventing Adolescent Pregnancy."

79. R. J. DiClemente, "Predictors of HIV-Preventive Sexual Behavior in a High-Risk Adolescent Population," *Journal of Adolescent Health,* Volume 12 (1991): 385–390.

80. Mildred Z. Solomon and William DeJong, "Recent Sexually Transmitted Disease Prevention Efforts and Their Implications for AIDS Health Education," *Health Education Quarterly,* Volume 13, Number 4 (Winter 1986): 301–316.

81. Denise Polit-O'Hara and Janet R. Kahn, "Communication and Contraceptive Practices in Adolescent Couples," *Adolescence,* Volume 20, Number 77 (Spring 1985): 33–43.

82. Grimley et al., "Preventing Adolescent Pregnancy, STD and HIV."

83. J. O. Prochaska, C. C. DiClemente, and J. C. Norcross, "In Search of How People Change: Applications to Addictive Behaviors," *American Psychologist,* Volume 47, Number 9 (September 1992): 1102–1114.

84. James Prochaska, Coleen Redding, Lisa Harlow, Joseph Rossi, and Wayne Velicer, "The Transtheoretical Model of Change and HIV Prevention: A Review," *Health Education Quarterly,* Volume 21, Number 4 (Winter 1994): 471–486.

85. Joan Helmich and Irene Peters et al., *Handbook for Delivering Family Planning Services in Chemical Dependency Treatment Centers* (Seattle: Washington State Division of Alcohol and Substance Abuse, 1995).

86. Project CARES Intervention Work Group, *Project CARES: Advocates' Guide to Stages of Change Counseling* (Atlanta, Ga.: CDC, Division of Reproductive Health and Division of STD/HIV Prevention, 1994).

Notes to Chapter 5

1. As it turned out, the father of the boy eventually was arrested and convicted of sexually assaulting his own son.

2. Peter Scales and Douglas Kirby, "Perceived Barriers to Sexuality Education: A Survey of Professionals," *Journal of Sex Research,* Volume 19, Number 4 (1983): 309–326.

3. Jacqueline Darroch Forrest and Jane Silverman, "What Public School Teachers Teach about Preventing Pregnancy, AIDS and Sexually Transmitted Diseases," *Family Planning Perspectives,* Volume 21, Number 2 (March/April 1989): 65–72.

4. Michael Young and Rod Roth, "Attitudes of School Officials toward Sex Education Programs: A Discriminant Analysis," ERIC Document #ED223543 (1982).

5. William L. Yarber and K. A. Pavese, "School Personnel Estimates of Community Support for Sex Education," *Journal of Sex Education and Therapy,* Volume 10, Number 21 (1984).

6. Madelon Zady and Kenneth Duckworth, "A Battle Lost," *American School Board Journal,* Volume 178, Number 2 (February 1991): 25–26.

7. Syble Brindley, "School Health Coalition Building—One State's Plan," paper presented at the Annual Meeting of the American Alliance for Health, Physical Education, Recreation and Dance, Washington, D.C., March 24–28, 1993.

8. Helen P. Koo, George H. Dunteman, Cindee George, Yvonne Green, and Murray Vincent, "Reducing Adolescent Pregnancy through a School- and Community-Based Intervention: Denmark, South Carolina, Revisited," *Family Planning Perspectives,* Volume 26, Number 5 (September/October 1994): 206–217.

9. M. Sedway, "Far Right Takes Aim at Sexuality Education," *SIECUS Report,* Volume 20, Number 2 (1992): 1–3.

10. Peggy Brick, personal communication, 1995.

11. Katie Meyer and Deanne Larsell, "Dealing with the Opposition," workshop presented at the Northwest Institute for Community Health Educators (NICHE), North Bend, Wash., November 1992).

12. Leslie Kantor, "Who Decides? Parents and Comprehensive Sexuality Education," *SIECUS Report* (February/March 1994): 7–12.

13. Webster's Unabridged Dictionary, 1989.

14. Peter Scales, "The New Opposition to Sex Education: A Powerful Threat to Democratic Society," *Journal of School Health* (1981): 300–304.

15. Patricia First, "Sex Education in the Public Schools: A Clash of Religious Freedom and the General Welfare," *The Educational Forum,* Volume 57 (Fall 1992): 76–83.

16. Vaughn vs. Reed, 1970, 313 F. Supp. 431, 443–444 (W.D.W.Va.); cited in First, "Sex Education in the Public Schools."

17. William L. Yarber and George P. McCabe, Jr., "Importance of Sex Education Topics: Correlates with Teacher Characteristics and Inclusion of Topics in Instruction," *Health Education* (February 1984): 36–41.

18. Cheryl A. Graham and Margaret Smith, "Operationalizing the Concept of Sexuality

Comfort: Applications for Sexuality Educators," *Journal of School Health,* Volume 54, Number 11 (December 1984): 439–442.

19. Evonne M. Hedgepeth, "Sexuality Comfort: Its Measurement, and Relationship to Other Variables in Sexuality Education," Ph.D. diss., University Microfilms, 1988.

20. M. Quackenbush and S. Villeareal, "*Does AIDS Hurt? Educating Young Children about AIDS*" (Santa Cruz, Calif.: ETR Associates, 1988).

21. Toni A. Campbell and David E. Campbell, "What's 'Verbil' Sex? An Analysis of Adolescents' Questions about Sex," paper presented at the 67th Annual Meeting of the Western Psychological Association, Long Beach, Calif., April 23–26, 1987.

22. Robert R. Troiden, "Walking the Line: The Personal and Professional Risks of Sex Education and Research," *Teaching Sociology,* Volume 15 (July 1987): 241–249.

23. Janie V. Ward and Jill M. Taylor, "Sexuality Education in a Multicultural Society," *Educational Leadership,* Volume 49, Number 1 (September 1991): 62–64.

24. Yarber and McCabe, "Importance of Sex Education Topics." 1984.

25. Historically, some schools have looked to local community health agencies to provide sexuality education they were unwilling or unable to offer themselves. However, the HIV/AIDS pandemic has increased demands on community health educators' time and resources, forcing reevaluation of this approach. Nowadays, many community health educators are changing their focus to assist teachers, rather than presenting programs themselves.

26. Ann Welbourne-Moglia and Ronald J. Moglia, "Sexuality Education in the United States: What It Is; What It Is Meant to Be," *Theory into Practice,* Volume 28, Number 3 (Summer 1989): 159–164.

27. Troiden, "Walking the Line." 1987.

28. *Ibid.*

29. Ann K. Welbourne, "A Review of the Current Status of Human Sexuality Training Programs for Professionals," *Marriage and Family Review,* Volume 6, Number 3–4 (1983): 61 77.

30. SIECUS, preliminary data from a review of college catalog course descriptions, to be published in fall of 1995. Contact SIECUS at 212-819-9770 for more information.

31. Dennis N. Thompson, "Sex Education Curricula in Teacher Education Institutions: A Survey," *Journal of Research and Development in Education,* Volume 16, Number 2 (1983): 41–44.

32. Welbourne-Moglia and Moglia, "Sexuality Education in the United States."

33. Pat Donovan, *Risk and Responsibility: Teaching Sex Education in America's Schools Today* (New York: Alan Guttmacher Institute, 1989).

34. Zady and Duckworth, "A Battle Lost."

Notes to Introduction to Part II

1. National Guidelines Taskforce, *Guidelines for Comprehensive Sexuality Education Kindergarten—12th Grade* (New York: Sexuality Information and Education Council of the U.S., 1991), 29.

Notes to Chapter 6

1. National Guidelines Task Force, *Guidelines for Comprehensive Sexuality Education Kindergarten—12th Grade* (New York: Sexuality Information and Education Council of the U.S., 1991).

2. Richard P. Barth, *Reducing the Risk: Building Skills to Prevent Pregnancy, STD & HIV* (Santa Cruz, Calif.: ETR Associates, 1993).
3. Peggy Brick et al., *Teaching Safer Sex* (Hackensack, N.J.: Planned Parenthood of Greater Northern New Jersey, 1989), 39–40.

Notes to Chapter 7

1. An excellent resource for information on group process in education settings is Gene Stanford and Albert E. Roark, *Human Interaction in Education* (Boston: Allyn and Bacon, 1974). In it they refer to many of the best writers on group process, including Bennis, Shepard and Schutz.
2. Joan Helmich and Jan Loreen, *Sexuality Education and Training: Theory, Techniques and Resources* (Seattle: Planned Parenthood of Seattle–King County, 1979), 13.
3. Stanford and Roark, *Human Interaction in Education,* 55.
4. Megan Monson, "What Is the Student's Role in Education about Sexuality?" *PTA Today* (December/January 1981–1982): 23–24.
5. Thanks to Gail Stringer, Planned Parenthood of Seattle–King County, Bellevue, Wash., for these suggestions.
6. Carolyn Cooperman and Chuck Rhoades, *New Methods for Puberty Education* (Hackensack, N.J.: Planned Parenthood of Greater Northern New Jersey, 1992), 33.
7. Dana McMurray, "When It Doesn't Work: Small Group Work in Adolescent Sexuality Education," *The School Counselor,* Volume 39 (March 1992): 385–389.

Notes to Chapter 8

1. Kathleen Middleton, ed., *Entering Adulthood: Coping with Sexual Pressures* (Santa Cruz, Calif.: ETR Associates, 1990).
2. Pamela Wilson and Craig Hollander, *When I'm Grown: Life Planning Education for Grades 3 & 4* (Washington, D.C.: Advocates for Youth, 1992), 25.
3. Carolyn Cooperman and Chuck Rhoades, *New Methods for Puberty Education* (Hackensack, N.J.: Planned Parenthood of Greater Northern New Jersey, 1992), 148.
4. *Ibid.,* 145.
5. Carol Hunter-Geboy, *Life Planning Education: A Youth Development Program* (Washington, D.C.: Advocates for Youth, 1994).
6. A source of material on guided imagery is the Academy for Guided Imagery, PO Box 2070, Mill Valley, CA 94942, 415-389-9324.
7. Hunter-Geboy, *Life Planning Education.*
8. Peggy Brick, "Sex and Society: Teaching the Connection," *The Journal of School Health,* Volume 51, Number 4 (April 1981): 42.
9. John Forliti et al., *Human Sexuality: Values and Choices* (Minneapolis: Search Institute, 1991).

Notes to Chapter 9

1. James O. Prochaska et. al., "The Transtheoretical Model of Change and HIV Prevention: A Review," *Health Education Quarterly,* Volume 21, Number 4 (Winter 1994): 471–486.
2. Elizabeth Reis, *9/10 F.L.A.S.H.: Family Life and Sexual Health* (Seattle: Seattle–King County Department of Public Health, 1989), 231.
3. Marion Howard and Marie E. Mitchell, *Postponing Sexual Involvement: An Educa-*

tional Series for Young Teens (Atlanta: Emory/Grady Teen Services Program, 1990).

4. Richard P. Barth, *Reducing the Risk: Building Skills to Prevent Pregnancy, STD & HIV* (Santa Cruz, Calif.: ETR Associates, 1993).

5. John Forliti et al., *Human Sexuality: Values and Choices* (Minneapolis: Search Institute, 1991).

6. *Ibid.*

7. *HIV/AIDS Audiovisual Resources: A SIECUS Guide to Selecting, Evaluating and Using AVRs* (New York: SIECUS, 1991).

8. Reis, *9/10 F.L.A.S.H.*, 5.

9. SIECUS reviews three texts in their resource guide, "Comprehensive Sexuality Education: A SIECUS Resource Guide of Recommended Curricula and Textbooks," *SIECUS Report* (August/September 1993). (Available from SIECUS as a reprint.)

10. In 1994, Holt, Rinehart and Winston pulled its high school text *Holt Health* from use in the Texas schools because of sex-negative censorship demands by the Texas Board of Education.

11. Howard and Mitchell, *Postponing Sexual Involvement,* 36.

12. Peggy Brick, "Sex and Society: Teaching the Connection," *The Journal of School Health,* Volume 51, Number 4 (April 1981): 42.

13. *Ibid.*

14. Reis, *9/10 F.L.A.S.H.*, 15.

15. A helpful review of sexuality education computerized learning programs is *A Review of Computer-Assisted Learning Programs Intended to Help Adolescents Make Good Life-Choices* (Austin, Tex.: James Bowman Associates, 1990). See also Steven Schinke and Mario Orlandi, "Skills-Based, Interactive Computer Interventions to Prevent HIV Infection Among African-American and Hispanic Adolescents," *Computers in Human Behavior,* Volume 6 (1990): 235–246.

Notes to Chapter 10

1. Gene Stanford and Albert E. Roark, *Human Interaction in Education* (Boston: Allyn and Bacon, 1974), 81–88.

2. Patti DeRosa, Laurie Prendergast, and Fran Smith, "When Race Is the Issue," *FLEducator* (Spring 1993), 26–28.

3. Richard P. Barth, *Reducing the Risk: Building Skills to Prevent Pregnancy, STD & HIV* (Santa Cruz, Calif.: ETR Associates, 1993), 55–56.

4. Carolyn Cooperman and Chuck Rhoades, *New Methods for Puberty Education* (Hackensack, N.J.: Planned Parenthood of Greater Northern New Jersey, 1992), 123–127.

5. Pamela Wilson, *When I'm Grown: Life Planning Education for Grades 5 & 6* (Washington, D.C.: Advocates for Youth, 1992), 51.

6. Marion Howard and Marie E. Mitchell, *Postponing Sexual Involvement: An Educational Series for Young Teens* (Atlanta: Emory/Grady Teen Services Program, 1990), 45–46.

7. Peggy Brick et al., *Teaching Safer Sex* (Hackensack, N.J.: Planned Parenthood of Greater Northern New Jersey, 1989), 17.

8. *Ibid.,* 1–3.

9. Thanks to Audrey Fine, The Center for Health Training, Seattle, for these suggestions.

10. Cooperman and Rhoades, *New Methods for Puberty Education,* III:3:A.

11. Elizabeth Reis, *9/10 F.L.A.S.H.: Family Life and Sexual Health* (Seattle: Seattle–King County Department of Public Health, 1989), 26–27.

1. Peggy Brick, "Actions Teach Better than Words: Teen Life Theater and Role Play in Sex Education," *Health Education* (February/March 1986): 49.
2. Richard P. Barth, *Reducing the Risk: Building Skills to Prevent Pregnancy, STD & HIV* (Santa Cruz, Calif.: ETR Associates, 1993).
3. These and many other ideas for warm-up activities preceding role plays are included in Gene Stanford and Albert E. Roark, *Human Interaction in Education* (Boston: Allyn and Bacon, 1974), 181–190.
4. John Forliti et al., *Human Sexuality: Values and Choices* (Minneapolis: Search Institute, 1991).
5. Peggy Brick, "Sex and Society: Teaching the Connection," *The Journal of School Health,* Volume 51, Number 4 (April 1981): 42.
6. Barth, *Reducing the Risk,* 51.
7. David Vaughan, "Communication Mixer I: Stating One's Needs" (Portland, Maine: Risky Zone Initiatives, 1994).
8. This list is adapted from Stanford and Roark, *Human Interaction in Education,* 172–174.
9. This list is adapted from Steven Paul Schinke and Lewayne D. Gilchrist, *Life Skills Counseling with Adolescents* (Baltimore: University Park Press, 1984), 15.
10. Forliti, *Human Sexuality: Values and Choices.*
11. Jane Stangle, *Special Education — Secondary F.L.A.S.H.* (Seattle: Seattle–King County Department of Public Health, 1991), 23.
12. Adapted from Schinke and Gilchrist, *Life Skills Counseling with Adolescents,* 16–17.
13. Carolyn Cooperman and Chuck Rhoades, *New Methods for Puberty Education* (Hackensack, N.J.: Planned Parenthood of Greater Northern New Jersey, 1992), 132–135.
14. We thank Gail Stringer, Planned Parenthood of Seattle–King County, Bellevue, Wash., and Paul Witt, Interlake High School, Bellevue, for the description of this simulation and for permission to reprint the worksheets.
15. Barth, *Reducing the Risk,* 13.
16. Linda Shaw, "Game Isn't Real, But the Grim AIDS News Is," *The Seattle Times,* May 5, 1994, B3. An information packet is available from Pat McCoy, Shoreline School District, 206-361-4246.
17. Richard P. Barth, Kathleen Middleton, and Ellen Wagman, "A Skill Building Approach to Preventing Teenage Pregnancy," *Theory Into Practice,* Volume 28, Number 3 (Summer 1989): 183–190.
18. *Ibid.*

Notes to Chapter 12

1. Pamela Wilson and Craig Hollander, *When I'm Grown: Life Planning Education for Grades 3 & 4* (Washington, D.C.: Advocates for Youth, 1992), 26.
2. H. Thornburg, "Adolescent Sources of Information about Sex," *Journal of School Health* 4 (April 1981): 274–277.
3. *Peer to Peer: Youth Preventing HIV Infection Together* (Washington, D.C.: Advocates for Youth, 1993), 9.
4. Marion Howard and Marie E. Mitchell, *Postponing Sexual Involvement: An Educational Series for Young Teens* (Atlanta: Emory/Grady Teen Services Program, 1990).
5. When we ask students about their needs for health education, they tell us how best to

utilize the peer education process. For example, many student comments on the Seattle School District 1993 Teen Health Survey were focused on how to improve the "Natural Helpers" program; they said that there should be a better selection process (not a "popularity contest") and more variety of students as Natural Helpers, people who are "good role models" to whom more students can relate, not just the "preppy," "snobbish," and "elite." They also asked for better safeguards for confidentiality, better training for peer educators, and "better adults leading" the program. Nancy Peterfreund and Karen Moe, *1993 Teen Health Survey: Report on Findings* (Seattle: Seattle School District Health Curriculum Office, March 1994).

6. *Peer to Peer.*
7. *Peer Education . . . a Little Help from Your Friends* (Grand Rapids, Mich.: Planned Parenthood Centers of West Michigan, 1993).
8. Peggy Brick, "Sex and Society: Teaching the Connection," *The Journal of School Health,* Volume 51, Number 4 (April 1981): 42.
9. Michael Rohd, "Hope Is Vital: A Prevention/Education Community Outreach Program for HIV/AIDS Awareness Utilizing Peer-Education and Interactive Theater," unpublished material; for information, contact Michael Rohd, 503-341-0747 or 410-363-6282.
10. Cited in *Peer to Peer,* 16.
11. Elizabeth Reis, *11/12 F.L.A.S.H: Family Life and Sexual Health* (Seattle: Seattle–King County Department of Public Health, 1992), 79–81.
12. Pamela Wilson, *When I'm Grown: Life Planning Education for Grades 5 & 6* (Washington, D.C.: Advocates for Youth, 1992), 156–158.
13. Carolyn Cooperman and Chuck Rhoades, *New Methods for Puberty Education* (Hackensack, N.J.: Planned Parenthood of Greater Northern New Jersey, 1992).
14. *Talk Listen Care Kit* (Brookline, Mass.: Harvard Community Health Plan Foundation, Inc., 1993).
15. Judy Drolet, "Games People Play," *Family Life Educator* (Spring 1991), 27–30.
16. *KNOW AIDS Prevention Curriculum* (Olympia: Washington State Office of the Superintendent of Public Instruction, 1994).

Notes to Chapter 13

1. Pamela Wilson, *When I'm Grown: Life Planning Education for Grades 5 & 6* (Washington, D.C.: Advocates for Youth, 1992), 204.
2. Elizabeth Reis, *9/10 F.L.A.S.H.: Family Life and Sexual Health* (Seattle: Seattle–King County Department of Public Health, 1989), 9–4, 553–556.
3. Carolyn Cooperman and Chuck Rhoades, *New Methods for Puberty Education* (Hackensack, N.J.: Planned Parenthood of Greater Northern New Jersey, 1992), 50–51.
4. Katie Meyer, Portland Public Schools, Portland, Oregon; unpublished material.
5. Richard P. Barth, *Reducing the Risk: Building Skills to Prevent Pregnancy, STD & HIV* (Santa Cruz, Calif.: ETR Associates, 1993), 197.
6. A touching example of a teen opening up in an anonymous note is reprinted in Steve Brown, *Streetwise to Sex-Wise: Sexuality Education for High-Risk Youth* (Hackensack, N.J.: Planned Parenthood of Greater Northern New Jersey, 1993), 93.
7. John Forliti et al., *Human Sexuality: Values and Choices* (Minneapolis: Search Institute, 1991), 207.

This bibliography represents only a small portion of the excellent resources available; we have tried to list a representative sample of materials in selected categories. Please also see the journals listed in Appendix C and the endnotes to all chapters for other references.

Data, Statistics, Research, and Other Sexuality Information

Brown, Sarah S., and Leon Eisenberg, eds. *The Best Intentions: Unintended Pregnancy and the Well-Being of Children and Families*. Washington, D.C.: Institute of Medicine, National Academy Press, 1995.

Haffner, Debra, ed. *Facing Facts: Sexual Health for America's Adolescents*. New York: The Report of the National Commission on Adolescent Sexual Health, SIECUS, 1995.

Hatcher, Robert A. et. al. *Contraceptive Technology*. 16th rev. ed. New York: Irvington Publishers, 1994.

Peterson, Lynn, et al. *Family Planning and Adolescent Health: Resource Guide and Model Programs*. Seattle: The Center for Health Training, 1994.

Readings on Teenage Pregnancy. New York and Washington, D.C.: The Alan Guttmacher Institute, 1989.

Sex and America's Teenagers. New York and Washington, D.C.: The Alan Guttmacher Institute, 1994.

Sex Education in America: AIDS and Adolescence (video). Boston: Media Works, 1993.

Teaching Methods

Corey, Gerald, and Marianne Schneider Corey. *Groups: Process and Practice*. Monterey, Calif.: Brooks/Cole Publishing, 1982.

Dietz, Susan, et al. *Guidelines for Health Education and Risk Reduction Activities*. Atlanta: Centers for Disease Control and Prevention, Division of STD/HIV Prevention, 1995.

Harmin, Merrill. *Inspiring Active Learning: A Handbook for Teachers*. Alexandria, Va.: Association for Supervision and Curriculum Development, 1994.

Shapiro, Marian. "Answering Anonymous Questions in Sexuality Education Class." *Family Life Educator*, Volume 13, Number 4 (Summer 1995): 8–13.

Learning Styles

Belenky, Mary Field, et al. *Women's Ways of Knowing: The Development of Self, Voice, and Mind*. New York: Basic Books, 1986.

Hale-Benson, Janice E. *Black Children: Their Roots, Culture, and Learning Styles*. Rev. ed. Baltimore: Johns Hopkins University Press, 1982.

Keefe, James W. *Learning Style Theory and Practice*. Reston, Va.: National Association of Secondary School Principals, 1987.

McCarthy, Bernice. *The 4MAT System: Teaching to Learning Styles with Right/Left Mode Techniques*. Oakbrook, Ill.: Excel, 1980–1981.

Samples, Bob. *Openmind/Wholemind: Parenting and Teaching Tomorrow's Children Today*. Rolling Hills Estates, Calif.: Jadmar Press, 1987.

College Sexuality Textbooks

Allgeier, Elizabeth Rice, and Albert Richard Allgeier. *Sexual Interactions*. Lexington, Mass.: D. C. Heath and Company, 1984.

Crooks, Robert, and Karla Baur. *Our Sexuality*. New York: The Benjamin/Cummings Publishing Company, 1990.

Katchadourian, Herant A. *Fundamentals of Human Sexuality*. Fort Worth, Tex.: Holt, Rinehart and Winston, 1989.

Kelly, Kathryn, and Donn Byrne. *Exploring Human Sexuality*. Old Tappan, N.J.: Prentice Hall, 1991.

McCammon, Susan L., David Knox, and Caroline Schacht. *Choices in Sexuality*. Minneapolis/St. Paul: West Publishing Company, 1993.

Sexuality Education

Cassell, Carol, and Pamela Wilson, eds. *Sexuality Education: A Resource Book*. Hamden, Conn.: Garland, 1989.

Cook, Ann Thompson, et al. *Sexuality Education: A Guide to Developing and Implementing Programs*. Arlington, Va.: Mathtech, 1984.

Drolet, Judy, and Kay Clark, eds. *The Sexuality Education Challenge: Promoting Healthy Sexuality in Young People*. Santa Cruz, Calif.: ETR Associates, 1994.

Kirby, Douglas. *Sexuality Education: An Evaluation of Programs and Their Effects*. Arlington, Va.: Mathtech, 1984.

National Guidelines Taskforce. *Guidelines for Comprehensive Sexuality Education Kindergarten — 12th Grade*. New York: SIECUS, 1991.

Sexuality Education within Comprehensive School Health Education. Kent, Ohio: American School Health Association, 1991.

Health and Sexuality Education Curricula

Barth, Richard P. *Reducing the Risk: Building Skills to Prevent Pregnancy, STD and HIV*. Santa Cruz, Calif.: ETR Associates, 1993.

Brick, Peggy, and Carolyn Cooperman. *Positive Images: A New Approach to Contraceptive Education*. Hackensack, N.J.: Planned Parenthood of Bergen County, 1987.

Brick, Peggy, et al. *Teaching Safer Sex*. Hackensack, N.J.: Planned Parenthood of Greater Northern New Jersey, 1989.

Brown, Steve. *Streetwise to Sex-Wise: Sexuality Education for High-Risk Youth.* Hackensack, N.J.: Planned Parenthood of Greater Northern New Jersey, 1993.

Browse, Deborah, and Pamela Wasserman. *For Earth's Sake: Lessons in Population and the Environment.* Washington, D.C.: ZPG Population Education Program, 1994.

Cooperman, Carolyn, and Chuck Rhoades. *New Methods for Puberty Education.* Hackensack, N.J.: Planned Parenthood of Greater Northern New Jersey, 1992.

Get Real about AIDS. Seattle: Comprehensive Health Education Foundation, 1995.

Here's Looking at You, 2000. Seattle: Comprehensive Health Education Foundation, 1991.

Howard, Marion, and Marie E. Mitchell. *Postponing Sexual Involvement: An Educational Series for Young Teens.* Atlanta: Emory/Grady Teen Services Program, 1990.

Natural Helpers. Seattle: Comprehensive Health Education Foundation, 1989.

Primarily Health. Seattle: Comprehensive Health Education Foundation, 1992.

Reis, Elizabeth, et. al. *Family Life and Sexual Health.* Seattle: Seattle–King County Department of Public Health, 1989–1994.

Skillwise. Seattle: Comprehensive Health Education Foundation, 1993.

Wilson, Pamela, and Douglas Kirby. *Sexuality Education: A Curriculum for Adolescents.* Arlington, Va.: Mathtech, 1984.

Annotated Bibliographies

Child Sexual Abuse Education, Prevention, and Treatment. New York: SIECUS, 1995.

Comprehensive Sexuality Education. New York: SIECUS, 1993.

Current Books on Sexuality. New York: SIECUS, 1993.

Current Religious Perspectives on Sexuality. New York: SIECUS, 1991.

Gay Male and Lesbian Sexuality and Issues. New York: SIECUS, 1991.

Global Sexuality. New York: SIECUS, 1994.

Growing Up. New York: SIECUS, 1994.

HIV/AIDS. New York: SIECUS, 1993.

Sexuality and Disability. New York: SIECUS, 1995.

Sexuality Education Resources for Religious Denominations. New York: SIECUS, 1992.

Sexuality in Middle and Later Life. New York: SIECUS, 1993.

Sexuality Periodicals for Professionals. New York: SIECUS, 1991.

Talking with Your Child about Sexuality and Other Important Issues. New York: SIECUS, 1994.

Miscellaneous

Community Action Kit: An Information Packet to Support Comprehensive Sexuality Education. New York: SIECUS, 1993.

de Mauro, Dian, and Carolyn Patierno. *Communication Strategies for HIV/AIDS and Sexuality: A Workshop for Mental Health and Health Professionals.* New York: SIECUS, 1990.

DiClemente, Ralph, and John L. Peterson, eds. *Preventing AIDS: Theories and Methods of Behavioral Interventions.* New York: Plenum Press, 1994.

How to Win: A Practical Guide to Defeating the Radical Right in Your Community. Washington, D.C.: PFLAG, 1994.

Winning the Battle: Developing Support for Sexuality and HIV/AIDS Education. New York: SIECUS, 1991.

INDEX

Abstinence: as curricular norm, 64; definition of, xviii; pledges of, 18; prevalence in curricula, 18

Abstinence-only curricula: characteristics of, 17; effectiveness of, 14

Active and interactive teaching methods, 110–12; and group process, 123

Administrators: need for training, 11; perceived support by, 37, 84

Affective domain, 109–10, 173–74

The American Association of Sex Educators, Counselors and Therapists (AASECT), 105

The Annual Workshop on Sexuality (Thornfield conference), 106

Anonymous questions, 92, 155–59; and confidentiality, 156

Anonymous statements method, 189–91, as evaluation, 238

Answering questions, 92–95; anonymous questions, 155–59; examples of, 92; experiential differences, 95; gender and developmental differences, 94; guidelines for, 157–59; improving skills in, 95; question box, 95; reasons why difficult, 93; value-based, 158–59

Asking questions. *See* Questioning process

Assessment, 113–16; with brainstorming, 211; as empowerment, 55–56; formal and informal methods, 56; by guest speakers, 115–16; methods, 55–56; on-the-spot, 124–26; rationale for, 55–56; "webbing," 56

Assignments, 162–63

Association for Sexuality Education and Training (ASSET), 105

Attitudes: assessment of, 55; and behavior, 28, 71, 81; correlation with sexual knowledge and comfort, 40–41; for democracy, 39; at different developmental stages, 32; and early sex-

uality education programs, xvi; educators', 37, 49, 97, 105; examination of, 14, 21, 28, 39; about HIV, 70; homophobia, 15, 53, 71, 99; impact of family and peers on, 35; impact of sexuality education on, 3; impact of socioeconomic inequities on, 8; media influence on, 9; and mental schemes, 70; non-competitive, 57; *Sexual Attitude Restructuring Workshop*, 105; and sexual pluralism, 21; of special populations, 73; and teaching methods, 109–10; and third-generation curricula, 64

Audience effect, 122

Barriers to effective sexuality/HIV education, 10–13

Behavioral domain, 109–10, 192

Behavior change theory, 80

Beliefs: and behaviors, 28; educator respect for, 42–43, 50, 87; educator's, 43; and fourth-generation curricula, 71–72; about HIV risk, 75–76; and mental schemes, 66, 70; and sexual pluralism, 21; and teaching methods, 109–10; tolerance for, in others, 40, 91

Books, as teaching method, 159–61; sexuality education texts and curricula, 159

Brainstorming method, 211–15; in discussions, 175

Case studies method, 187–89

Classroom. *See* Learning environment

Cognitive domain, 109–10, 147

Collaboration, between classroom teacher and community health educator, 100–101; questions to ask in, 115–16, 216; and other sources of sexuality information, 35–36, 85–87

Comfort, among learners, 44, 46–47; and establishing trust, 124; with what happens in class, 54. *See also* Sexuality comfort

Community health educator. *See* Educator

Competitive learning, disadvantages of, 57

Computerized learning programs, 172

Conceptually-based sexuality/HIV education: description of, 68; discerning key concepts, 112–13, 116; examples, 68–69; rationale for, 69

Condoms: misinformation/omissions about, 18, 77; and prevention of pregnancy and HIV, 76–78

Confidentiality: educator maintenance of, 37, 42; and educator liability, 96; for educator's safety, 104; as ground rule, 44; and learning, 21

Continuum method, 183–85

Cooperative learning groups, 131, 167–68; benefits of, 57

Co-teaching and training, 249

Credibility. *See* Educator: credibility

Criteria for Evaluating an AIDS Curriculum, 58

Critical thinking in sexuality education, 19, 21

Cultural pluralism: definition of, 21; fostering in classroom, 22, 96; in physical environment, 59; rationale for, 22

Dale, "Cone of Experience and Learning," 26

Debate, 225–26

Declarations, 234

Deductive lessons, 117–19

Democracy in sexuality education, 19, 20, 22, 39

Denmark, S.C., program, 35, 85

Designing sexuality education and training sessions, 112–20

Developmental differences, 32–33

Dewey, John, 39, 63

Directing groups, 129–38

Disclosure: guidelines for, 99; learner, 98; educator, 94, 98–100

Discussion, 129–30, 174–76

Disequilibration, 62, 78; definition of, 66

Display of contraceptives, 152

Documentation of programs, 238

Double entendres, 50

Drawing activities, 142

Dyads and triads, 133–34, 178–79

Educator: as "coach," 63; comfort with sexuality, 37, 89–91; credibility, 41–44, 76; desirable qualities, 36–37; feelings about preparation, 37; introductions, 42; limitations, 95–97; training, 11, 37–38, 104–6; values, 24, 97

Educator Trainer Assessment Tool (ETAT), 244–50

Efficacy, 71, 76–78, 81

Empowerment: definition of, 20; fostering, 20, 21, 55

Entering Adulthood: Coping with Sexual Pressures, 141

Environment. See *Learning environment*

Erotophobia, 15

Ethical standards, for sexuality educators and trainers, 250; and philosophy, attitude, 249–50; and limitations of educator, 95–97; and transference, 102

Evaluation: of educators and trainers, 236–38, 244–50; formative, 228; forms, 236–38; methods for, 228–38; planning for, 119; reasons for, 227–28; self-evaluation by learners, 234–35; summative, 228

Facilitation. *See* Group facilitation

"Fair witness," 104

Family: definition of, xvii; diverse configurations of, 6–7, 54; role in sexuality education, 35

Family Life and Sexual Health (F.L.A.S.H), 150, 153, 163; *11/12 F.L.A.S.H.,* 222; *9/10 F.L.A.S.H.,* 156, 171, 189, 230; *Special Education F.L.A.S.H.,* 199

Fear-based curricula. *See* Abstinence-only curricula

Feedback, guidelines for giving, 235–36, 247

Feedback forms, 236–38

Feelings: and dyads/triads, 178–79; and sexual decisions, 173; and teaching methods, 109–10

Field trips, 171–72

Fishbowl method, 181–83

Focus writing, 140–41

Forced choice method, 185

Freire, Paulo, 63

Games, 223–25; evaluative, 229–30

Gay/lesbian youth: and self-efficacy, 78; and self-esteem, 18, 78

Gender differences in sexuality education, 19, 21, 26; bias in language, 50; girls and "generic" male pronoun, 22; in questions asked, 94; and self-efficacy, 78

Generations of sexuality education programs, description of, 64–65, 83

Grief, of educator, 103

Ground rules: definitions of, 44; examples, 44, 127–29; methods for developing, 46, 126–28; purpose, 45

Group dynamics, 121–23

Group facilitation, 129–38; assigning groups, 132, 134; dyads and triads, 133–34; flexibility, 135–38; large groups, 129–30; of problem situations, 137–38; process interventions, 135–38; reporting process, 133; small groups, 131–34; task groups, 167–71

Group process, 121–23; and discussion, 129–30; and giving directions, 129; and interventions, 135–38; and member roles, 131, 137; stages of group growth, 122–23

Group size: ideal, 58; impact on group cohesion, 58; impact on learner comfort, 55

Guest speakers, 215–17

Guided imagery, 143–45; in self-talk, 199

Guidelines for Comprehensive Sexuality Education, 107, 112

Heterosexism: definition, xviii; role in youth risk-taking, 18

HIV/AIDS: and behavior change, 80–83; and beliefs about susceptibility, 61, 75–76, 78; and condom efficacy, 76; impact of social problems on, 13; and loss, 68; and lowered self-efficacy, 78; and media campaigns, 79; misinformation about in fear-based curricula, 17; and peer support, 79; and related professional disciplines, 29; relationship to knowledge and behavior, 61, 70; and respectful language, 50; and social norms, 79

HIV/AIDS Audiovisual Resources, 155

HIV education: and abstinence, 18; and assessment, 39; barriers to, 10–13; and behavior change, 28; collaboration among sources of, 35; conceptually-based, 68; and cultural/sexual diversity, 22; evaluation of, 35; as form of "prophylactic" sexuality education, 3; ideal group size, 58; impact of homophobia on, 15, 53; infusion approach, 29–31; interdisciplinary approaches, 29–31; key concepts in, 69; and learning domains, 28; minimum recommended hours, 12; modern realities in teaching, 6–9; omissions in, 12; parental comfort in teaching, 4; and personalization, 72; and Piagetian theory, 65–68; public support for, 4; sex-positive, 15; and social learning theory, 70–80; and special populations, 73–74; state mandates for, 12; student recommendations for, 5; teacher preparation for, 11, 37; tone and character of, 11

Homophobia: activities for decreasing, 53; definition, xviii; impact on learning, 53; role in youth risk-taking, 18

Hope is Vital, 219

Human Sexuality: Values and Choices, 146, 153, 154, 193, 199, 238

Humor: in introductions, 48; spontaneous, 51

Inductive lessons, 119

Infusion approach, 29–31; impact on teachers, 37

Integrating "across the curriculum." *See* Infusion approach

Interventions, in group process, 135–38

Interview method, 179–81

Introductions, 124–25; of educator, 42–43, 124–25; of learners, 46–49; of lesson, 124–25

Introspective methods, 140–46; defined, 139; facilitating, 140

Jemmott curriculum, as culturally specific, 22

Journal writing, 145–46

Kinesthetic methods, 220–22

KNOW AIDS curriculum, 225

Leadership, by participants, 130

Learner: characteristics, 6; as co-evaluator, 56–58; as co-planner, 56; introductions, 46–49; as leaders, 123, 130; recommendations for sexuality education, 5

Learner-centered teaching: and discussion, 130; and group process, 123

Learning domains, 28, 63, 109–10

Learning environment: definition of, 39; educator introductions, 42; flexibility in, 59; group configuration, 58; learner introductions, 46–49; learner preferences for, 59; on-the-spot adjustments, 123–24; physical aspects, 58–60; physical interventions, 124; and planning lessons, 117; pluralism in, 59; educator location, 59; workshop introductions, 48

Learning styles, 24–28; active vs. passive, 24; modalities, 24; multiple intelligences, 24; social interaction preferences, 25

Lecture, 147

Legal considerations, 96; and questioning of students, 173

Life Planning Education: A Youth Development Program, 144, 145, 159

Limitations of educator, 95–97

Listening, 125; uninterrupted listening technique, 134; and whip method, 176

Methods: affective, 109–10, 173–74; behavioral, 109–10, 192; cognitive, 109–10, 147; definition, 107; and teacher evaluation, 248

Models of anatomy, 151

National Coalition to Support Sexuality Education, 4

New Methods for Puberty Education, 127, 143, 159, 160, 162, 163, 180, 189, 205, 222, 233, 237

Norms: community, 23; curricular, 64; and media campaigns, 79; and peer education, 79; and popular opinion leaders, 79; social, 9, 71–72, 79, 81–82; and teen theater, 79; youth perceptions of, 79–80

Northwest Institute for Community Health Educators (NICHE), 105–6, 244

Opposition: as barrier, 10, 13, 84, 87; key national groups, 85; one-on-one confrontations, 86–87; organized, 84–85, 87; strategies to counteract, 85–89
Overhead transparencies, use of, 153

Panel presentations, 215–17
Parent: barriers to communications with own children, 5; involvement in school sexuality education, 35–36; as primary sexuality educators, 4–5, 35; of school-aged children, 85; support for sexuality education, 4, 84
Passive learning: and group process, 123; and presentations, 150; and teaching methods, 110–12; and videos, 154
Peer education, 217–18; to empower learners, 21; role in personalization, 72
Peer Education . . . a little help from your friends . . . , 218
Peer support, and maintaining health-positive behaviors, 79
Peer to Peer: Youth Preventing HIV Infection Together, 217, 218
Personalization, 62, 71–72, 74–75, 81
Personal safety. See *Safety*
Physical environment. *See* Learning environment
Piaget, Jean, 65
Piagetian cognitive theory, 65–70; accommodation, 65–66; assimilation, 65; concepts, 67–68; crystallization, 69; disequilibration, 66, 78; elaboration, 69; figurative vs. operative knowing, 66–67; mental schemes, 65; other applications, 70
Pictures, in activities, 143
Planning sexuality education sessions, 112–20
Pluralistic ignorance, 122
Polls, 166–67
Portfolios, 233–34
Positive Images: A New Approach to Contraceptive Education, 159
Posters, 152–53
Postponing Sexual Involvement, 34, 64–65, 79, 151, 167, 175, 184, 217
Presentations, 148–53; and assessment, 148; key concepts, 149; language, 149–50; by learners, 162; scripts for, 150–51
Problem solving method, 202–5; interpersonal problem solving, 203–5
Protecting learners, 137; during disclosure, 98
Psychological environment. *See* Learning environment
Public support for sexuality education, 4

Quadrant method, 185–86
Questioning process, 215; asking about behaviors, 166, 215; asking for feelings, values, beliefs, 136, 173; in brainstorming, 215; and

discussions, 130; in interviews, 179–80; and legal considerations, 173
Questionnaires, 141–42; for evaluation, 233

Real life homework, 208–10
Reducing the Risk, 28, 34, 52, 64–65, 74, 118, 151, 180, 193, 195, 207, 234
Referrals, 95, 161–62; after learner disclosures, 98
Rehearsal method, 196–98; in self-talk, 199
Reporting process, from small groups, 133, 168
Research by students, 162–63; student presentations, 162
Resources, 161–62
Role play method, 192–98

Safer sex: definition of, xviii; relative risk, 78
Safety, of educator, 104
Schinke-Blythe-Gilchrist curriculum, 34, 64
Secular humanism, 87–88
Self-care, of educator, 89
Self-talk, 198–199
Self-efficacy, 71, 78, 81–82
Sequencing activities, 117–20
Sex Respect, on gender roles, 21
Sexual Attitude Restructuring (SAR) Workshop, 105
Sexuality, definition of, xviii, 1
Sexuality comfort: correlation with knowledge, attitudes, and behaviors, 40, 53, 55; as developmental task, 91; educator's, 41, 89–91; evidence of, 90; facilitating for learners, 44, 49, 52, 55; in gender-segregated groups, 54–55; general vs. personal, 91; and privacy, 54; role in learning, 40–41, 55
Sexuality education: abstinence-only, 17; advocating for, 106; barriers to, 10–12; collaboration among sources of, 35; comprehensive, 1–2, 12, 15, 17, 19, 83; and the courts, 89; definition of, 1; effectiveness of, 15; effects of, 3–4, 19; evaluation of, 35; generations of, 64–65, 83; goals of, 2; history of, 10; infusion approach to, 29–31; interdisciplinary approaches to, 29–31; learner needs for, 38; learner recommendations for, 5; opposition to, 10; prophylactic, 2; rationale for, 4; school-based, 2; sex-negative, 16, 19; sex-positive, 2, 15–16, 19, 83; support for, 4
"Sexuality guru" effect, 95–96
Sexuality Information and Education Council of the U.S. (SIECUS), 105
Sexual orientation: definition of, xviii; misinformation about, in fear-based curricula, 17; why teach about it, 18
Sexual pluralism: definition of, 21; fostering in classroom, 22; in language, 50; rationale for, 22
Sexual risk-taking: among adults, 75; impact of

social inequalities on, 8; among long-term couples, 76; media influence on, 9; among young gay men, 75; among youth, 7–9, 75

Simulation method, 205–8; in kinesthetic activities, 220–22

Skills, 71, 80–82; and teaching methods, 110

Skits method, 199–202

Slides, of STDs, 152

Social learning theory, 71; cognitive behavioral theory, 71; key concepts in, 71–80; social cognitive theory, 71; social influence theory, 71; social inoculation theory, 71; weakness of, 83

Social norms. *See* Norms: social

Society for the Scientific Study of Sex (SSSS), 105

Sociofugal arrangement, 58

Sociopetal arrangement, 58

Special populations, special needs, 73, 115

Stages of change, 81

Stem sentences, 142–43

Stigma, of teaching sexuality/HIV education, 103

Story telling method, 187, 189

Stream-of-consciousness writing, 141

Streetwise to Sex-Wise: Sexuality Education for High Risk Youth, 159

Stress, for educator, 102–4

Surveys, 166–67

Susceptibility, 62, 71, 75–76, 81

Talk Listen Care Kit, 224

Task groups, 167–71

Taught Not Caught, 153

Teacher. *See* Educator

Teaching Safer Sex, 76, 118, 159, 185, 223

Teen Aid, on gender roles, 21

Teen theater, 219–20

Tests, 230–32

Theory-based sexuality education, rationale for, 62, 65

Training of educators and administrators: comfort and preparedness of teachers, 37–38; in-service methods, 105–6; lack of, 11; recommendations for, 38; training needs, 104

Transference, 102; and countertransference, 102

Transitions, 135

Transtheoretical Model (TTM), 81

Universal values: balancing with pluralism, 23; definition of, 22–23; examples, 23

Values: of conflicting groups, 23; discussion in dyads and triads, 178–79; of educators, 24, 97; teaching methods, 109–10

Videos: evaluation of, 155, 241–44; use of, 153–55

Vocabulary: building group vocabulary, 49–50; double entendres, 50; glossary of terms, xvi–xix; politicized, 50; sexually pluralistic, 50

Webbing, and planning, 113

When I'm Grown: Life Planning Education, 153, 159; *for Grades 3 & 4*, 143, 214; *for Grades 5 & 6*, 181, 222, 230

Whip, 175, 176–78

Whitehead, Alfred North, 63–64, 67

Worksheets, 163–64; for evaluation, 233